Living & Dying with Strokes, Alzheimer's, Diabetes, & Congestive Heart Failure

Roy Lique

(This book is also available in Kindle (mobi) format at Amazon.)

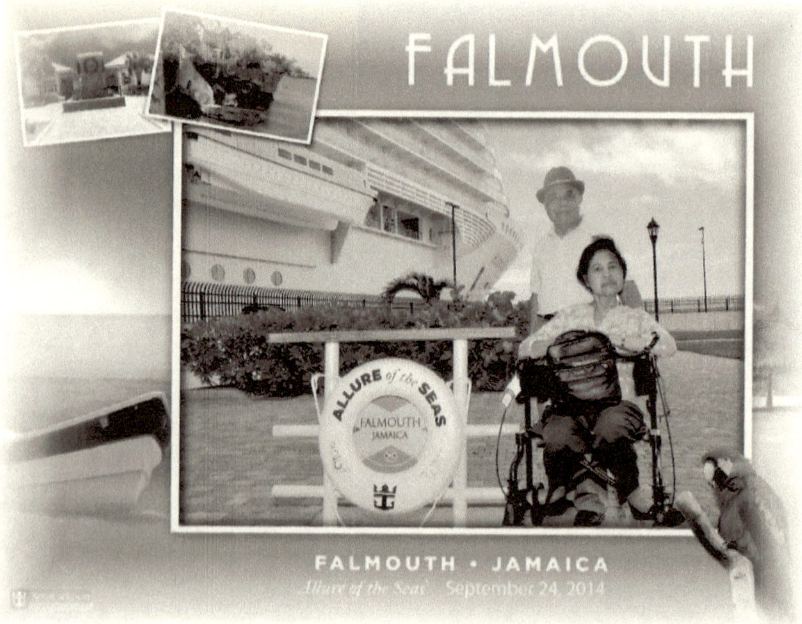

My special thanks to the members of the staff and crew of the following cruise ships, who might have helped Amelia while she was a passenger on their ship:

Carnival Elation, Carnival Inspiration, Golden Princess, Sapphire Princess, Dawn Princess, Regal Princess, Norwegian Star, Norwegian Sun, Celebrity Century, Voyager of the Sea, Allure of the Seas, and Queen Mary II

ISBN-10: 1536833940
ISBN-13: 978-1536833942

ACKNOWLEDGEMENT

I acknowledge the influence and support of the following when I am writing this book:

Elizabeth Ann Seton Church,
For providing a place for Amelia to pray and console with God,

Dr. Quian Zhang and other Staff of Kaiser Permanente Hospital,
Pomona Valley Hospital Medical Center and Staff,
La Palma Intercommunity Hospital and Staff,
for the emergency and post-emergency care for Amelia,

Dolly Dominguez and Dennis Dominguez,
whose alert thinking averted some dire consequences for Amelia, and whose company we enjoyed while traveling,

Olga Campion and Edmond Campion,
for suggesting cruising as an excellent form of therapy, and a safe and healthy source of enjoyment for strokes, Alzheimer's, diabetic, and with congestive heart failure, patient like Amelia,

Elvie Villamor and Erlindo Villamor,
who actually led and helped Amelia to eat,

Linda de la Rosa and Bobby de la Rosa, Sonia Tanchoco and Douglas Tanchoco, Shiony Tolentino and Albert Tolentino, Flora Pineda and Isidro Pineda, Flor Bautista, Marie Bautista, Zenie Bautista, and Mariza Soriente
whose friendship and encouragement keep Amelia's hope and spirit high,

Norma Apalit and Jimmy Apalit and members of their families,
whose alert disposition averted a tragedy, and whose continuing support keeps Amelia brave and vigorous,

family members,
Mary Secor and Zachary Secor, Samantha Secor, Alison Secor, Kimberly Lique and Homer Lique, Dominique Lique, Mariah Tapia, Kenady Lique, Amelita Solorzano and Rich Solorzano, Jesseca Solorzano, Justin Solorzano, and Erlinda Abundo,
whose constant support keeps the family's spirit high and forward-looking.

Special Thanks to:

Dr. Ted Shih-Yu Chen

In behalf of Amelia's family, I thank Dr. Chen for his professional service. Throughout her employment and retirement years, Amelia has not preferred a personal physician other than Dr. Chen.

Because of Dr. Chen's advice, Amelia remains active despite her ailments. She feels more at ease and comfortable discussing her problems with Dr. Chen than with other doctors.

Dr. Chen's assuring affirmation that she is still active and healthy makes Amelia hopeful and determined to prevail against strokes, Alzheimer's, diabetes, and congestive heart failure.

Dr. Wulur, Arlaine Hansaputri

I personally thank Dr. Wulur for advising me about my health status and for making sure I keep my medical appointments to ensure that my medical history is up-to-date and that I am getting the right medications to keep me strong and healthy so that I could perform my caregiving duties to Amelia.

Dr. Wulur advised me about what possible options including financial, were available to us to alleviate the hardships inflicted by the diseases that felled Amelia.

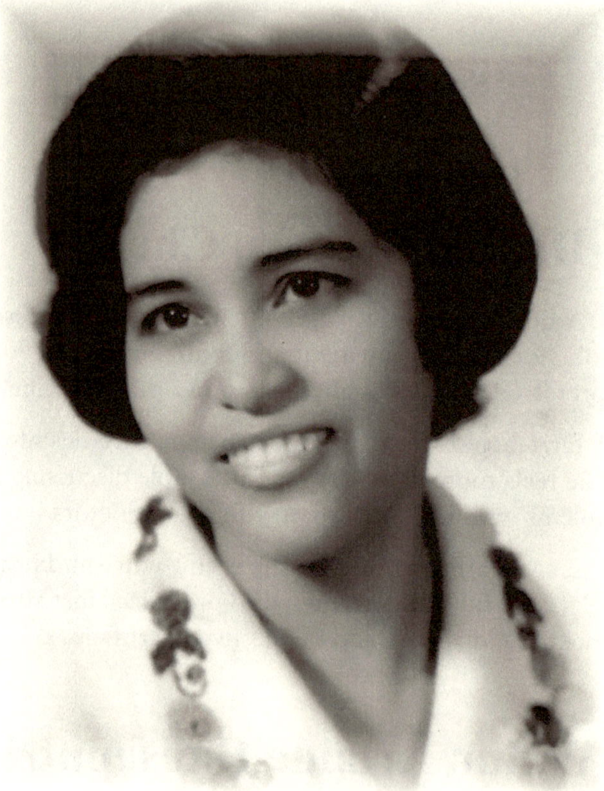

DEDICATION

To you Amelia, my wife, I dedicate this book, inspired by your struggles with strokes, Alzheimer's, diabetes, and congestive heart failure. Herein, are described the happy and sad moments that molded me into a compassionate self-made caregiver whose mission is to prolong your life if ever possible. You may not even read the book before you succumb to the diseases that have befallen you, but those who may, will find helpful hints on how to take care of a loved one.

Table of Contents

Table of Contents

Introduction

My wife, Amelia, has been struggling with strokes, Alzheimer's, diabetes, and lately just two weeks before her 78th birthday, with congestive heart failure. That her life may be taken away anytime is already a reality that is sadly accepted by my family.

This book recounts and chronicles the activities associated with taking care of a patient plagued by the diseases above. The subjects of caregiving, entertaining, and physical and mental workouts are narrated from experience.

Following the initial strokes, caregiving was a task that I thought I would never be able to perform. With limited options, however, and after fourteen years of doing it, I have the job reduced to second nature, allowing me and my wife to concentrate on the more entertaining activities. Aware of her dire condition, my wife's idea of entertainment is cruising while she is still capable of moderate movements.

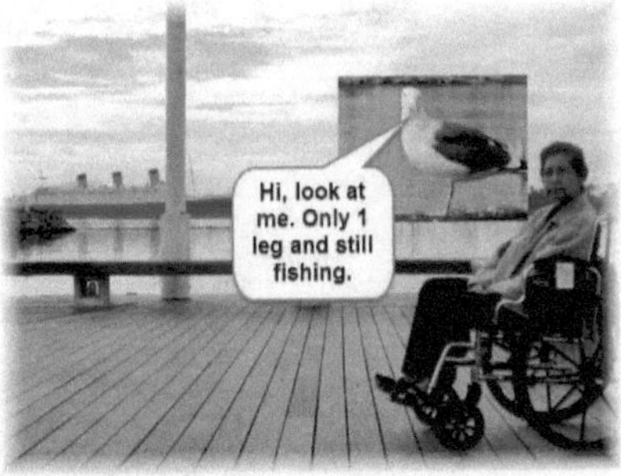

And cruising we did, both locally and internationally, following her retirement that was accelerated by the first two strokes. A cruise is less strenuous, safe, and relaxing. Combined with land tours, it is in my belief, to be the best form of entertainment and exercise for her.

Caring for a victim of strokes, Alzheimer's, diabetes, and congestive heart failure is hard but not impossible as I show in this book. The book is published the way I want it without embellishments beyond the actual events, and devoid of potential change in tone resulting from too much editions.

I hope that the experience I have with taking care of my wife be not replicated in anyone else's case, for it is humbling, demanding, and at times, challenging to the point of exhaustion. As the book indicates, I add pages at appropriate places to accommodate different phases of caregiving and entertaining occurring at different times

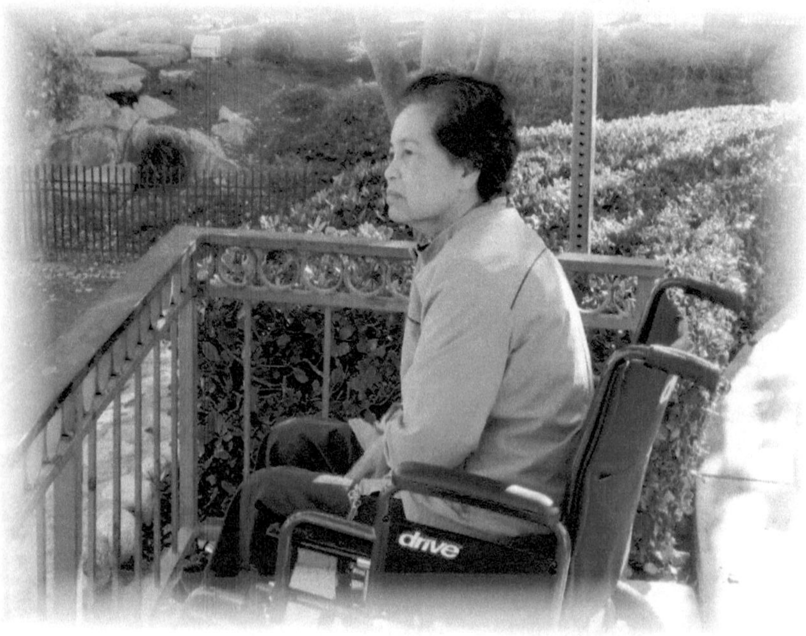

Chapter 1 – Progression of Bodily Disorders

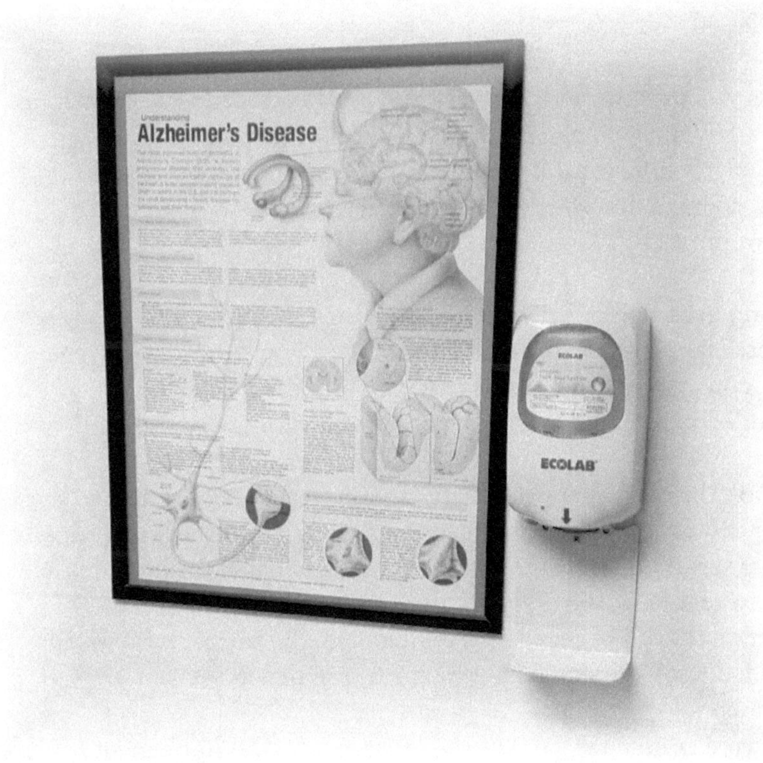

Diabetes

Although diabetes plagues millions of people all over the world, it did not concern Amelia because she felt that she did not have it. Her thought was more occupied by how she was taking care of the family, the home, and her job. That was the state of her health and physical condition until a strange thing happened one day, perhaps after her 40th birthday.

Amelia was driving, and as a passenger, I was directing her where to make a few turns to reach our destination. Freeway onramp signs are highly visible, yet she was unable to read them. She would not even recognize the overhead signs directly above us; of her, that was not normal.

Heading back home, we switched positions; I drove while she was the passenger. I asked her to read the freeway overhead signs; she barely could, even when I was driving at moderate speeds. I concluded then that something was wrong with her.

She took the earliest appointment that she could have with a doctor. Because she had been feeling healthy up to this time, trips to a physician's office were infrequent. She was not even aware that every patient has been assigned to a personal physician of the patient's choice. I believed that henceforth, the doctor who initially examined her had become her personal physician.

Tests were conducted on Amelia. For her who did not expect to contract an ailment as debilitating as diabetes, the results were shocking – she already had one. And she had to change her eating habits and her daily exercise routine abruptly and to adapt to a few new medications for the first time.

Diabetes

Amelia was able to control diabetes by diligently following the doctor's orders and observing strict dietary recommendations. However, diabetes started to change her outlook, particularly the way she picked her food and the way she dressed up to compensate for the loss of weight resulting from medications. These changes would become fixed with her for as long as she lives.

Diabetes is just the first of her ailments. I believe that it is the cause of her other ailments that will continue to plague her for the rest of her life. However, at this stage of her physical downturn, she was not yet ready to give up her job and her responsibilities towards her family. She was still ably taking care of herself.

She self-administered her medications, and caregiving was not yet a critical issue. The family was not too concerned about her condition, her case being type II diabetes which is controllable. If nothing else would change, her circumstance was considerably not alarming. But as the reader will find out later on, most of Amelia's ensuing physical disorders are suspiciously attributable to diabetes.

First Two Strokes

First Two Strokes

Strokes happening to a patient in a hospital under the watchful eyes of nurses and doctors are unlikely. That was what I believed until Amelia had two strokes almost fifteen years ago. Stroke detection may have improved since then; what I now understand is that if a stroke patient is brought to the hospital within four hours of the initial symptoms, the effects of the stroke can be reversed leaving the patient with almost unnoticeable consequence.

Amelia's first two strokes happened at the same time in June 2002. As she was not familiar with the symptoms of strokes, she thought that on the day she was not feeling well she would just call her employer, requesting to be excused from work. Left alone in the house, Amelia also called her sister-in-law, a registered nurse, to describe her condition. Together with Amelia's brother, the nurse took her to the hospital where she threw up while getting out of the car.

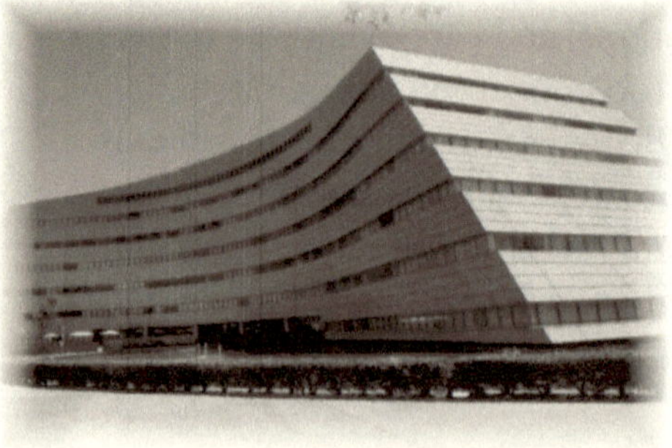

Amelia was admitted to the emergency ward of the hospital and placed under observation. Having health coverage under said hospital's plan, I assumed that the medical staff was able to deduce the right treatment of her symptoms, based on her medical history.

Amelia was still in the emergency ward when I visited her after work. I was told that everything was fine with her and that she would be transferred to one of the non-emergency rooms for careful overnight observation. I did not even bother to stay long, knowing that Amelia was in good hands.

First Two Strokes

What happened the following morning when I visited Amelia was out of ordinary. I talked to her, and she just stared at the ceiling without responding. I thought she was just feigning and making a fool of me. Because it was still very early in the morning, I left to eat breakfast at the hospital cafeteria. I was taking all the time to get out of the way while shift change was in progress. In fact, I leisurely read some newspapers to catch up with the news of the day.

In the elevator on my way back to Amelia's room, the night doctor, sensing that I am Amelia's husband, asked if I was visiting a particular patient. When I said 'yes,' she asked me if it was Amelia I was visiting. I said, 'yes' again.

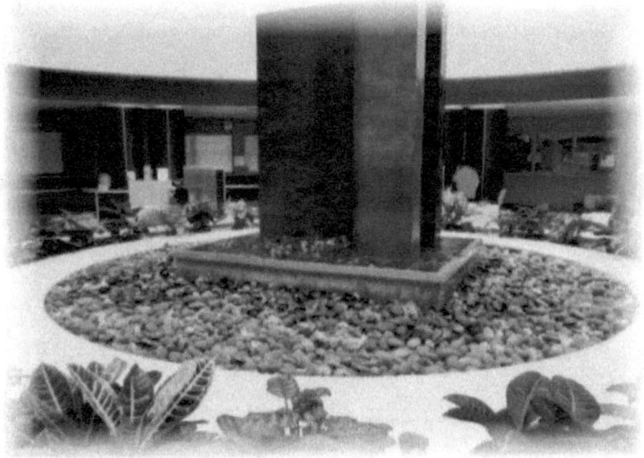

The doctor broke the sad news to me that Amelia suffered strokes during the night. That was the occasion when I first learned about Amelia's grievous condition. As I then recalled, the strokes were the reasons why Amelia was not responding when I talked to her earlier. She suffered two strokes, one at the back of her head and one at the left side.

I was in tears when I alerted our children and Amelia's brother and his wife, about Amelia's serious medical condition. My quizzical and restrained reaction was why the strokes happened while Amelia was being cared for at the hospital. Upon inquiry, I was told that a stroke could occur any time at any place, sometimes with warning signs and sometimes without. A stroke may even occur without the patient knowing it.

First Two Strokes

Her condition now dawning on me, Amelia appeared very pathetic; she used to be cheerful and fun to be with especially when the family gathered for some celebratory occasions. Her health seems to be slowly slipping, but hope was instilled in me by the doctors at the hospital.

Following the doctors' recommendation, I committed Amelia to an aggressive therapy program. Her right side was completely paralyzed, and her mental capacity was diminished to a fourth-grade level. Using building blocks, she had to be taught again how to count numbers and how to recite the alphabet. Handling utensils such as forks and spoons was a struggle owing to her right hand and arm having been rendered limp and useless. She was in a state of disequilibrium like a child just learning how to walk. Amelia was released from the on-site therapy program after one month.

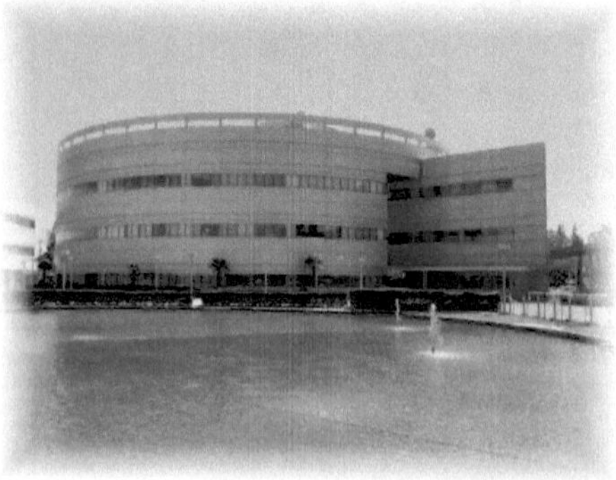

Aggressive Therapy, Not What I Thought

The first two strokes had all but left Amelia completely immobile on the right side, speechless, and unable to communicate coherently. Her left side, to some degree, was affected as well. She needed help turning her head with a blank stare in her eyes. The hospital already did as much as they could with her. It was time to discharge her for therapy.

Two days before her release, a member of the hospital staff handed me a list of four possible treatment facilities. I had to make a choice to which of the four I would like to have Amelia taken.

The first I checked out was the one closest to home. It was a moderately sized contracting facility admitting most types of patients. Were Amelia admitted there, she would be mingling with patients recovering from substance abuse and other criminal histories. I discounted the facility right away.

The second one about fifteen miles from home, was a hospital-administered facility but was no longer admitting patients since they were in the process of being closed. Indeed it was closed not too long after I talked to them.

Based on my telephone conversation with them, the third facility was similar to the first one, so I did not bother to check it out because it was slow going there, it being reachable only by surface streets from home.

I reserved the rest of the day to see the fourth facility since it was more than twenty miles from home and located where traffic was notoriously heavy in the afternoon. It turned out to be very close to a huge hospital, adding peace of mind in case of medical emergency. They were admitting only certain patients with strict

Aggressive Therapy, Not What I Thought

admission criteria. The facility was where Amelia would be having therapy, I concluded.

Back at the hospital the following day, the day of Amelia's discharge, I was congratulated by the hospital staff for making the right choice where Amelia would be undergoing "aggressive therapy." Based on the selection, the paper works were initiated, and transportation was readied. In the haste that ensued, I had no time to think about the term "aggressive therapy," until I was driving to the facility to where Amelia was already taken, and until I gathered myself and thought about the events that rapidly occurred during the day.

It was already evening when Amelia was admitted to the facility by a night duty nurse who appeared to be in control of the place. Looking muscular and appearing to weigh one and a half times as much as Amelia does, in my mind she was the kind who would not hesitate to whip an unruly patient given the assignment of aggressive authority.

She showed me where Amelia would be sleeping during the night, a location several beds away from the nurse station. That worried me even more. I hesitated to leave, but it was the end of the visiting hours, so I left. Before I did, I cautioned Amelia, still in her confused state, that she should not dare give the nurse a hard time lest she would treat her unkindly.

Thinking about Amelia and what "aggressive therapy" meant, I did not sleep at all during the first night of her stay at the facility. I was up very early in the morning to return to the place to check on Amelia. The first thing I did was to examine Amelia for bruises. She had a small one on her elbow. That was a confirmation, I felt, of aggression towards her.

Aggressive Therapy, Not What I Thought

I waited for the head nurse and confronted her with Amelia's bruise. Upon checking, it turned that it was caused by falling from the bed in Amelia's attempt to get down. She thought she could get down by herself, not realizing that her right side was completely paralyzed. She made few similar attempts only to be warned and put back on the bed each time, by the nurse. If she would not stop trying to get down from the bed, the facility would have no choice, I was told, but to belt Amelia down to the furniture. That was cruel and unkind, but it was necessary to avoid further injuries to her.

To keep a closer watch on Amelia, the nurse planned to move her closer to the nurse station, when a bed became available. In time for the second night and just across the nurse station, a bed was vacated and became available for Amelia.

Still confused by the term "aggressive therapy," I was told to discuss it with the therapist. The therapist explained to me what procedures were involved in "aggressive treatment." Nothing of the proceedings was the kind I had in mind, not even close, not to mention illegal. The procedures involved among others were: learning the alphabet, learning how to count, speech development, memory training, how to use the muscles, and how to maintain balance. Each day, the intensity of each procedure was raised until Amelia was able to repeat it independently.

Every day that I visited to check on Amelia's progress, I graced the therapists, the nurses, and other members of the staff, with candies, flowers, and snacks. On the day before her discharge from the facility, I brought enough snacks for an hour of pick-and-eat, thanking the staff for their kindness and professionalism in treating Amelia and the other patients. Finally, I learned what "aggressive therapy" meant.

Dementia or Alzheimer's

The first two simultaneous strokes that befell Amelia left her physically weakened. She lost a good percentage of her ability to move her right arm and leg. Her right cheek drooped and her speech slurred. Evaluation by the therapist suggested that Amelia's cognitive capacity dropped to a fourth-grade level, down from a school teacher's level.

An aggressive in-facility therapy program lasting one month was initiated for Amelia. When released from the facility, she was only able to recover a small percentage of what she lost in her ability to move and speak. I was advised that a continued in-home therapy program with follow-ups from the therapist would allow Amelia to recover some more of the deficits. The program indeed helped Amelia. In the meantime, out of eagerness, she went back to work taking only very light duties.

I was overwhelmed with excitement at her rapid recovery until I learned that while driving, she was ignoring traffic signals including red lights. Then she had the unfortunate accident described in this book under the title, "Taco Bell Accident." Because of the crash, she was required to take a neurological test by the Department of Motor Vehicles. She, failing the test miserably, was asked to hand over her driver's license to the Department, and it was never returned to her. The neurological test somewhat signaled memory failure.

Just after release from the therapy facility, Amelia's personal physician required her to consult with a neurologist. The neurologist diagnosed Amelia with dementia which I assumed, was the cause of her forgetfulness which in turn caused her to fail the Department of Motor Vehicles test. Understanding nothing about

Dementia or Alzheimer's

dementia, I immediately associated forgetfulness to Alzheimer's. As I learned later, Alzheimer's is a form of dementia after all.

Regardless of the source of dementia or Alzheimer's in her – be it triggered by the strokes or already in progress before the strokes - Amelia has to bear it for as long as she lives. It has been ironic, however, that in Alzheimer's, Amelia has found a natural ally in forgetting that she has other dreadful bodily disorders.

Sometimes when asked if any part of her body hurts, her response has been mostly none even though pain is evident in her facial expression. Embarrassing behaviors in public like talking to complete strangers have now been a common occurrence. She now has to be reminded to swallow her food and not talk with food in her mouth.

Amelia is not alone in fighting Alzheimer's, the disease that slowly gnaws at one's dignity down to the point of utter shamelessness and helplessness. I hope and pray that no one else suffers from it like Amelia does. I also wish and pray that no one else is a witness like I have been, to the sufferings of an Alzheimer's patient. One more Alzheimer's patient is one too many already, a reason to decry the slow progress in finding a cure, a real one that not only slows it down but completely eradicates it. Education, research, and intervention from the scientific world and the governments – we need all of these to fight the disease.

Third Stroke

The third stroke that happened to Amelia traumatized me more than the first two did. Whereas the first two strokes happened at the hospital at night when not a single family member was in attendance, the third one happened under my eyes.

At about 5:30 in the morning Amelia tried to get up from bed. When she rose she fell back and collapsed, waking me up with a thud on the floor. Immediately I went around the bed to check on her. There she was, flat on her back on the floor, having uncontrollable convulsions and spasms on her legs. She was stuttering quite heavily; only inaudible words were coming out of her mouth when she attempted to speak. In reality, I was witnessing a stroke in progress - the third one for Amelia.

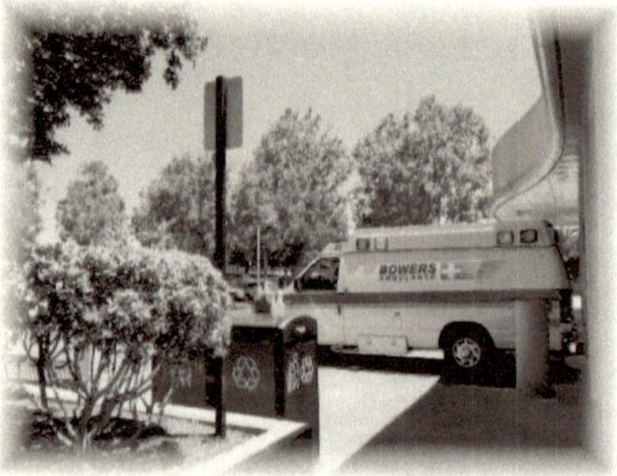

After calling 911 I tried to pick her up. She was limp and cold and was perspiring profusely. It took me a few attempts to raise her back up to the bed where she lay still, speechless, and motionless except for the spasms on her legs. She was not responding to my questions. Her neck appeared to be twisted a little bit, and her lips were pale.

When the paramedics arrived, they asked her a few questions; she was not responding to them either. The paramedics were in communication with someone on the telephone. I assumed that they were describing Amelia's symptoms and condition. When they asked for her current medications, I handed them the list. While the scene was not chaotic, anxiety was making me restless.

Third Stroke

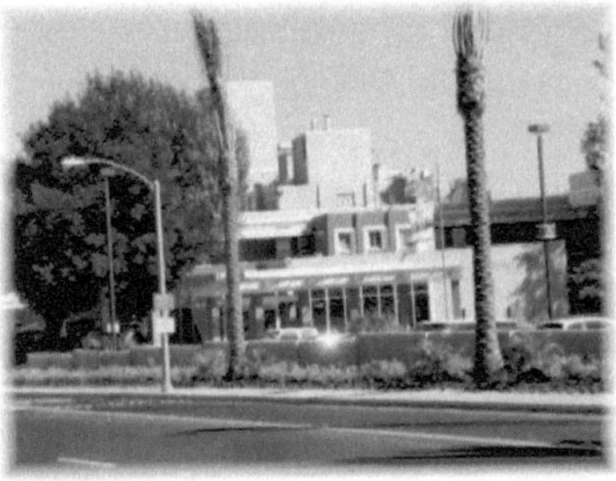

The paramedics checked Amelia's blood pressure and other vital signs. I told them that Amelia has diabetes; they took a reading of her glucose level too. They said that it was very low. It was then that I suspected that the low glucose level was the culprit for her condition; the paramedics would not confirm that it was.

They took Amelia to the nearest hospital. Other than placing her on a precautionary status, the hospital would not treat her until they got her medical history and instructions from the hospital of which Amelia is a plan member. While we were waiting, the doctor at the hospital indicated, but not with certainty, that Amelia was having a stroke and that the precautionary measures she was placed under would prevent any further damage.

Four hours later Amelia was transferred to the hospital of which she is a plan member. It was in this hospital that confirmation was made that Amelia did indeed suffer a stroke. The doctors said that the stroke was a mild one, but from what I could tell, it was more debilitating and weakening than the previous two.

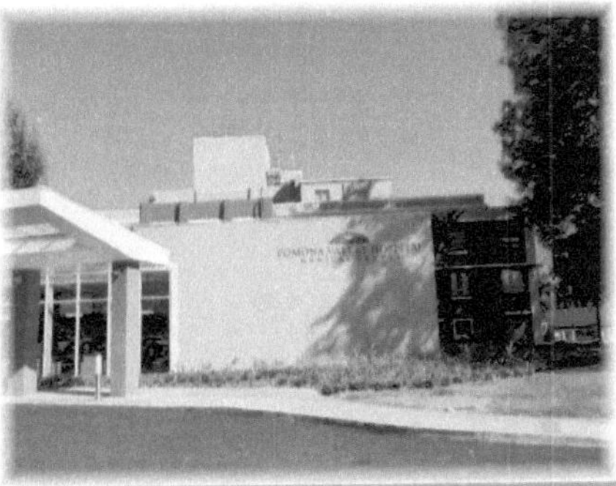

Irrespective of the severity of the stroke, plans for taking care of Amelia had to be reviewed and revised. I informed all the family members about Amelia's condition. Her status was far from being comparable to

Third Stroke

what she was before the stroke. To compound the problem, Alzheimer's appeared to be well on its destructive course.

As Amelia's condition has been worsening each time a bodily disorder like a stroke occurs, my function as a caregiver is getting more and more defined accordingly. Only time will tell what will happen next.

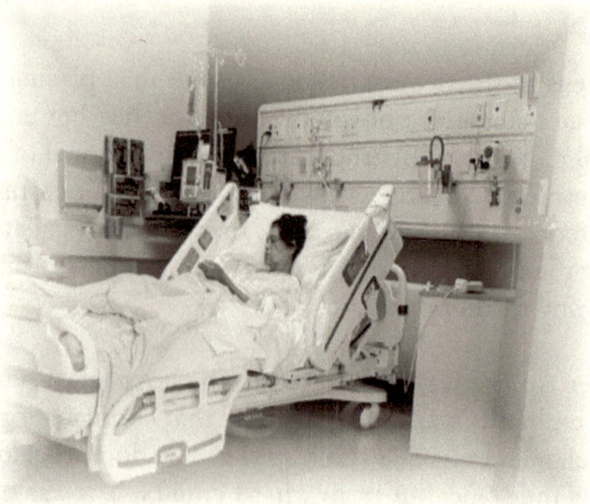

Congestive Heart Failure

Congestive Heart Failure

The Shocking Diagnosis

The morning after a routine checkup by her personal physician and just two weeks before her 78th birthday, Amelia felt confident and relaxed. The tests performed on her returned negative results. It was a cause for light rejoicing considering that Amelia had not seen her physician in more than six months.

As has been the case already till this book's publication, her blood pressure was on the high side. Not a cause for alarm, the doctor decided to adjust it through medication. Also, Amelia was given the anti-pneumonia vaccine. Nothing appeared to be ruining Amelia's day, but as I found out later, all was everything but rosy.

Towards midday Amelia started to feel general weakness on her body which caused her to be unstable; she could not pick up herself and stand as she normally does. The anti-pneumonia vaccine was the culprit, I first assumed. When she started feeling drowsy and would not talk, I decided to take her to the hospital.

Results from the initial tests at the emergency room indicated that Amelia was probably suffering from slight dehydration and the anti-pneumonia vaccine probably was causing the pain that she was complaining of on her shoulder. Also, urine tests indicated that she contracted urinary tract infection. I expected that results of various other tests would yield nothing worse.

However, the doctor who read the results had shocking news for me the following morning. He disclosed that Amelia has been suffering from severe stenosis of the heart, a condition characterized by the narrowing of the heart valves in both the right and left sides. As his was only an initial assessment, he said he would be conferring with the cardiologist who is a specialist in heart cases.

Confirming the sad news that the first doctor discussed with me, the cardiologist made the same assessment of Amelia's heart. He went on to explain the different options available to alleviate her condition. Bypass surgery was one, and the other was through medication. Even sadder was the reality that at any minute within a year Amelia's life may be taken away.

Due to Amelia's frail condition and her age, surgery is no longer a viable option. The success rate of cases like hers is less than fifty percent. Even if it is successful, the result may not be long-lasting enough to prolong Amelia's life. Left with medication as the sole option to alleviate Amelia's condition, the family agreed with the doctor's recommendations under the circumstance.

The drugs in Amelia's case will be designed to slow the occurrence of death by regulating the heart's functions to utmost possible efficiency. It is up to the doctors to prescribe the necessary medications to help her. I am prepared to follow their instructions to prolong her life

Medication necessitates that I understand what congestive heart failure is, to appreciate the need to follow the doctors' instructions strictly. Without being technical, congestive heart failure is a serious condition that occurs when the body becomes congested with extra fluid resulting from a weakened heart. It does not mean that the heart has stopped functioning.

To prevent Amelia from accumulating fluid in her system, I have to weigh her every morning just after waking up, before breakfast, on the same scale, and she wearing same-weight clothes. If there is a gain of two or more pounds between days, I have to add precise dosage to her medications. Additionally, strict diet control is to be observed, and moderate exercises are to be performed. Not too much of a chore, I have been following the exact instructions conscientiously.

I am unable to tell if the medications and the doctors' instructions are having an impact on Amelia's health. I hope they have and that everything I am doing has been helping her to stay alive a little bit longer. The sad news of her having a severe heart condition is being felt with anxiety and fear, by the family. I pray that no one else has to suffer the fate that Amelia suffers, and that no one else has to have the misfortune of attending to a sick member of a family like I have.

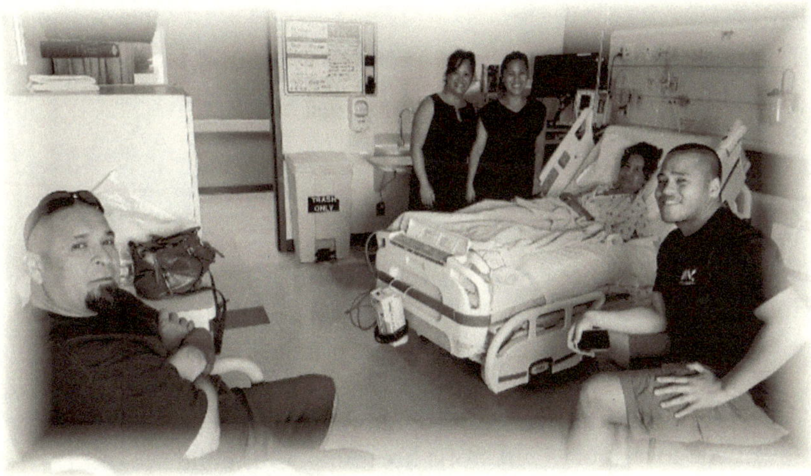

The Physician Orders for Life-Sustaining Treatment

The shock of learning that Amelia has severe stenosis of the heart had barely subsided. We were evaluating the seriousness of the disease, its impact on Amelia, and the necessary steps to cope with it. As the doctor explained, the potential for sudden death within a year is a reality that the family has to accept.

The Physician Orders for Life-Sustaining Treatment (POLST) is a parallel form to go with Advance Directive. In the absence of the latter, I had to make tough choices to complete the form so that members of the medical staff are empowered to perform necessary life sustaining treatment of Amelia should the need arises.

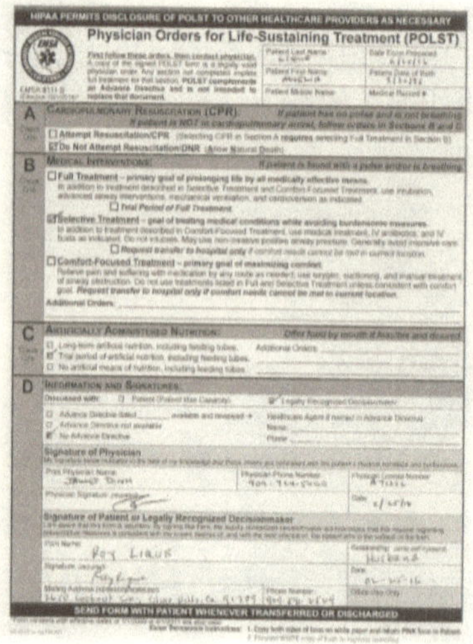

HIPAA PERMITS DISCLOSURE OF POLST TO OTHER HEALTHCARE PROVIDERS AS NECESSARY

Physician Orders for Life-Sustaining Treatment (POLST)

A Cardiopulmonary Resuscitation (CPR)

☐ Attempt Resuscitation/CPR

☑ Do Not Attempt Resuscitation/DNR

B Medical Interventions

☐ Full Treatment – primary goal of prolonging life by all medically effective means.

☐ Trial Period of Full Treatment

☑ Selective Treatment – goal of treating medical conditions while avoiding burdensome measures.

☐ Request transfer to hospital only

☐ Comfort-Focused Treatment – primary goal of maximizing comfort.

Request transfer to hospital only if comfort needs cannot be met in current location.

Additional Orders:

C Artificially Administered Nutrition

D Information and Signatures

Signature of Physician

Signature of Patient or Legally Recognized Decisionmaker

SEND FORM WITH PATIENT WHENEVER TRANSFERRED OR DISCHARGED

Having to fill the form in front of Amelia while she was innocently smiling and conversing with people in the hospital ward was a scene I hope no one else has to witness. She was relatively in good spirit, oblivious of the fact that she has been very ill and that her very temporal existence was the topic of discussion.

Part A of the form deals with cardiopulmonary resuscitation (CPR) in case Amelia loses pulse and stops breathing. Our children and I unanimously agreed that at her condition, CPR is doubtful to succeed. Regardless of our reluctance and indecision, I had to make a hard choice to complete the form.

Congestive Heart Failure

Before I checked off my choice, I glanced at Amelia who was smiling while trying to convince the doctor that she was well and healthy enough to be released from the hospital, if the doctor would only say so. It was very melancholic when I checked off "Do Not Attempt Resuscitation/DNR (Allow Natural Death)." What was I doing letting her die, I kept saying to myself. I felt like I was an executioner of some kind, committing her to death.

Part B of the form deals with Medical Intervention in case Amelia is found with a pulse and is breathing. Engulfed by the same level of sadness as when I made a check mark in Part A, I chose "Selective Treatment – goal of treating medical conditions while avoiding burdensome measures." Only to delay an imminent death, the choice was a tough one as well.

Part C of the form deals with artificially administered nutrition. Again the family was unanimous in choosing "Trial period of artificial nutrition, including feeding tubes." I felt that this would only prolong Amelia's misery, but it was the least painful and horrifying one among the choices.

The rest of the form was merely informational that did not evoke emotional strain on me. I included the form in this book to illustrate the real difficulties a victim of strokes, Alzheimer's, diabetes, and congestive heart failure, has to endure. Likewise, the caregiver suffers as much if not more. These diseases do not recognize boundaries; anyone is a potential victim. I hope and pray that cure for them be discovered in the very near future.

Fourth Stroke

Fifty-five years of marriage of which fourteen have been spent as a caregiver of Amelia, are enough for me to develop a keen awareness of her unpredictable health status. In few past occasions, intense grief was averted by my appropriate actions of taking her to the nearest medical facilities for emergency treatments.

Like most previous emergencies, the recent stroke that befell Amelia was prevented from becoming a potentially tragic and sad occurrence in her fight to prolong her life. The stigma from the stroke is noticeable, but I still felt lucky when I caught the symptom that alerted me to take her to the hospital in time.

As is our customary practice, on the night of the stroke we delayed our sleep time by listening to music and watching television. The following morning seemed to be a continuation of the previous night – it was pleasant – until I noticed that when Amelia spoke, her speech was slurred. The slur was especially noticeable when she pronounced a two- or more- syllable words. Suspecting that a stroke was in progress, I hurriedly took her to the hospital.

Upon learning of Amelia's slurred speech, the hospital emergency staff did not waste any time attending to her. A CT scan (computer tomography) was immediately performed on her while her medical history was being reviewed.

The result of the CT scan came out so fast revealing that Amelia did not have a stroke. It was assuring that there was no clot in her head. It was too early to relax though, because the problem of Amelia's slurred speech still existed.

I was told that a CT scan does not reveal all that is wrong with a patient; it is an emergency procedure to detect where a head clot is

Fourth Stroke

located if there is one. A more thorough process – a Magnetic Resonance Imaging, MRI for short - was necessary.

An MRI was not performed until the later part of the day because reversing the effect of a stroke was no longer urgent in the absence of a clot on Amelia's head. By then she was already admitted to the hospital, waiting for the results of several other tests.

The result of the MRI was not revealed to me until the following morning. It was a reversal of the favorable CT scan and a confirmation of my original suspicion that Amelia was having a stroke. The stroke did not show up on the CT scan.

Had I not noticed the symptom of a stroke, Amelia could have ended in a far worse situation. Without the tests, it was impossible to know if her case was or was not a prelude to a more serious medical condition. Taking her to the hospital was the right decision I made.

This stroke being Amelia's fourth has eroded her strength further resulting in her health status to be more unpredictable and dire. I hope that the medications prescribed for her, work as well as anticipated.

Caregiving has been all I can do for her; that has been what she was getting the past fourteen years. Only time will tell when Amelia, a fighter as she is, will succumb to one or more of her ailments. She already survived four strokes, each one progressively rendering her weaker and more debilitated.

Profound Change on Independence Day

July 4, 2016, was the cutoff date of an uncontrolled change relating to food preference by Amelia, who had multiple strokes, is diabetic, has Alzheimer's, and lately, diagnosed with congestive heart failure. The fact that this date of the change happened on Independence Day made the coincidence all that strange and worth noting.

The significance of the date was not being discounted; its celebration was still in keeping with the jubilation for the attainment of the United States independence. Personally though, the major significance of this date was, more than the attainment of independence, the change in Amelia's food preference and her diminished ability to move.

This book is strewn with accounts of unusual behaviors that a patient like Amelia, unconsciously reveals in ostentatious manner. Amelia is struggling with four of the most deadly diseases, so I understand and accommodate the strange behaviors that she thinks are discreet.

People who are not familiar with the kind of diseases that Amelia has may think that she is vulgar and is lacking refinement. That is perfectly all right; Amelia is ill and medical science has yet to discover the perfect cure for even one of her illnesses, not to mention four.

What was normal with Amelia for ten years. For close to ten years Amelia would have nothing for breakfast but pancakes with sugar-free syrup, fruits, coffee with cream, eggs, and short slices of sausage. Strange as it may seem, Amelia expected to have a handful supply of napkins as if it was part of the menu. Absent the napkins, she would not start eating breakfast.

Profound Change on Independence Day

For lunch and dinner, her preference was one of the fast food dishes with exceptions of certain brands. In familiar places it was easy to find her preferred food because I know the locations; in unfamiliar localities however, I had to drive around to locate a place where she liked the food.

Between lunch and dinner, Amelia had to have a snack of coffee and preferably apple pie; sometimes she liked pumpkin pies, pastries, and pretzels. For close to ten years she seldom missed snacks albeit of different makeup. When we were away from home, like being in an excursion, I always had snacks carried around for her. If the length of time that she had to indulge in her food preferences - 10 years - was strikingly odd, equally odd and stranger, was the sudden change of her choices.

What happened on July 4, 2016, Independence Day. Which of the four major ailments - strokes, diabetes, Alzheimer's, and congestive failure - caused her to change behavior is unclear to me. Perhaps one, a combination of two or more, or all of them simultaneously, caused the sudden change.

On this Independence Day, sharing Amelia's menu of pancakes, et al, we ate breakfast before we drove to Palm Springs to celebrate the day by taking the Aerial Tramway ride. Nothing appeared to be abnormal to indicate a change in Amelia's food preference. Her love of pancakes was still very much evident.

The tramway ride that took us 8,500 feet up the San Jacinto Mountain Range was enjoyable and did nothing to possibly cause the change either. We drove back home to escape the summer heat in Palm Springs and hoped to eat lunch locally. I knew where to take her for lunch because we had been to the place a few times previously.

Profound Change on Independence Day

Strangely, Amelia would not eat her preferred lunch; at night, against my supplication, she would not eat dinner either. She would rather sleep than eat. No abnormal behavior was evident in her sleep; I stayed awake for as long as I could to monitor her while she was sleeping. I did not blame her at all; she might be tired from the more than 4-hour drive round trip.

Even stranger though, in the morning she would not eat her menu of pancakes which she had been enjoying for close to ten years, even cringing at the mention of it. She used to like stopping at the restaurant to eat breakfast even close to midday; now she would not even mention the place.

Instead, from a different eating place, she asked to have rice porridge called 'Champorado', thickened with cocoa products and sweetened with brown sugar, similar to but soupier than a rice pudding. In addition, she also wanted 'Arroz Caldo,' a chicken rice porridge with ginger, and a variety of flavor enhancers.

Since July 4, 2016 until the publication of this book, early January 2017 and may be even later, Amelia has been eating Champorado and Arroz Caldo for breakfast, lunch, snack, and dinner. I tried to cheat and change her preference by serving other soft food to limited avail. Sometimes I am successful; most of the times I am not.

Soft food is my choice for her also because she now needs to be told to chew and swallow her food. The change in her food preference is abrupt, and appears to be causing her to lose energy thus weakening her to the point of needing more assistance and care.

The change happening on Independence Day, July 4, 2016, is strangely odd. Amelia is not even aware of it. With her not expected to live much longer, she needs to eat what she likes. I follow her wishes as much as possible, avoiding food that exacerbates her physical and mental disorder.

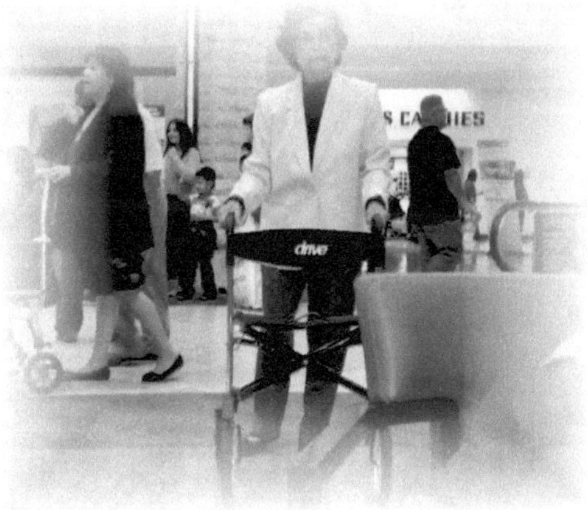

Chapter 2 – Caregiving

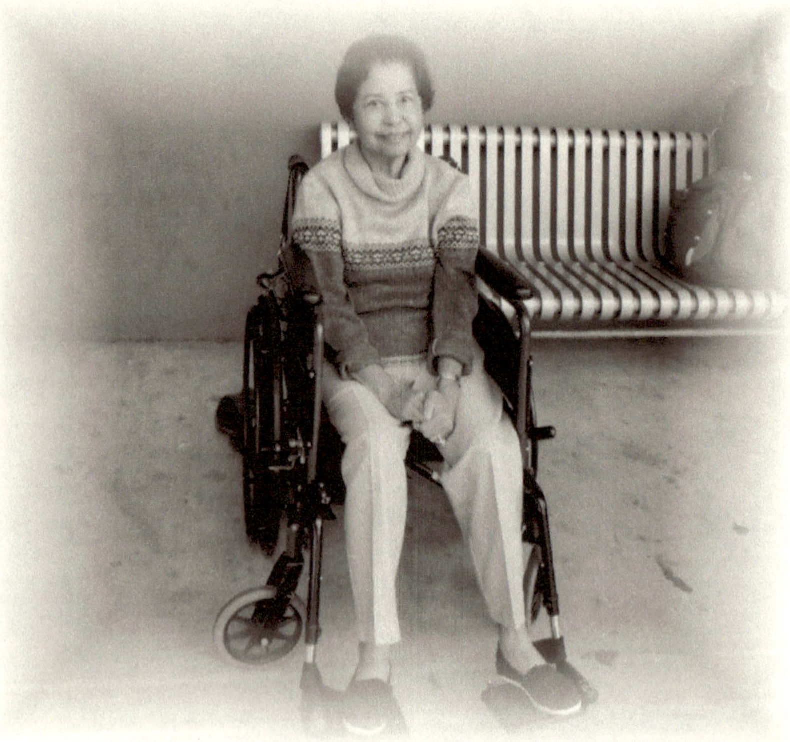

Hazards at Home

Strokes changed the way we utilized certain areas in our house particularly in heavily traveled ones like stairs and hallways. Where it was never done before, traits of practicing protective caution started to be observed since Amelia's first strokes. Consequently, the excitement of owning a home, an American dream, was dampened and made less intense.

During the first few years of ownership, I made some improvements to the house without ever thinking that someday the house itself would pose a danger to a person with a handicap like Amelia. For example, we replaced the floor coverings with

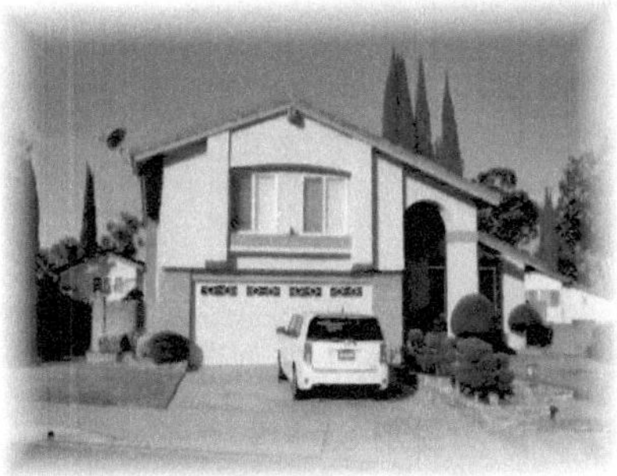

hardwood, and in particular areas, with shiny porcelain tiles. The improvements certainly made the house look good, even improving its value. Little did I anticipate that they also would threaten Amelia's physical wellbeing.

The house was tri-level. There were eleven steps on the stairs from the living room to the second story. Even though handrails were installed on both sides of the stairs, each step that Amelia had to take posed a danger to her. A misstep could mean a very hard fall with a sad or even tragic result. I saw to it that she did not climb the stairs without me watching and being ready to assist her. Nevertheless, in her stubborn way, she would exactly try it when left alone. This act of stubbornness caused me to admonish her repeatedly.

There were other steps, namely, steps between the family room and the living room, and steps at the entrance to the house. Just waiting

Hazards at Home

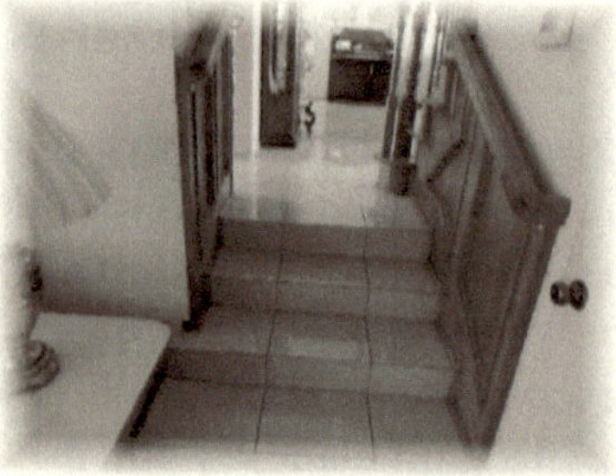

to be tripped on, these steps were potential hazards to Amelia. Although they were less likely to cause severe injury as the steps leading to the second story, they were my source of much concern and state of worry most of the time.

As mentioned earlier, the floors of the house were either tile or hardwood. When polished after a thorough cleaning, they could cause a healthy person to fall due to slipperiness. The frequency of the fall happening is higher if one like Amelia, has a physical handicap, and the result could be worse. Placing area rugs did not ease the danger because they too moved on slippery floors. So I would usually instruct the cleaning person not to apply polish to the floors.

Then there were the moving parts of the house including swinging doors, shutters, and furniture. Amelia tended to hold onto swinging doors and shutters or even window blinds for support. She also tended to support herself by using table tops, chairs, or any furniture close by, when she attempted to stand up or sit down. To avoid accidents caused by her dependence on moving objects for support, I would keep a close watch on her while she was in motion.

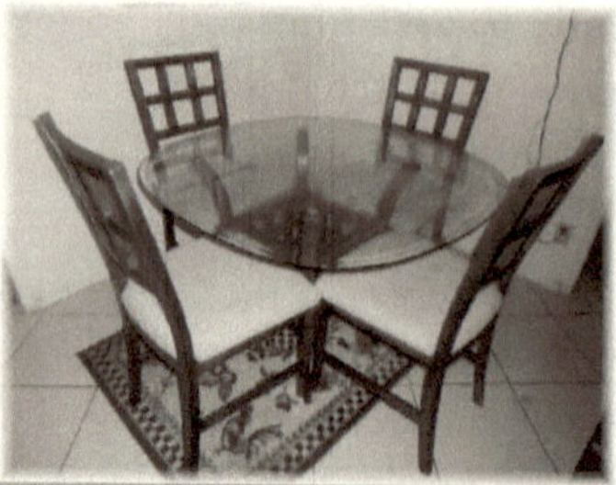

I would also point out to her the danger of accidentally falling, resulting in broken bones and the possibility of being bedridden. Like a child, she would heed my advice for a while, only to disregard it again when I was distracted.

Hazards at Home

The ordinary stepladder we had been using at home was a hazard as well. Before she had the strokes, Amelia would use it to organize shelves, her altars, and stuffs at hard-to-reach areas of the house. She still thought that she could use the stepladder safely. With her condition she could not, without the risk of accidentally falling. By keeping the stepladder away from sight, I diminished the risk.

Cooking used to be Amelia's preoccupation, but during the first few days after the strokes, she would not feel and realize that the skin on her right hand would be burning. Because of partial memory loss, the range would be left on until it would glow and emit burnt smell. To avoid her from being burned we stopped cooking in the house. The arrangement prevented potential fire hazard from a range left on for an extended period.

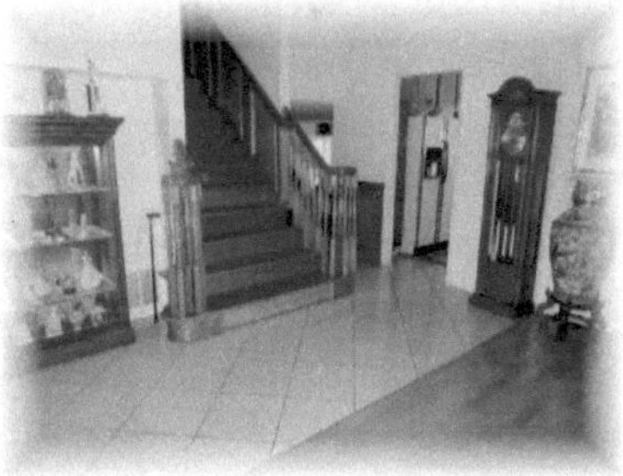

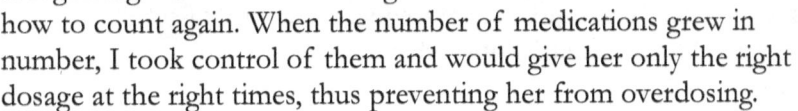

I allowed Amelia to take her prescribed medications herself, hoping that it would help her in recognizing them and in learning how to count again. When the number of medications grew in number, I took control of them and would give her only the right dosage at the right times, thus preventing her from overdosing.

We observe the same traits of protective cautions in our current residence. But, as Amelia's case continues to degenerate, more hazards will become apparent and needed to be avoided. Protective cautions will have to be adjusted accordingly, and as husband-turned-caregiver, I am responsible for the adjustments.

Measuring Food Intake

Cooking healthy food was Amelia's pastime before she suffered the first two massive strokes. With some help, she could cook meals for as many as two hundred guests on a single occasion. She was always proud to talk about her home economics diploma earned in college.

Knowing that she has type II diabetes made her very meticulous about the kinds of food that she ate. I did not have to worry about her feeling hungry because she was very accurate on the times she had to eat meals and the times she had to take her medications. She even advised her friends who have the same type of ailment how to take care of themselves without starving.

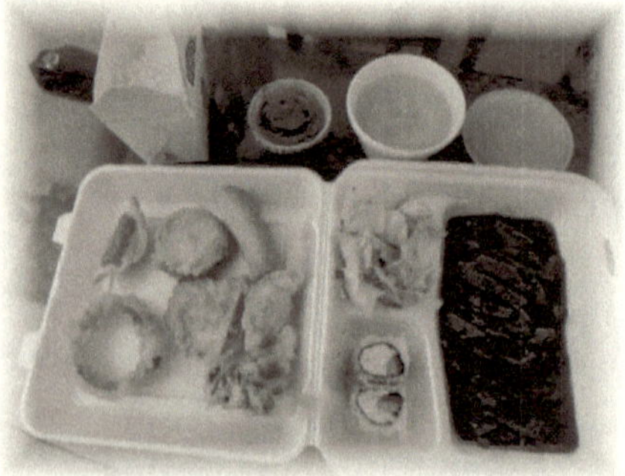

Things changed when the first strokes occurred. Some food that Amelia used to like became offensive. For example, she used to like steaks with vegetables, but now, we frequently discard tastefully cooked ones. She eats a little bit of them and pushes them aside, her excuse being that she is already full and that she is done eating.

Her eating habit has become a major problem. When I am not looking, she would wrap her food and discard it as trash. I am concerned that if she is not eating enough, her physical and mental conditions will exacerbate rapidly.

She lost her appetite perhaps due to medications, so I devised a ridiculous method for measuring her food intake, a method that I still practice to date of publication of this book. I split every meal

Measuring Food Intake

that we eat in half. If after eating my half I feel full, and I see that nothing of her half is left, I just assume that she is also satisfied with the meal and that she eats well. If I see something left of her half, I keep coaxing her to keep on eating until her half or most of it is gone.

Taking her words that she eats enough is not conclusive and accurate; she tends to lie about the amount of food she eats. It is hard to know how many hours she can sustain herself with little or no food at all. If the food we eat is the type that offends her, I just keep note not to order it again next time. Otherwise, I just go along with what she likes even if it is the food that I, myself, dislike.

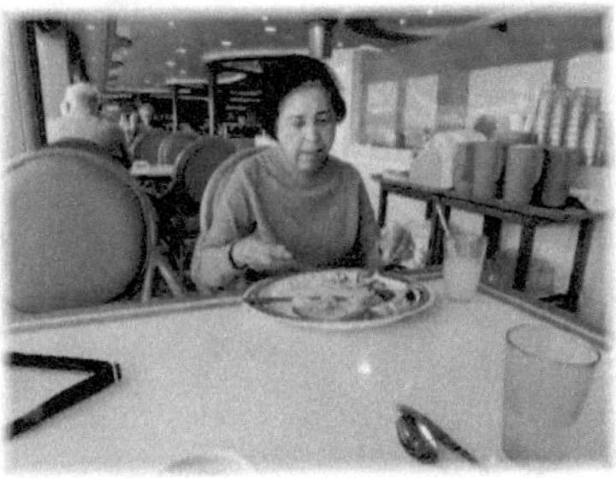

The choice of food that she likes has dwindled to very few. Lest I offend her, I just offer her whatever she wants, but trying to stay with the type that I learned to be good for her such as fish, fowl, brown rice, vegetables and poultry products. She verges on throwing up when she tastes food that is not familiar to her.

Alzheimer's has a way of tricking the victim's mind into accepting a dubious thing as truth. In Amelia's case, for example, her taste bud has been reconstituted to like nothing but pancakes for breakfast. So, up to the date of publication of this book – more than ten years – pancakes have been Amelia's regular food for breakfast, except when she is far away from the pancake place. Owing to the split arrangement of food we order, I have been eating pancakes myself to make the food attractive to her, but with an option to vary my part.

Measuring Food Intake

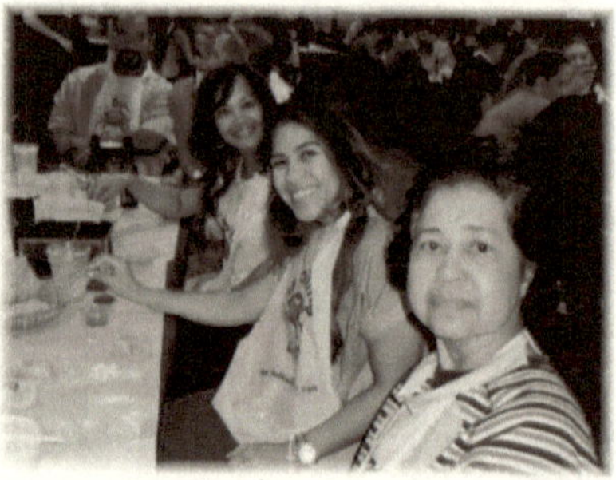

I miss Amelia's cooking, but with her condition, we are disposed to eating at restaurants every day. Eating outside of the home for more than ten years appears to relieve me from stress imposed by caregiving. At first, getting used to the arrangement was very irritating and annoying, but left with not much choice, I learned how to adjust.

Medical Alert

I started looking into the so-called life alert system after a friend of ours fell from the stairs and was unable to summon help due to injuries. He was found unconscious and unresponsive, dying a short time later. The critical period for surviving the fall was lost due to the late arrival of the paramedics. Were he able to call the medical emergency number immediately, perhaps the fall would have a different ending. Alternatively, if he had one of the so-called life alert gadgets his chance of surviving the fall would have improved significantly.

The system I was looking for was one that would enable Amelia or me to summon help in case of emergency. The system must not tie me up to a long contract so that in case there are better ones in the market, I would be free to change service. I was not prepared to pay for options that I did not need; so, over and above my simple requirements, would be considered as bonus features and must be free.

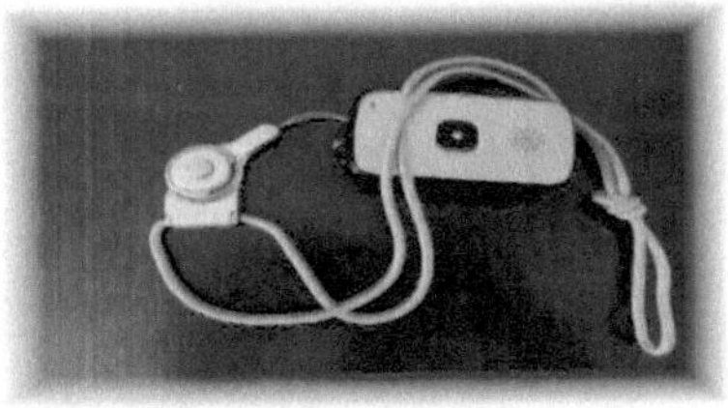

It turned out that after a simple search, the system I found and liked has more features than what I required, namely:

- is waterproof,
- allows us to call in case of a mix-up in Amelia's medications,
- gives us direction in case we get lost while driving,
- alerts someone we designate if Amelia stumbles and gets hurt,
- alerts someone we name if Amelia feels dizzy, disoriented, and needs help,

Medical Alert

- signals the service to help us in case we got locked out of the house,
- alerts someone we designate if we feel unsafe walking to the car at some locations at certain times,
- allows someone we choose to know where we are all the time,
- alerts Amelia's doctor in case of emergency,
- informs Amelia's caregiver of her medical conditions,
- and is light and easy to carry.

To ensure that if Amelia has an emergency and needs to alert someone, I designated our daughters and Amelia's brother as primary contacts. The system does not require that the selected contact be outside of our residence, but I figured that the chance of reaching someone else besides me outside our home is better, since I am with Amelia most of the time.

The system is very simple to set up, but if one finds difficulties in doing so, the support staff is ready to help 24/7. Once it is configured, one of the largest cellular phones and internet services providers provides the 24 hours of emergency alert service.

The hardware itself costs $49.95. I choose the premium plan which costs $19.95 per month. Since Amelia no longer uses a cell phone, I drop the line to save $40.00 per month. Applying $20.00 of our savings from the discontinued line, to the cost of the life alert service still leaves us $20.00 in extra savings.

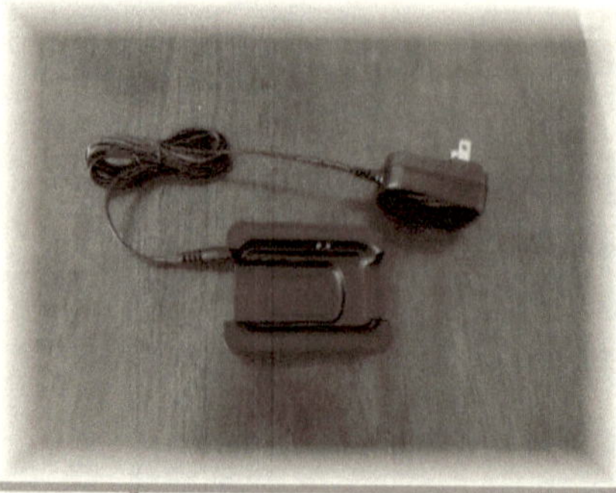

Medical Alert

The system does not require a contract; I am free to discontinue the service at any time without penalty. Unlike some systems which are bundled with other products, discontinuance of the service does not affect our other accounts with the phones and internet services provider.

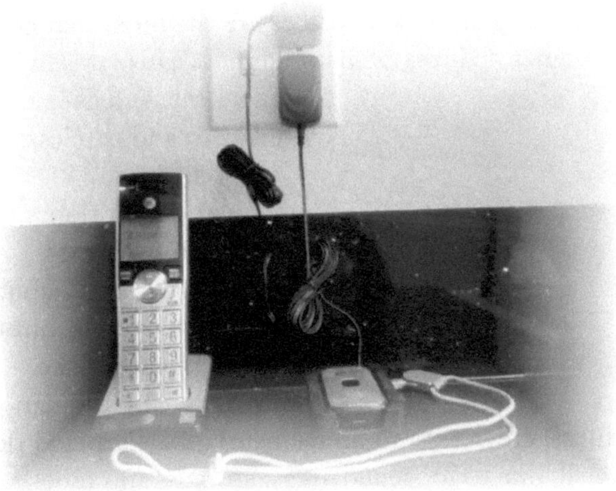

Preventing Near Falls

The falls being laid out here are less likely to cause severe injuries as do falls from elevated platforms, stairs, ladders, and steep slopes. Using my terminology, I call this type of falls as "near falls."

Amelia's many admissions and releases from the hospitals always carry warnings from the medical staff against all kinds of falls. Apparently, an accidental fall can inflict severe injuries including broken bones, total incapacity, or even death, to any one specially Amelia, whose physical strength has been compromised due to strokes. Falls occurring at unlikely places are the most that concern me. They have higher chances of happening because it is in those places where Amelia is more complacent and careless.

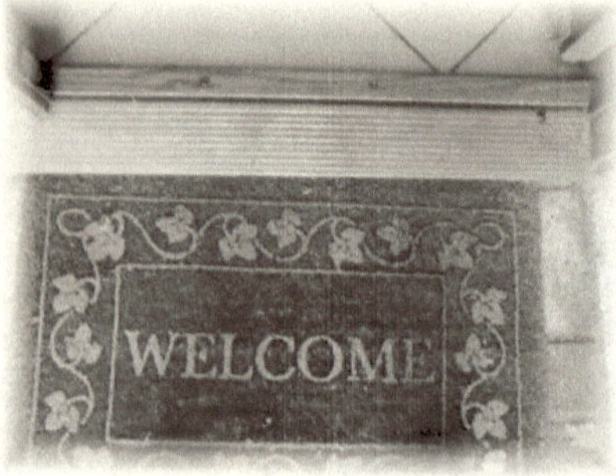

Wooden and tiled floors that are common to homes, shopping malls, and public places look harmless, but to a weakened physique like Amelia's, they pose a danger due to slipperiness, crevices, and uneven surfaces. Carpeted floors pose a risk as well, due to loosened areas, strands, and tapes.

Near falls exist practically everywhere, both indoors and outdoors. The transitions between the curbs and streets are significant challenges to Amelia. Their many damaged joints and uneven surfaces can easily trip her off balance. On drizzly days, they pose an even treacherous path for Amelia, utmost care notwithstanding.

Preventing Near Falls

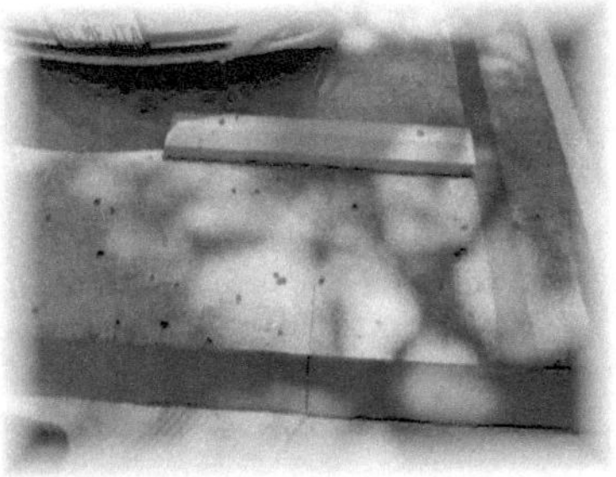

Amelia's effort to move around also contributes to the likelihood of falling. She still feels that she can do the things that she used to do before the strokes. She tends to overextend her arms beyond their reach, throwing her off balance. Her mind tells her how to do one thing while her body refuses to cooperate.

When she walks, she tends to bend forward throwing off her center of gravity. Consequently, it does not take much to trip her into a bad fall. Owing to the strokes, she drags her right foot instead of lifting it making it susceptible of being caught on an uneven surface, creating yet another possibility of falling.

The bathtub fall is one I have Amelia avoid from being a potential victim of easily. Disabling the shower-on-tub discourages Amelia from getting into the tub; she ultimately stopped using it. Nevertheless, I am still leery that not knowing what she is doing, she might still use the bathtub.

The bathroom shower fall is the unavoidable threat that I have to protect Amelia from regularly. Even when the shower area is thoroughly cleaned, it tends to be slippery and can potentially cause Amelia to slip and fall. However, realizing the danger and even with her compromised awareness, Amelia does not want to step into the shower area without me watching her. I minimize the threat by standing close by while she is taking a shower, ready to assist her if the need arises.

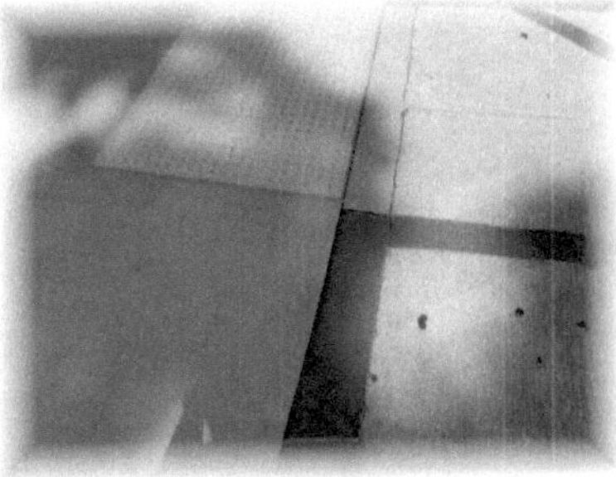

Preventing Near Falls

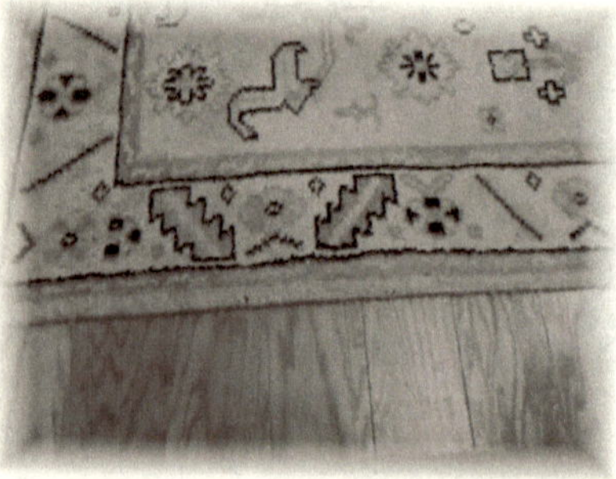

Staying close to Amelia most of the time to lessen the chances of her falling has been paying off. Up to the date of publication of this book, she has not had a serious fall despite one stroke after another rendering her vulnerable and helpless. Raised awareness of her surroundings significantly contributes to the safety record. However, the demand for heightened vigilance over her will grow as her health slowly deteriorates.

Glucose Tracker

Tracking Amelia's glucose level is one of the activities I undertake every day to control her diabetes. From what I learned, glucose is energy, but its presence in the blood stream in exceedingly high level is harmful and can lead to other health complications. On the other hand, the low glucose level is just as damaging, if not more, which can also result in an even worse condition. Maintaining an ideal glucose level requires that I measure and monitor it consistently, if possible at certain times of the day before or after meals, and make a note of any significant spike or drop which might require medical attention.

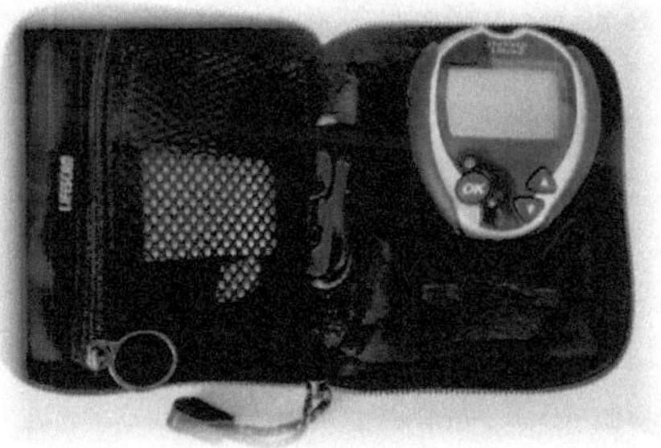

An inexpensive glucose meter is all I need to measure Amelia's glucose level. Different glucose meters are available from pharmaceutical and electronic stores; I procured Amelia's kit for free with a doctor's prescription based on her medical plan. Proficiency in the use of the meter is achieved in just one or two attempts. The meter automatically displays the glucose level which varies each time a measurement is taken.

It is impossible to get consistent readings of Amelia's glucose level every time. The best I can do is to keep the glucose level between 90 and 200, the latter number being suggested by the doctor based on Amelia's age. A reading of 90 or lower is a signal for me to give Amelia orange juice, ensure, apple juice, or candies designed to raise her glucose level. A reading of 200 or over indicates that Amelia needs to be told to lessen her sugar intake through the food she eats and fluids she drinks. Though I have not had an occasion

Glucose Tracker

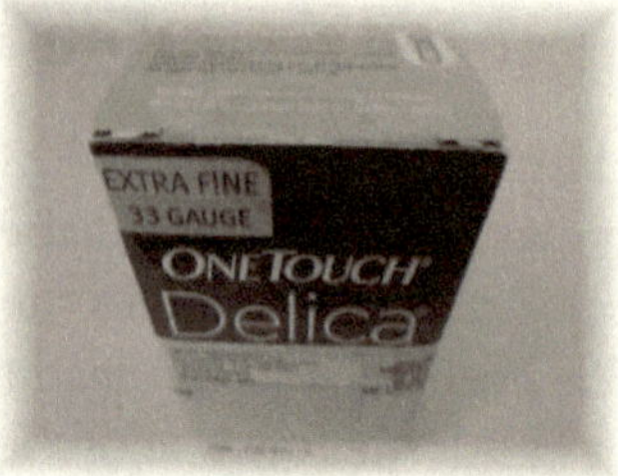

to consult a medical professional based on consecutive very high or very low readings, the option is always open in case the need arises, to allay my fear and anxiety.

Upon inquiry from the hospitals, approximately six hours is how long I should allow her medications to be fully absorbed and circulated in her system. To monitor fluctuations in her glucose level, I take readings at around 7:00 AM and 5:00 PM just before she takes her medications. If she shows any sign of abnormality in between those hours, I take more readings as necessary. This arrangement ensures that Amelia's glucose level does not go too far below or too far above the target levels especially while we are asleep.

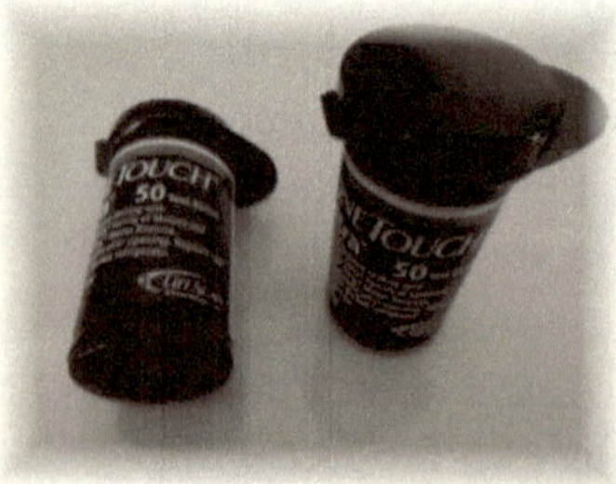

I learned that the symptoms of severe glucose level spike or drop include weakness, confusion, nausea, discoloration, shaking, and stuttering. When any of these occurs, I take a glucose level reading, and if the symptom is confirmed, I sit Amelia down comfortably and give her medications or sugar aids as necessary. Otherwise, I prepare her for a possible trip to the hospital.

When we expect to be away from home for an extended period, I always carry the tote bag that contains Amelia's glucose meter and other glucose levelers including her medications, juices, and other personal stuff.

Surveillance Cameras

One has to experience the trauma and emotional strain of taking care of a diabetic patient who had multiple strokes, Alzheimer's, and congestive heart failure, to appreciate any hint of relief from the constant chore. The case I have with Amelia is ongoing making me open to ideas that ease the stress within me. One such idea is the use of cameras – surveillance cameras in particular.

What does a camera have to do with a patient like Amelia? First of all, I have to admit that after fourteen years of singly taking care of her, I need to be away from her sometimes but still being able to monitor her movements. As I realized, surveillance cameras will allow me to do just that, specifically watch Amelia regularly without being nearby. The benefits of installing surveillance cameras are numerous; the most important ones in Amelia's case are specific.

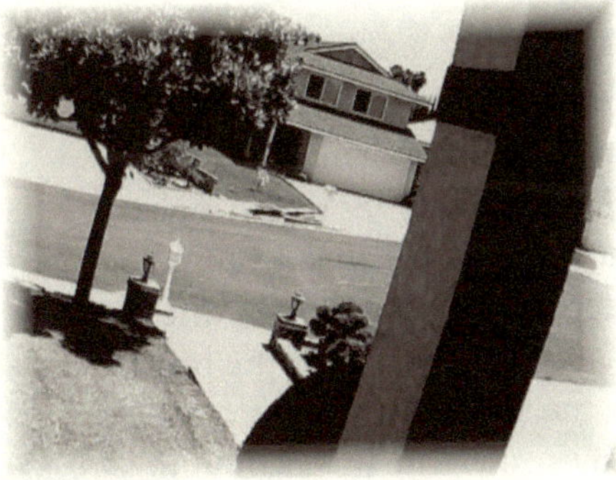

Regarding diabetes, her glucose level fluctuates between an acceptable low and an acceptable high. I am at ease when it stays within the target levels. However, many times it drifts below and exceeds the fair high measurements. Either level affects Amelia in a negative way. For example, when the glucose level is very low she shakes, feels disoriented, and becomes nauseated. Catching the symptoms in time through observation minimizes the chance of further health complications.

After three strokes, Amelia has been physically debilitated to the health state that makes her susceptible to falls at the slightest

Surveillance Cameras

disequilibrium. Her memory is failing as well, rendering her unable to help herself in case of emergency. She is incoherent on the telephone making an urgent call almost ineffective. Keeping her in sight makes calling for immediate medical assistance fast and easy.

Finally, because of Alzheimer's, Amelia does not readily remember names of even the close members of the family including children and grandchildren. The telephone is no longer an emergency tool for her; she does not have any idea who to call in case of emergency. Though she does not step out of the house and roam around like some Alzheimer's patients do, the thought of it happening is haunting me. The house, as well as its surroundings, needs to be watched and monitored as well.

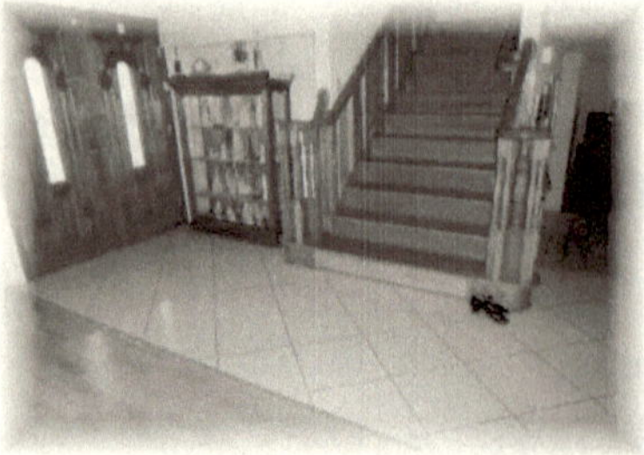

I shopped around for surveillance cameras that would allow me to follow at least 75% of Amelia's movements because I cannot keep her in sight all the time. For example, I may be in the backyard or the store or the post office at which time she is out of my sight physically. The installation does not have to be expensive and elaborate.

I found one for less than $500. I installed two fixed cameras to monitor the front and back yards, one panning camera to catch what is going on in the living area, kitchen, and stairs, and another panning camera to watch the family room including the patio door and the garage door.

The cameras allow me to take photos and videos of the covered areas, from anywhere in the world that I have a connection to the internet, with a cell phone, a tablet or a computer. Also, the panning cameras accept voice messages from the mobile phone.

Surveillance Cameras

The cameras are Wi-Fi enabled through a router which I already own with my computer. No television or computer connection is necessary.

I can monitor Amelia's movements even if I am away from home. If an emergency occurs, I can quickly summon assistance and help. Furthermore, the sight of the cameras alone deters some people who might be thinking of doing us harm. My sense of security is improved, and the tension within me has certainly subsided to a large extent.

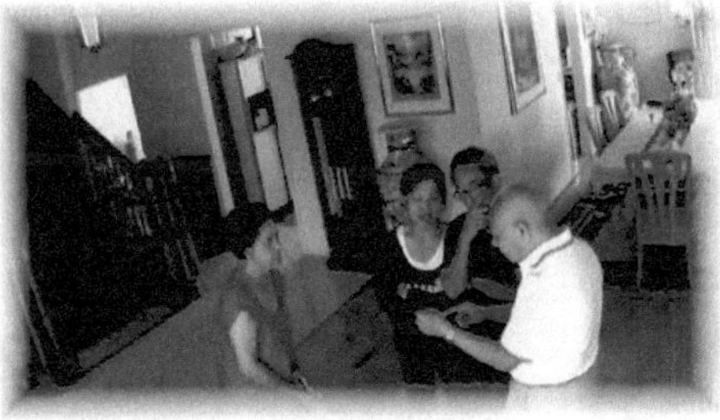

Amelia is Home – Not Nursing Home – Bound

Amelia is home, not nursing home, bound! This statement will forever be right as long as I can take care of her. After the third stroke, my children and I evaluated the options opened to us for taking care of her, including placing her in a nursing home. The children were concerned about the toll on me having to provide constant assistance when Amelia moves around the house, like going to the bathroom, getting into the car, following up on appointments, so on so forth.

Our research and inquiries about nursing homes revealed some information that discouraged the family from pursuing the option. A nursing home has specially designated units for Alzheimer's patients. If a couple signs up for residency, the facility separates the pair for certain aspects of their stay. The one without Alzheimer's has all the freedom to move around, while the one with Alzheimer's would be grouped with Alzheimer's patients only, whose freedom of movement is within a limited area. That is not the option I want to take for Amelia. I am not willing to sign her in alone either.

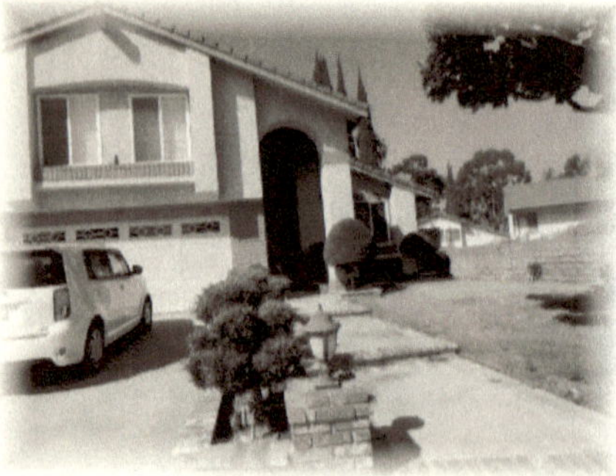

The horror stories about nursing home patients being abused and maltreated send shivers to me and paint a picture in my mind of Amelia being beaten. I feel that the members of the staff at nursing homes have their limits too, regarding having to accommodate patients' needs and complaints. Not too long ago, a video was posted on YouTube showing how one patient was being beaten mercilessly by an emotionally hardened member of a

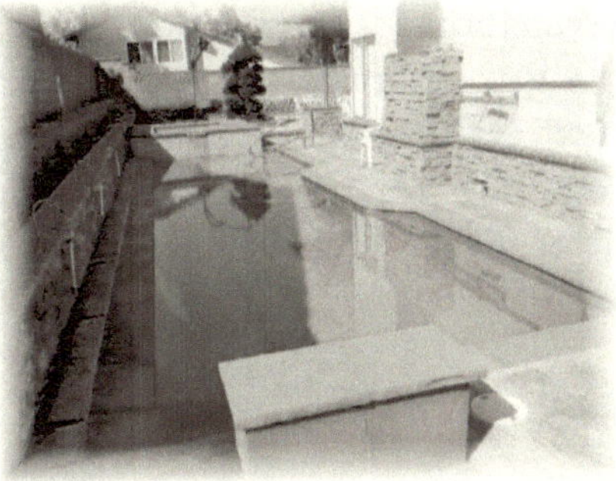

nursing home staff. The video always comes to my mind when I think of Amelia being in a nursing home.

Amelia is obstinate and acts like a kid sometimes, her mental capacity having been downgraded to a fourth-grade level because of the strokes. Now that Alzheimer's has taken a grip on her, the mood is often unpredictable. Leaving her care to members of the nursing home staff who handle several patients with the same or worse condition than Amelia's, is an invitation for abuse. She will tend to be a victim more than other patients because of the number of her ailments, and her inability to respond. Sometimes I tend to lose control myself, and for brief moments I am tempted to abuse her. I surmise that the same emotion can overcome caregivers in the nursing home facility. They too are susceptible to being burnt-out as I am.

From experience I have with taking care of Amelia for more than fourteen years, I can tell that she still has normal senses, but because of her inability to communicate, she endures pain and suffering silently. I can clearly imagine her poor condition being in a nursing home and being abused and maltreated without someone around to help her. She is too fragile already that a slight instance of physical and mental abuse will certainly make her condition worse. If I can help it, I want her health to improve, not to worsen.

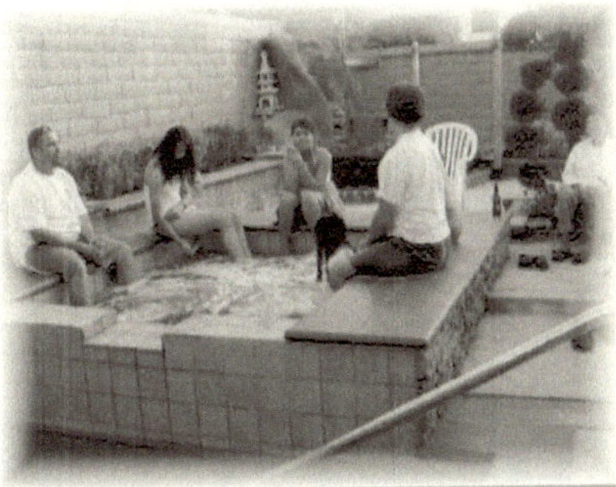

Amelia is Home – Not Nursing Home – Bound

A nursing home is not the preferred option as far as taking care of Amelia is concerned. Search for other options has virtually stopped, because, with attention and perseverance, I can take care of her. I only hope that my health remains stable while she still needs my help. Caregiving as I know it now is not as difficult as I feared it to be before.

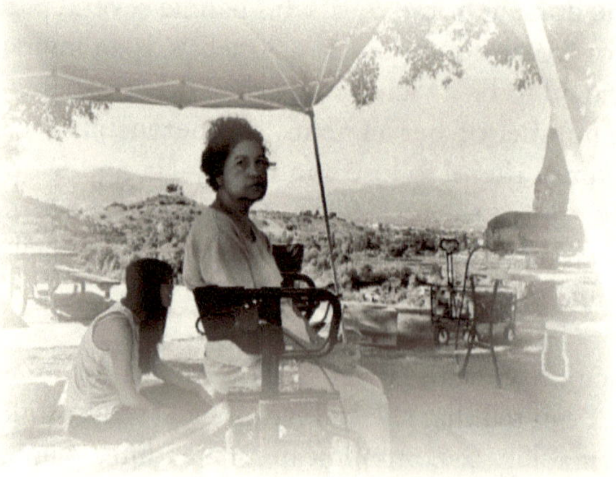

Travel Ease and Care

Strokes inflict different levels of discomfort and deformity on a victim. A mild one may even occur without the victim knowing it, while a severe one may cause severe physical deformity or even death. The first two strokes, I was told, that Amelia suffered at the same time were massive. The right side of her body was completely paralyzed and immobile for a while. Her mental capacity was diminished to a fourth-grade level, while her speech slurred, and only incoherent words would come out of her mouth.

With obvious difficulty and sheer determination, Amelia slowly recovered her mobility, allowing her to move around the house provided someone was along to hold her. Initially, she needed assistance in most of the things she tried to do in motion. Her comfort level in most physical and mental activities went up though, after more than two months. Very slowly she was able to walk again on her own, thanks to aggressive therapy and constant exercise. Her speech started to come out more audible and understandable.

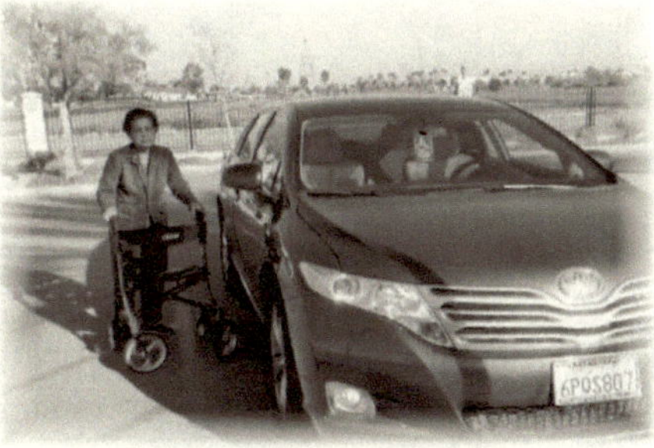

Like clockwork, however, almost to the day in the 10th year after the first two strokes, Amelia suffered another one. Although the doctors characterized the stroke as mild, it seemed that it debilitated Amelia more than the first two did. Once again most of the damage was inflicted on the right side of her body. Ability to move from place to place appeared more forced than natural. Fatefully, the stroke seemed to have triggered Alzheimer's into action to subdue Amelia, complicating her case even more.

Travel Ease and Care

As a result of the stroke on top of the previous two, Amelia started to have difficulty getting on and off the car we had, the so-called cross between a sports utility vehicle and a sedan. Most of the time she struggled letting her right leg in, requiring her to lift it with her right hand which was also weakened by the strokes. Though I observed the pain from the expression on her face, she was not complaining, haplessly accepting her condition as normal.

With Amelia's comfort in mind and with her agreement, we decided to get rid of the car and opted for one with smaller tires. The smaller tires meant easier access for Amelia, allowing her to slide her leg in. I test-drove one brand after another; all the models offer the same convenience for Amelia. The prices differ only on the options we wanted of which, I only had a guidance system installed, principally for use in unfamiliar places.

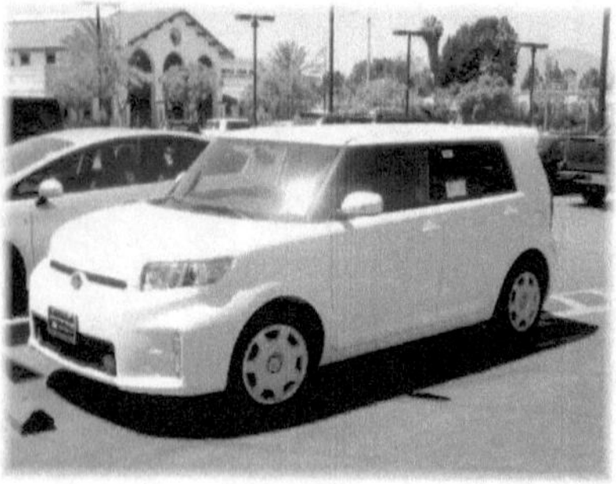

I have been with Toyota Leasing for as many years as I could remember. Time was the essence, so I decided to stay with them to shorten the lease application process. I leased the Scion XB which Amelia likes and which provides the comfort that she desperately needs. Getting in and out of a car bigger than the Scion XB would impose too much difficulty on her. Should a better model appear in the market, I can terminate the lease and get a more comfortable vehicle to suit Amelia's needs.

Medications and Paraphernalia

After the first two strokes but before Alzheimer's overwhelmed her, Amelia was comfortable in scheduling and taking her medications on time. My sole responsibility was placing the orders for her when prescribed drugs start to run low. I had to watch her closely, though, when she was bundling them to ensure that she did not miss taking certain medications while overdosing on others. The arrangement worked very well because she was forced to learn how to count again and remember the times of the day that she had to take them.

Regaining her confidence, Amelia insisted on being completely left alone and unwatched, to handle the medications herself. After assuring me of her accuracy, I stopped interfering with her. The arrangement worked smoothly well for a while until the pharmacist called my attention about having to fill an order too soon. The pharmacist indicated that Amelia was perhaps overdosing on certain medications while missing on others; Amelia denied doing it.

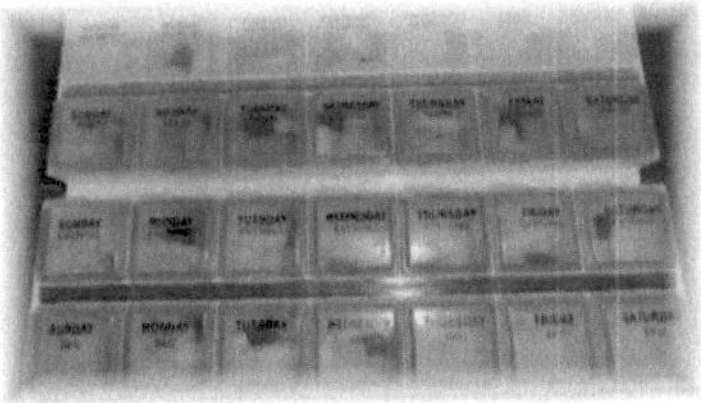

I took control of all her medications including placing the orders, populating the plastic medication receptacle, and giving them to her only at scheduled times. After the third stroke and the just recently diagnosed severe stenosis of the heart valves, the number of prescribed drugs frequently changed, requiring a simple tracking method. A tabulation of the medications as of May 2016 follows:

Medications and Paraphernalia

Medication	Time Taken	Dosage	Frequency
Centrum Silver	AM	1	Daily
B-12	AM	1	Daily
Caltrate	AM	600mg	Daily
Memantine	AM/PM	10mg	2 Daily
Atorvastatin	PM	20mg	2Daily
Metformin HCL	AM/PM	1000mg	2 Daily
Glipizide	AM	5mg	Daily
Carvedilol	AM/PM	40mg	Daily
Aggrenox	AM/PM	200mg	2Daily
Furosemide	PM	20mg	1Daily but varies

When populated, the plastic medication receptacle alerts me which medications are running low and requiring reordering.

To complete Amelia's medical paraphernalia, I keep the glucose level measuring kit and the blood pressure meter within easy reach in case I have to use them. I do not know what to do with an elevated blood pressure, but I hope that if someone asks me to take it and wait for instructions, I should be able to do it.

Medications and Paraphernalia

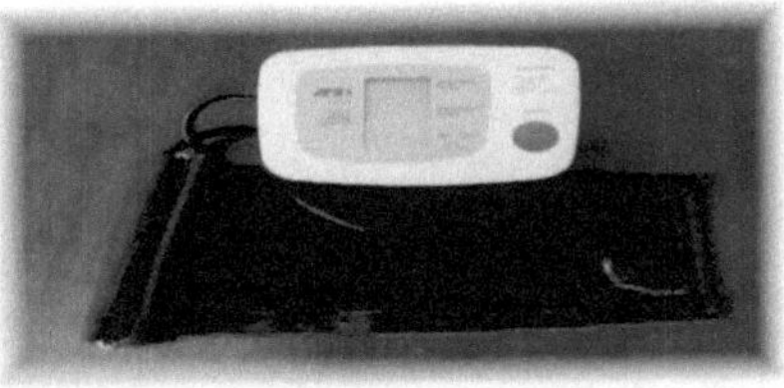

Additionally, I keep a detailed list of Amelia's medications with our travel documents. In case of an emergency away from home, members of the medical staff shall be able to prescribe the right prescribed drugs based on the list.

Before we embark on a trip, I populate the plastic medications receptacle with the exact number of prescribed drugs for each day that we expect to be gone. When fully filled and at the rate Amelia is taking them, the receptacle provides for a fourteen-day supply of medications. To meet additional days' supply, I pack an extra amount for seven days in a separate container. Amelia's medical alert system also lists her medications, providing additional emergency readiness.

Last Line of Defense

This book is about compassion, empathy, humility, survival, and caregiving. Sadly, though, these distinguishing features of human nature are easy to preach than to emulate and practice. A significant number in our society are shielded from these feelings. Greed in many forms appears to be more prevalent than kindness. Many are driven to harass others who are minding their own business, by financial gains and plain callousness. One only needs to watch the news about crimes to check the accuracy of these statements.

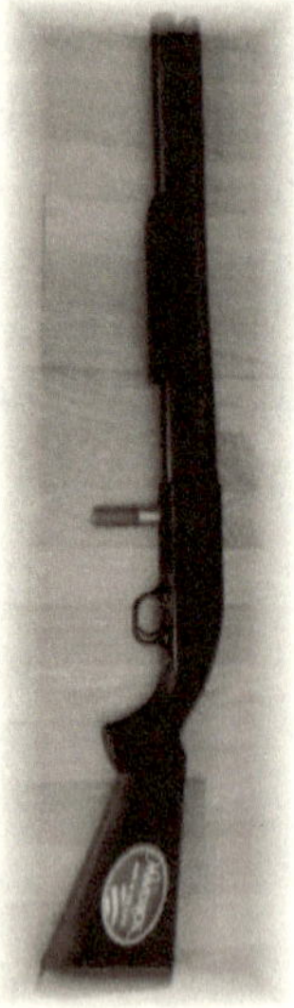

Initially, we did not pay attention to calls from people offering general services and merchandise. Our attitude changed after Amelia suffered strokes; we started getting calls from people offering merchandise and services for stroke victims. It changed again after Amelia was diagnosed with Alzheimer's; we have begun getting calls from people offering similar services and merchandise for Alzheimer's patients.

The change of offers from one type of merchandise and services to a different kind corresponding to Amelia's physical disorders, was swift and simultaneous, indicating that we are in a database of some sort. The calls are non-stop. It is impossible to tell which calls are important and which ones are not; they come at different times of the day. What irks me most is that some calls are from unattended machines designed to annoy and harass legitimate subscribers.

Last Line of Defense

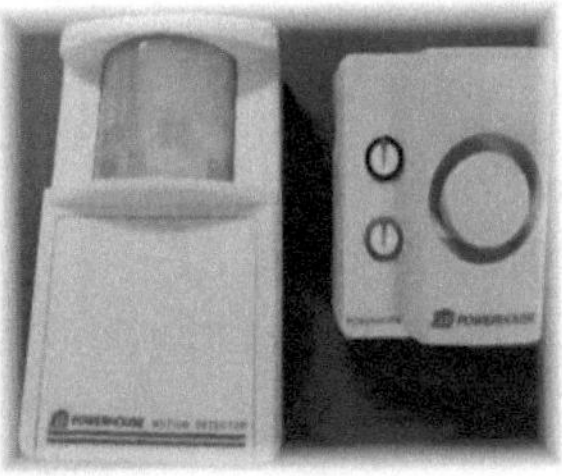

I understand that some calls are to find out if anybody is at home, to hatch a plan to commit a crime. There is probably no truth to it, but I heard that some are from people freshly out of prison being offered jobs to start a new life. If my understanding is correct, this type of people will not hesitate to commit another crime.

Home security companies offer their services because of the number of burglaries in certain areas, according to them. They pressure residents to buy their services under the pretext of rampant crimes in the neighborhood. They even offer to put their signs on yards for free, to convince potential customers to buy their services. To bolster their claim of numerous burglaries, they even provide statistics.

Internet services providers and telephone and cable companies are somewhat complicit as well, in violating privacy. They call to announce new products and services and to secure answers to surveys that could end up in indexed databases which are shared with their subsidiary companies.

Collection agencies leave messages on our answering machine. I have no reason to deal with them because my credit rating is beyond reproach. Nevertheless, I am forced to subscribe to a credit reporting agency to alert me of possible intrusion into my private files.

We even get calls from oil drilling companies with which we have no dealings at all; they offer shares of stocks at discounted prices,

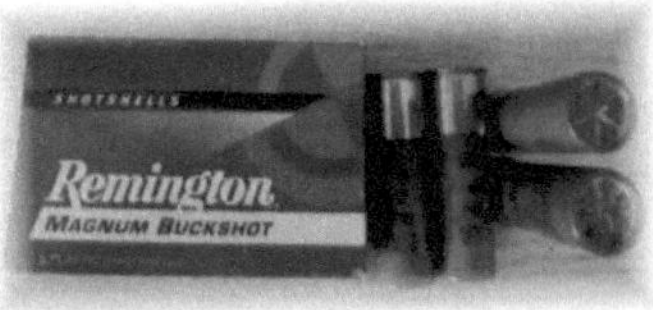

Last Line of Defense

promising better than average returns on investment.

Similar activities are happening on my computer. Solicitations eclipse my legitimate emails, for donations and offers for sale of merchandise and services. Spams and legitimate emails are hardly distinguishable from each other.

The list of unwanted calls and unauthorized electronics access is endless, strengthening the argument that it is up to me to protect our privacy when nothing else works to protect it. Apparently, the no calls legislation is useless; it does not stop the calls even when our telephones are in the registry. Evidently, our vulnerabilities are of public record. What privacy we had - we no longer enjoy, it is gone.

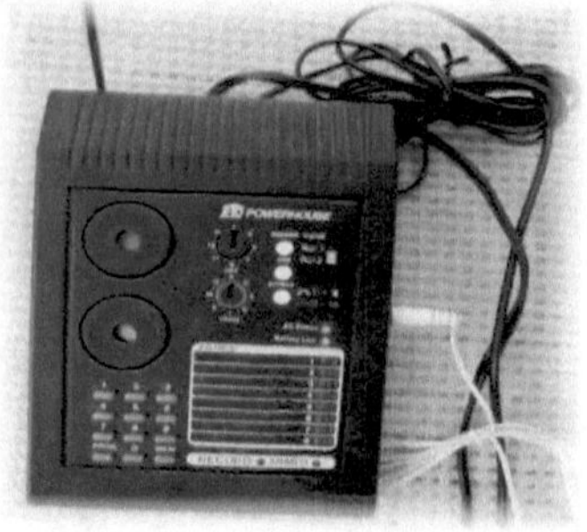

I installed surveillance cameras outside and inside the house. Floodlights automatically turn on when someone is within the cameras' viewing angles. I bolted our windows and doors; motion sensors turn on the alarms automatically.

Our last line of defense is a bolted door in the room where we sleep at night. Amelia cannot run or jump; neither can she yell for help. We are an easy prey if someone is intent on doing us harm.

However, when all the precautions I installed do not deter one from harming us, and our last line of defense is breached, I will not hesitate to use a gun which I keep within reach at all times at night. Our need for a protective firearm is real, considering Amelia's physical and mental condition.

Mercy Move

Early in the book, I made a vow that Amelia was not going to a nursing home as long as I am physically able to take care of her. Here, I affirm the pledge notwithstanding my advancing age, but with luck and perseverance. She, frail and with failing health, greatly appreciates my commitment. Our final move was a necessity which I did not anticipate when I made the promise.

The house that we had been calling home for thirty-seven years was well-built, so, other than for Amelia's convenience, we were somber to bid goodbye to it. The primary consideration for buying it in the first place was Amelia's requirement that the main door opened to the east facing the sun in the morning. That requirement was not important to me at the time we purchased the house; the practical floor plan attracted me more than anything else after having seen few other models.

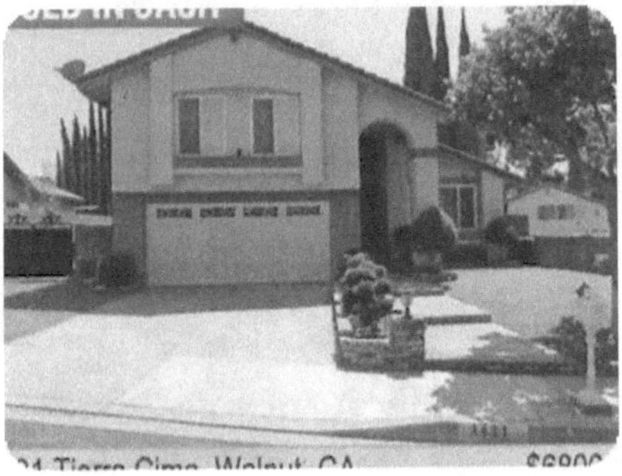

Our children grew up in the same house since their elementary and early adulthood years; our grandchildren spent their early childhood days in it as well. Moreover, about 40% of the improvements in the house were done by me – by my hands. So the loss of the home was nostalgic and with an enormous degree of reluctance.

The lack of a bedroom and a bathroom in the downstairs area of the tri-level house did not discourage me from staying in it until the later part of the year 2015. By then Amelia was in the thirteenth

Mercy Move

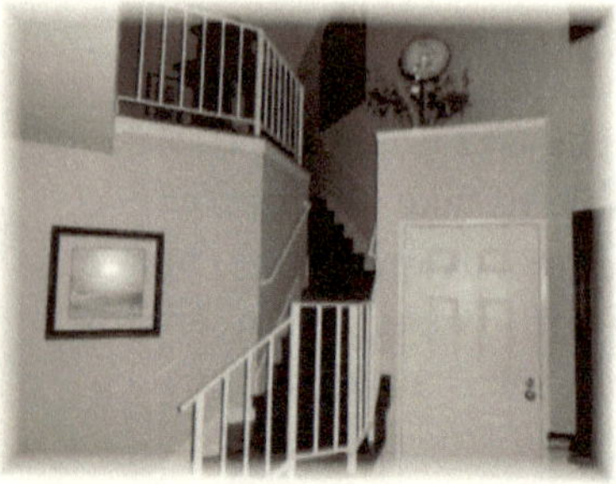

year of her ailments of strokes, dementia, diabetes, and lately-diagnosed severe stenosis of the heart valves.

As Amelia's physical condition continues to deteriorate, I started to become desperate for a solution to her commute between the rooms downstairs and the rooms upstairs where the full bathrooms are located. Finding a house with a bedroom and a bathroom downstairs at a price consistent with our combined income as retirees is not easy. I was ready to reconsider my pledge, exploring the idea of moving Amelia to a nursing home.

Alternatively, I leaned towards moving to an apartment unit where she would not have to climb stairs. The alternative led me to sell the house first and to take a chance of finding an apartment unit later.

Luck was with us starting at the time we listed the house for sale. The house sold in two weeks with an escrow stipulation that we be allowed to stay in it for three months until final construction of the apartment we were planning to rent. In the meantime, we had to move thirty-seven years of accumulated household stuffs to a public storage. I anticipated donating or throwing away stuffs that would not fit in a 2-bedroom apartment unit – refrigerator, washers, tools, pool table, dishes, clothes, work benches, and much, much more – what a waste that would have been!

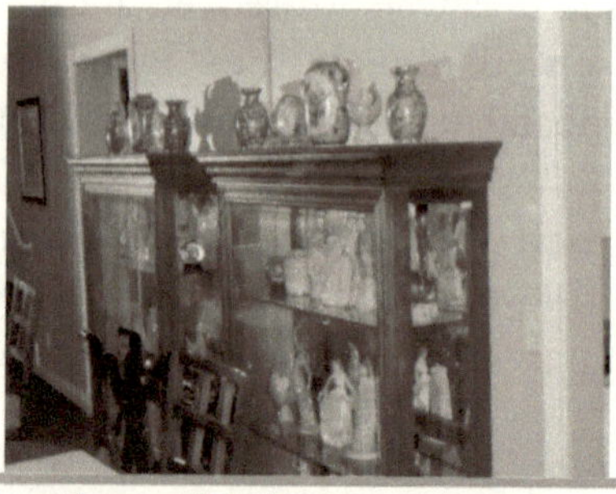

Mercy Move

On the last month of the extension of our stay in the house we sold, a jewel of a townhouse came into the market. The townhouse has two upstairs suites each complete with a full bath, and a loft as large as another bedroom. More important, it has a bathroom and a bedroom downstairs, both extremely necessary for Amelia's needs. After viewing and inspecting the townhouse, I made a purchase offer right on the spot through the agent who helped us sell our original house. I learned later that there were two other pending cash offers for the townhouse, which were being considered by the seller.

We moved into the townhouse in one month. It has big enough closets and utility spaces for most of the stuffs we brought along from the old house. The garage is big enough for me to build a work table after giving away the old one in the house we sold. Our son took the pool table which I dearly liked for recreation.

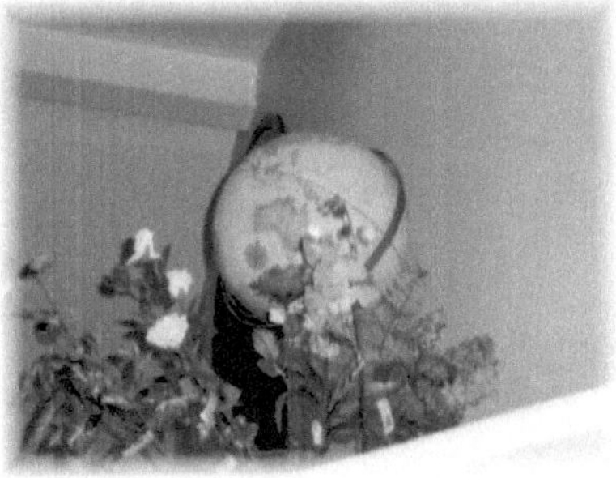

To carefully avoid hurting Amelia's feelings for possible disposition of some stuffs dear to her, I maintain three closetsful of her clothes even though she is not in a position to wear them anymore. We gave away a China and a dining set. The cupboard which contains Amelia's souvenirs and mementos she acquired during our travels and cruises finds a beautiful spot in the house.

Except for installing optional pavers on the walkway and shutters on the windows, there is not much more to do for Amelia and me to comfortably inhabit the townhouse. Should Amelia desire to go upstairs to enjoy the views of the sparkling lights at night and the valley during the day, I had a few grab bars installed for her to hold on to while climbing the stairs.

The move lessens my work associated with home ownership – no more yard work and no more pool maintenance, for example – while reaping the benefits of tax shelter and a possible increase in home value. Amelia's easy access to a bathroom is the most urgent and important aspect of our final move which I call a "mercy move."

The pride of still owning a home more than offsets the regret of losing our old house. While the move is difficult, its consequence is an enormous relief to me from not having to deal with Amelia's difficulty in locating a full bathroom.

Chapter 3 – Protracted Living

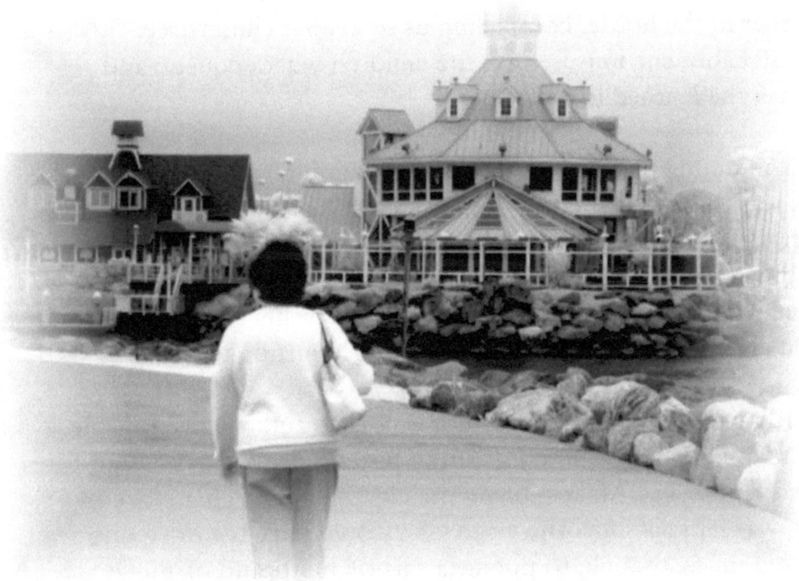

Quality of Life in Ruin

This part of the book deals with the idiosyncratic behaviors that Amelia exhibits as a victim of strokes, Alzheimer's, diabetes, and congestive heart failure. A contrast of her personalities before and after contracting the diseases provides insights of how the maladies affect her.

Earning a college diploma in home economics, she was a stickler for order in the house, compelling us to keep it clutter-free. Unmistakably, she imposed on the children what etiquette and theories she learned in college.

It was in dining places though, that her training was more evident for it was there that she was very keen in even the simple activities of arranging tableware and in the order of which food was being consumed. Irked as I was by her precision, I was astonished at how far she would go to make dining enjoyable for her family. She would always suggest a short prayer before starting to eat.

Regarding dressing up, she was not excessive and too fashionable, only adapting changes to conform to pseudo dress requirement for regular employees. Macy's, being the closest store to her place of work, was Amelia's favorite store. She would have me drive one hundred miles, though, to pursue a sale of her brand of purse.

Her distaste of disrespectful manners particularly against the elderly was absolute. She was friendly and devoid of ill feelings against others. Amelia felt obligated to go to church every week, her faith in God virtually handed to her by her mother. She was as normal as anyone could be, having similar frustrations, disappointments, and triumphal moments.

Quality of Life in Ruin

After Amelia contracted the previously mentioned diseases, her personality completely changed, leaving me aghast with diminished hope and faith.

Now Amelia has difficulty recognizing her children and grandchildren. Her inability to identify our daughter's house despite our frequent visits reveals a state of disorientation. In absolute nonsense, she tells of her parents living close by our house when in fact they have never been to the United States.

She now has to be told to swallow her food and not to talk with a full mouth. Occasionally against my admonitions, she would carry conversations with complete strangers, some with different languages and apparent race orientations. Her speech opens her to potential ridicule because it is limited to few garbled words resulting in incomplete sentences.

For unexplained development in her mind, she now has the tendency to say the exact opposite attributes of what she means. For example, when water is already too hot for a shower, she would yell to turn the hot water on more, when she means to turn it slightly down. Meaning to raise the room temperature up because of cold weather, she would ask to turn it off instead. Frequently she asks me to close an already closed door.

On certain occasions she feels hungry and asks for food, not remembering that she just had one just moments ago. Once she likes a particular food, she does not readily give it up; it becomes the essential staple that sustains her for days until she tastes a replacement food that she likes. Lunch and dinner no longer have timelines; when she feels the need to eat, she eats regardless of the times.

Quality of Life in Ruin

Another perplexing phenomenon is her ability to remember events that occurred oceans away, more than fifty years ago. High school activities that she participated in years and years ago are still vivid in her mind. Without hesitation, she could name some relatives she had not seen, and I had not known either, in more than fifty years. In perfect rhythm with music, she could break into few folkloric dance steps, activities she did as a teacher years ago.

Amelia has to live with her changed personality throughout her remaining life. Her physical handicap does not show until she moves around. Her diminished mental capacity is evident only when she communicates and carries a conversation with other people. With enough support, we hope to prolong her life a little longer; having her still – that is what counts the most.

Food Dilemma

In a separate title, I described the manners Amelia exhibits while eating breakfast. Apart from breakfast, she eats lunch, snack, and dinner at certain times. Lunch and dinner are the times when my problem occurs because I have to coax Amelia to eat before hunger syndrome makes its presence known, making her feel uneasy and nauseated.

Amelia has an unpredictable mood regarding food preference. Whether the changing preference is due to diabetes, Alzheimer's, strokes, congestive heart failure, or all of them, is impossible to tell. To avoid her from getting sick, I go along with her preference, picking only the food that is balanced and nutritious. However, since we share our food all the time, her choice may turn out to be one that I dislike.

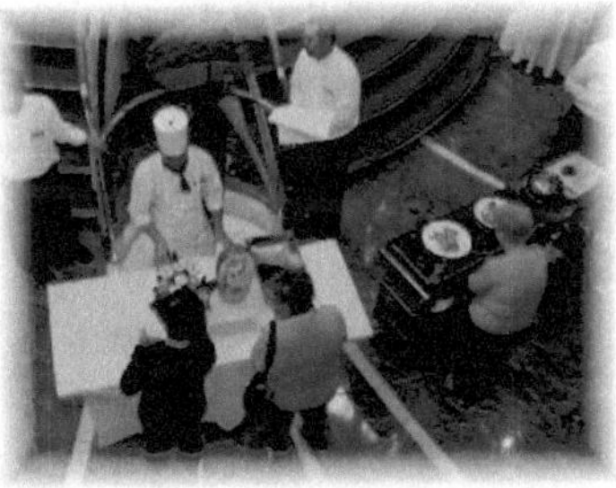

Broiled chicken, Amelia's favorite for lunch or dinner at the start, was also the one I liked because it was the easiest one for me to order. Suggested by nutritionists and shed of fat, it freed me to customize and make it savory by the addition of some condiments. Everywhere we went Amelia would seek the place and had me order the same food. My opposition to it was my having to share and eat with her all the time. When it dropped out of Amelia's favor, I sighed with relief.

She complained about her food not having any taste at all. Against the suggestion that she ought to eat food with less sodium, I tricked her into liking teriyaki burger. The teriyaki burger I had in mind was being prepared with vegetables which Amelia needed but stopped eating. To my surprise, she loved the teriyaki burger,

Food Dilemma

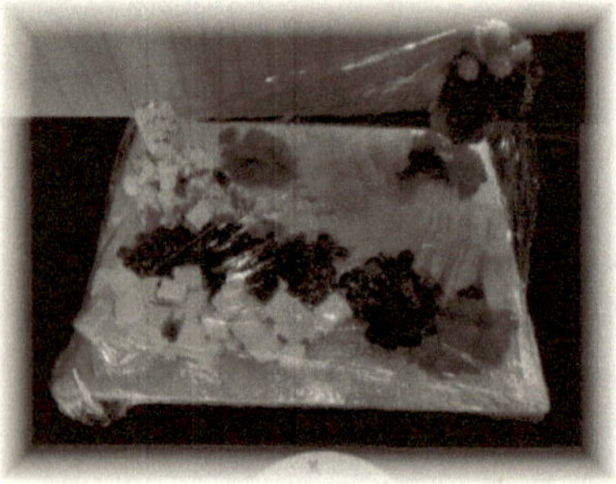

making it the essential staple that sustained her for a while. We would then be on the lookout for the teriyaki burger place whenever we made short trips. For no reason other than a change in her sense of taste, she abandoned the teriyaki burger.

I hoped, in exasperation, that a very popular and well-reviewed Japanese restaurant close to us was an alternative place where Amelia could dine without the dreaded uneasiness. I was furious that even with all the inducements to fine dining, Amelia did not like the food either; she was feeling uneasy, I could tell. Rather than risk her throwing up in the place, I ate as fast as I could, paid the bill, and we left with a package of leftovers. Surprisingly, she loved to eat the food at home. Intrigued and irked, I kept ordering the same food once or twice a week until it dropped from her favor again.

The choice of possible eating places near our home was endless, but few of them satisfied Amelia's liking. For taste variation, I took her to a popular eating place where I ordered a steak with baked potato, salad, and vegetables, for dinner. To my dismay, Amelia only tasted the steak, ate a small amount of salad, sipped some soup, pushed the food away, and told me she was done eating. Except for certain pastries, she did not like the restaurant making it among the dining places we sought to avoid in the future.

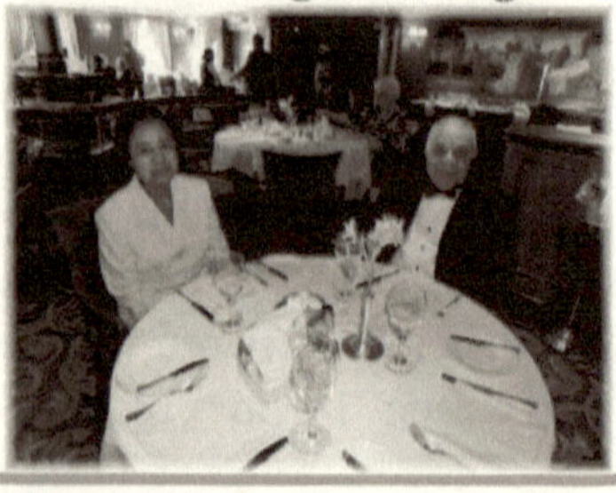

Before her bodily disorders, Amelia's love for Chinese food was insatiable. Concluding that perhaps she still liked it, I took her to the Chinese restaurant where she used to enjoy the food, a place we had been to a few times before. As soon as we walked into the place, Amelia threw up at the lobby because of the odor emanating from the kitchen. Helpless and embarrassed, I apologized to the people in the hallway, but no amount of apologies made up for the angry looks and comments among the customers. We left without eating and probably totally maligned.

Rotating through all the fast-food places one after another is all we have been doing to sustain Amelia and maintain her strength. A more formal eating place is not an option for fear of embarrassment in case Amelia feels uneasy and nauseated. We also shun away from buffet style eating places because of the same apprehension. Luckily, because of Alzheimer's, Amelia does not remember which food is coming from which source.

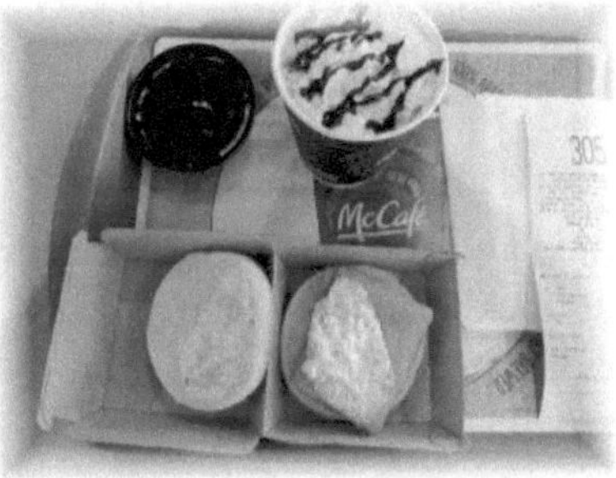

Fearing that Amelia might get sick due to lack of food, I adopt a dynamic default menu which she has to eat. Otherwise, I threaten to completely cut off her food supply. Apropos, she does not want to drink water either unless told to do so, making my caregiving obligation even more challenging.

Since the onset of Alzheimer's, Amelia has been behaving in this manner. Left alone with no one to encourage her to eat and unaware of the consequences, I believe she can go on for days without food. It is not fair to ridicule and make fun of her eating habits, but sometimes I have to, to see if I can slightly redirect her manners towards normalcy. No, my attempt does not work; her bodily disorders prevail, having already overwhelmed her.

Incontinence

My one night's sleep at the hospital where Amelia was confined served as a harbinger of what I should be expecting when she was released. Some members of the hospital staff told me that Amelia developed an incontinence problem. I did not understand what the term was, but watching them cleaned her up was enough explanation.

The day after she was released, one of the topics discussed in the family was about Amelia's involuntary urination and defecation. None of our children would be able to help me in this regard because they do not live with us. Obviously, that was an excuse to avoid dealing with the problem. I ended up, naturally, having to deal with it.

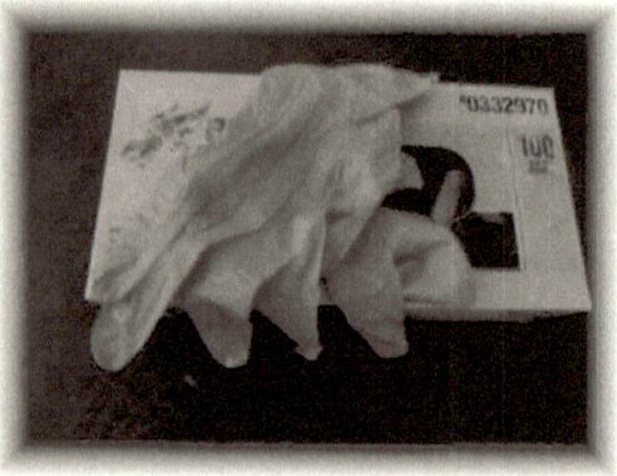

I considered the first month that I had to tackle the gross chore, as the worst period in our married lives of 53+ years. I did not have any idea what to do with her involuntary urination and defecation. I could not exonerate her for what she was doing. I was barely sleeping; I begged, screamed, cursed, and cried, to no avail; she would uncontrollably urinate and defecate at any time

No readily available bed liners would prevent her urine from penetrating into the comforters and the mattress. I had to throw a couple of relatively new comforters away. I had to replace our 8-year old mattress too. My nose was getting very sensitive that even if there was no scent, it kept sending signals to me to start ranting and cursing.

Incontinence

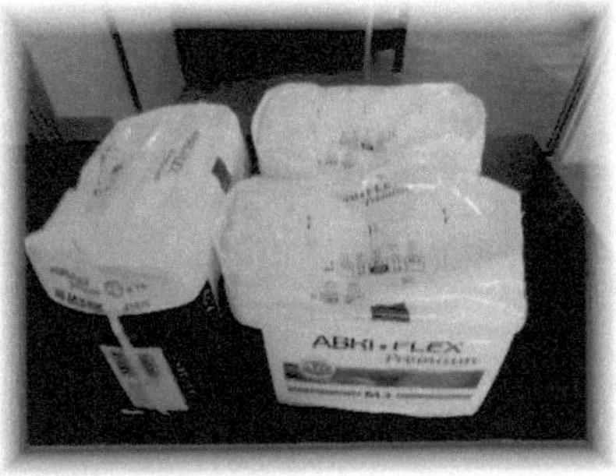

I looked at various options that could relieve me of the vile chore. One option which our children and I immediately implemented, was hiring a caregiver who helped us eight hours a day. The choice did not last long and work out as hoped because Amelia's modus operandi of urinating and defecating was mostly happening at night when the caregiver was gone; I was still stuck with the chore. If we did not want to live in filth, I must find an easier and cleaner way to handle Amelia's incontinence problem.

Finally, I remembered the news about a woman astronaut who drove from Texas to Florida without bathroom stops because she was wearing a special kind of diapers for adults. I googled 'diaper' in the internet; diapers of different qualities and makes were displayed. I placed an order with Amazon for the most appropriately described diapers. The diapers that came with the first order of 84 pieces were slightly tight for Amelia, but we forced them to fit until they were all used up. Next order of another 84 pieces was for the next higher size which perfectly fits her. At last, I found the solution to Amelia's incontinence problem.

The diaper works fittingly well; it is very soft, durable, and absorbent. It does not allow urine and defecation to penetrate to the comforters and mattress. We still do use bed liners but only as a precaution against leakage; leakage has not happened even once. Although the diaper is relatively expensive, cost is not an

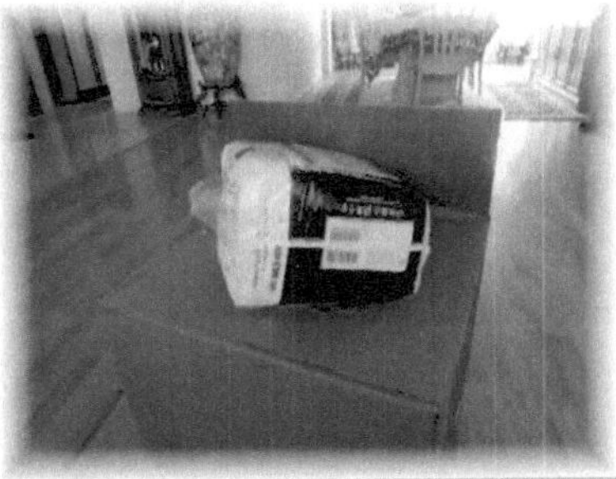

Incontinence

item I quibble with when what I get in return, is control of involuntary urination and defecation.

In the meantime Amelia has regained enough control of her incontinence; she now alerts me when she is ready to go to the bathroom. Incontinence appears to be not a problem anymore, allowing me to recover from temporary derangement.

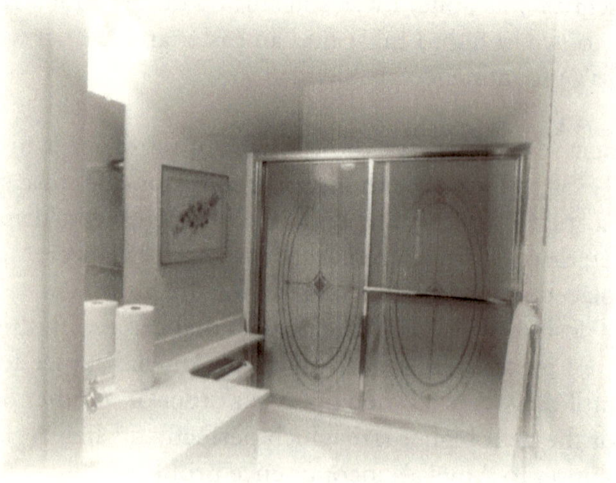

Breakfast Scene

If one keeps a record for most consecutive days and years of having the same food for breakfast, ours will be at the top, for who would think that that it is possible to eat pancakes at the same place for almost ten years? Amelia and I have that record. This part of the book is as much about nutrition as it is about the depiction of the personal behaviors that strokes, Alzheimer's, diabetes, and congestive heart failure inflict on Amelia.

What the restaurant calls as grand slam slugger is what makes up the staple of our breakfast for most of the past ten years until the publication of this book? With an unshakable appetite for it, Amelia is not showing any sign of diversification, preferring to go hungry, if needed, with empty stomach until the next meal time.

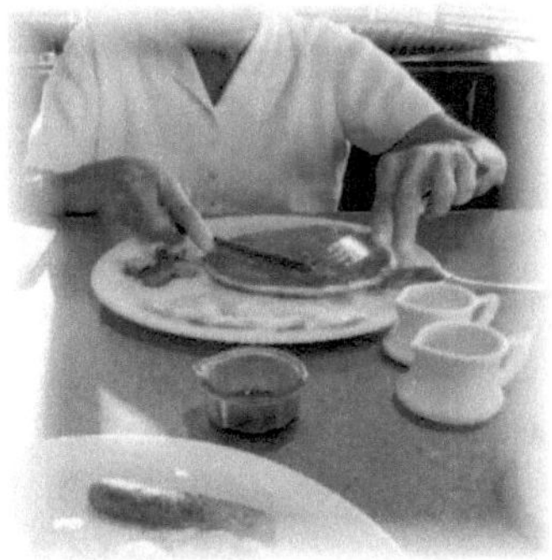

The grand slam slugger comes with two pancakes, two sausage links, two eggs cooked to specification, two coffees, two small bowls of fruits, and regular and sugar-free syrups. The arrangement is perfect for us because we split our meals in half most of the time. The drawback is the monotony that I have to endure consuming the same food every morning because Amelia feels uneasy and nauseated when offered an unfamiliar food.

To test Amelia's appetite for different food for breakfast, sometimes I order one other than pancakes, which she, more often than not, turns down and declines. If she relents and allows me to order one for myself, we have to discard half of the grand slam slugger; Amelia expects to eat only her half of it.

Breakfast Scene

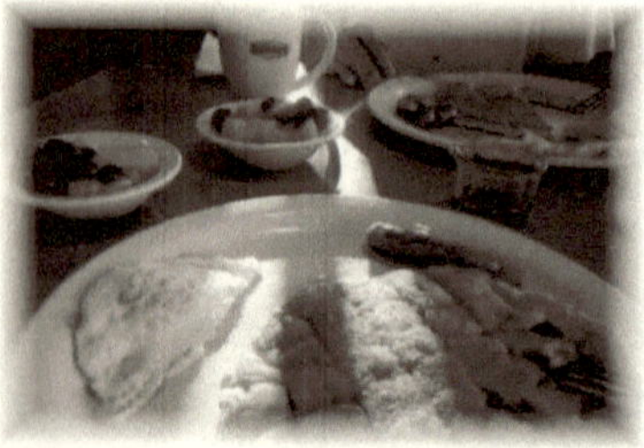

Fifteen to twenty minutes is all it takes me to eat my half of the grand slam slugger, whereas Amelia takes thirty minutes to an hour to finish hers even with my constant coaxing to eat faster. She eats very slow and modest, triggering an argument if I try to rush her. The scene is repeated daily in the same pancake place as long as we are within a 10-mile distance from it. The restaurant servers automatically prepare the grand slam slugger as soon as they see us pulling into the parking lot.

As Alzheimer's gradually overwhelms Amelia, her appetite appears to be waning, limited only to certain types, pancakes for breakfast in particular. From what I heard, Alzheimer's has a way of leaving only certain cells capable of limited taste selections. If it is true, I am witnessing the effects now, forcing me to adjust my caregiving duties accordingly.

One of the unusual things that Amelia also does during breakfast is every time she sips her coffee she wipes the cup clean. Then she also demurely rubs her nose and lips with napkins even though they are clean. She repeats the habit until she finishes eating. Nothing is unusual about the behavior except that it looks too formal for the occasion and the place, and that she is doing it more frequently now. She appears to be emulating what she does in a formal dining seating.

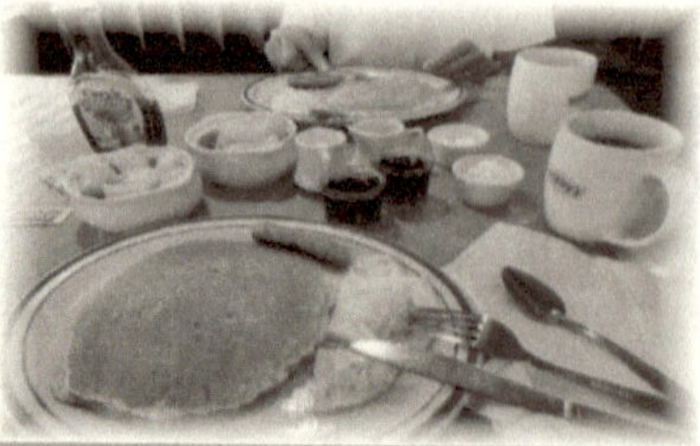

I find it interesting though, that our daily kind of breakfast allows me to maintain an ideal weight without starving. Our meal, when described to friends who know

Breakfast Scene

about food and nutrition, is healthy indeed, not requiring any change to avoid confrontation with Amelia who has an impaired ability to rationalize.

Whether it is strokes, Alzheimer's, diabetes, congestive heart failure, or the combination of all four, which causes Amelia to like a particular food and dislike others, is unclear. She has been through tests that the doctors ordered; nothing seems to be the matter, and that is the welcome news.

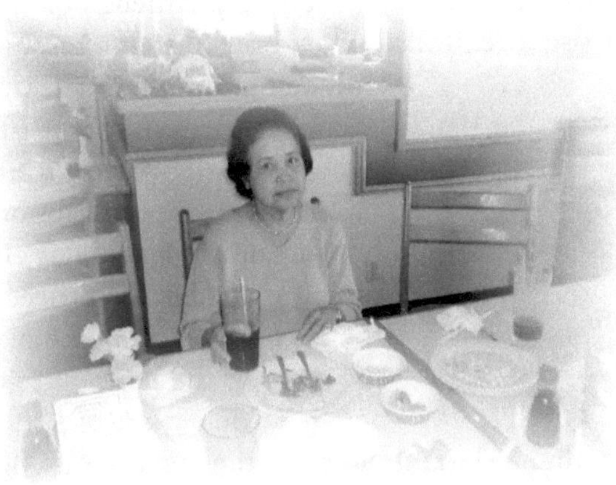

My Daily Tasks

Each time that Amelia was in the hospital for any treatment, the members of the hospital staff emphasized the need for her to exercise. Nothing was extraordinary with the suggestion as Amelia had been exercising regularly without being told. However, whereas the training at the gym was casual and leisurely before, the current requirement is with a more sense of purpose, to prolong her life after she had massive strokes, and after the diagnoses of Alzheimer's, diabetes, and congestive heart failure.

Our day starts with measuring and recording Amelia's blood pressure and glucose level, followed by breakfast at a restaurant

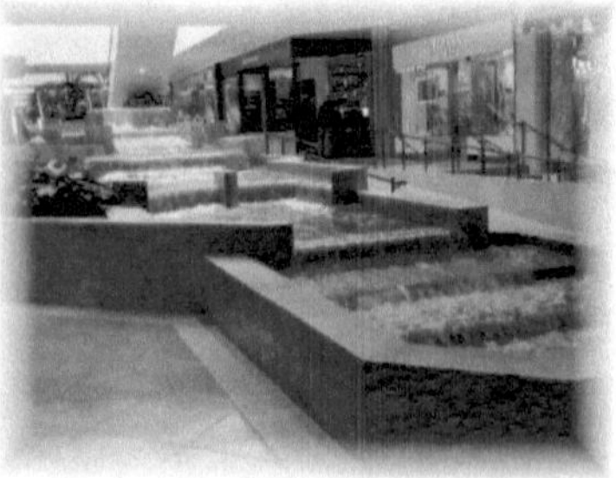

only ten minutes away from our residence. Breakfast consisting of pancakes, eggs, coffee, fruits, and sausage takes us only about an hour to finish, leaving us enough time to relax before proceeding to the exercise place, be it the gym, the mall, or the park.

Some malls are within a short drive from the restaurant where we eat breakfast daily. Amelia likes the mall with the central oval-shaped and clutter-free area. With gentle urging, she makes a few rounds of the area with her walker and without straying away from my sight, before she gets tired and needs to rest. Without encouragement, she would just sit down and watch other people working out.

We have active memberships with a gym that has a few locations close by and that carries all types of exercise equipment. If the gym is the place where we decide to work out during the day, I set up the exercise equipment for Amelia.

My Daily Tasks

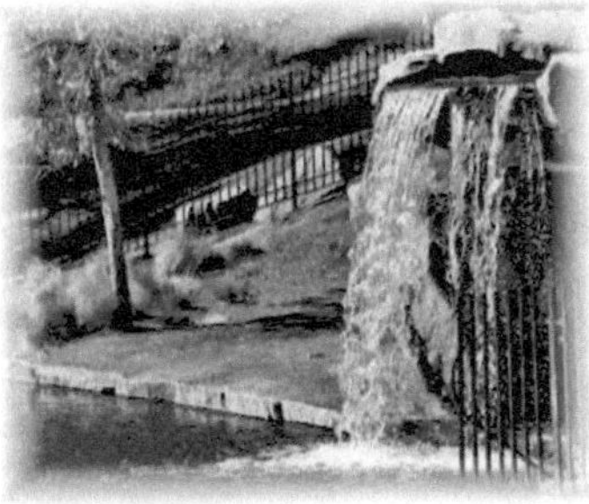

Before she had the third stroke, swimming in the pool and soaking in the health spa were her preferred routine after the exercise equipment, with my assistance of course. The preference has since been discarded owing to her diminished strength and mobility, and my inability to hold and stabilize her in the pool.

Lunch time is when I always have a conflict with Amelia because of her dislike for a particular food. Under threat of starvation, I try to force her to eat whatever I think is right for her. Sometimes the threat works, sometimes it does not, in which case out of sympathy and disgust, I let her eat whatever she likes even when the food is not appropriate for the time of day.

To enliven her in the afternoon, I take her to a mall of my choice where we have snacks. The short period at the mall allows me to unwind and if for only a brief moment, to catch up with badly needed rest. The distractions at the mall help Amelia from looking depressed and low-spirited. Her impatient look and expression are signals for me to bring her home.

Coming home from the mall, I pick up her food for dinner, the kind we agree upon after a slight persuasion. Amelia is aware of the adverse consequence of sleeping on an empty stomach, making it easy for me to win her over to a particular food, in contrast with her objections to certain food during lunch.

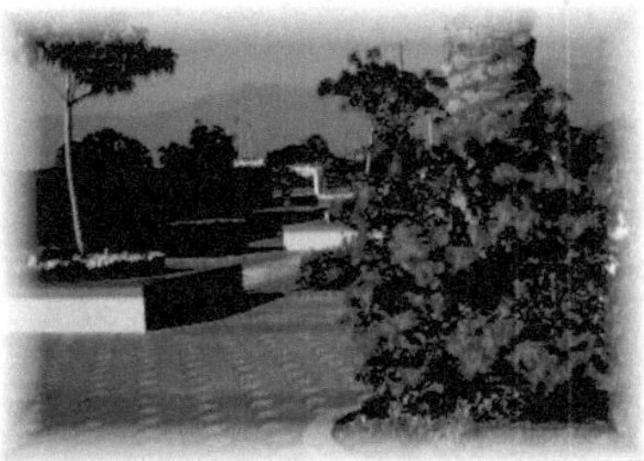

My Daily Tasks

Dinner over, I measure and record her blood pressure and glucose level. Next, under my watch, I have her accurately take her medications; Alzheimer's causes her to miss some medications and overdose on some. Able to do most personal hygiene herself, she needs less attention in this regard, but I am always nearby in case she needs assistance. She gets ready to sleep at around 6:00 PM. But my day is not completely over yet, only lightened, because I always look out for signs of discomfort on her part even when she is sleeping.

Other places available for working out are parks of which there are few in our area. Seldom do we go there, however, owing to Amelia's fear of developing rashes caused by exposure to the sun. Villages close to the beach are also within driving distance, where we eat and dine at some restaurants sometimes.

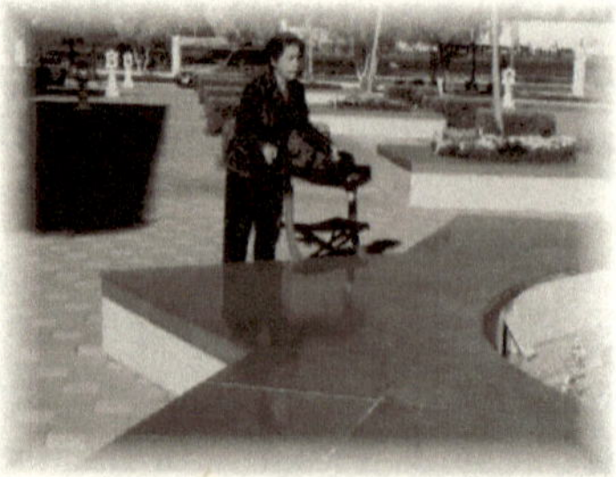

At home, if I observe Amelia being depressed and looking hopeless, I initiate some activities that draw laughter from her. Sometimes I start a conversation about her days as a teenager or any day which she likes recalling, to create a back and forth conversation. I do everything I can to take her mind away from depression because the sight of her being depressed concerns and depresses me too. I am forced to dedicate my day taking care of her exclusively, Strokes, Alzheimer's, diabetes, and congestive heart failure having rendered her sadly helpless.

Spiritual Commitment

Her upbringing molded by Catholicism, Amelia extended her faith to the whole family with absolute firmness, annoying the children and me sometimes with her constant sermon. Either Saturday or Sunday of each week was a day of obligation for going to church. If we missed going to church on a Saturday, the following Sunday was a church day by all means.

Be it Saturday or Sunday, church day was always a special forward-looking day for Amelia, calling for modest early planning. She would take the time to dress up, similarly requiring the children to do the same, to be presentable in the church. Being tired from working during the week was not an excuse for not going to church. The church was not the only place of worship for Amelia. The home as well was a place for prayers before eating, before going to sleep, and before rising in the morning.

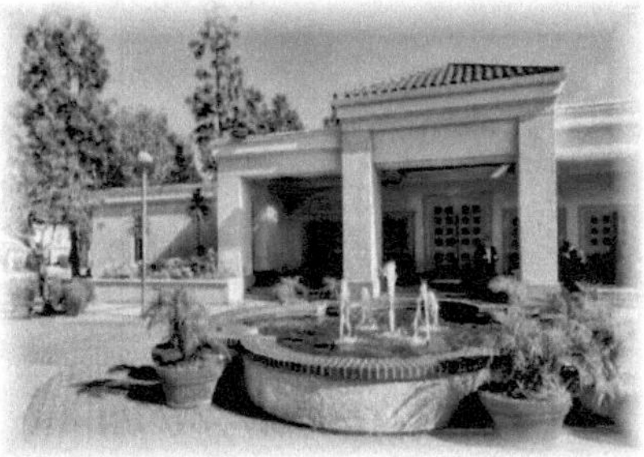

On the first day on board a cruise ship, as we occasionally went cruising, Amelia would inquire about what time and in which deck would mass be solemnized. Knowing where it was and at what time was not enough; she would still ask to double check to be sure that we have the right schedule.

At the church, her memory not yet showing any sign of declination, she would say her prayers by heart with the right pauses and timing in unison with the other churchgoers. She would readily identify and greet friends, even remembering those she encountered from short meetings. The church was where she derived consolation as it was where she met friends.

Spiritual Commitment

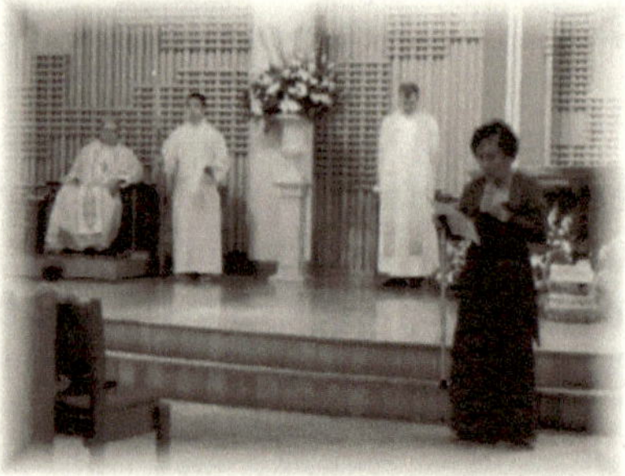

The preceding description of Amelia's faith covers the period before the occurrence of the third stroke; she already had two previous massive ones. Profound and disconcerting changes were about to happen to Amelia and her relationship with the church and the religion she indeed espoused. Strokes, Alzheimer's, diabetes, and congestive heart failure forced the changes onto her.

She has forgotten what day of the week is church day. The frequency of going to church noticeably declined although the eagerness still exists. What is unusual is that she prepares for going to church more than four hours ahead of the mass, a unique trait that Amelia starts to exhibit. For example, if the mass is at 5:00 PM, Amelia begins preparing just after lunch and by 1:00 PM she is ready to leave for the church. She knows that it only takes ten minutes to drive to church; she does not care, she wants to be at the church early. Anxiety is replacing rationality, perhaps due to Alzheimer's.

She likes to meet friends at the church even though she stops remembering their names, making the encounters somewhat an expression of sympathy for her rather than natural friendly greetings. Sometimes she greets and talks to complete strangers who she thinks she knows, but does not, requiring me to apologize for the rudeness.

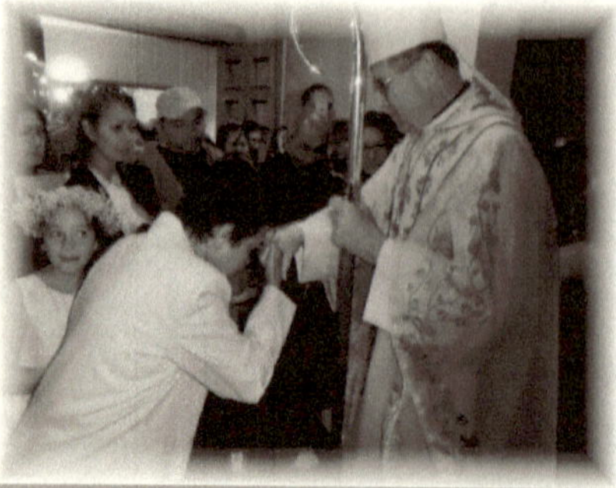

Spiritual Commitment

Her faith may have changed slightly owing to her ailments, but it is still unshakable. Her prayers are coming out garbled, but they are as sincere as they were when she was healthy. May God help her in her fight against strokes, Alzheimer's, diabetes, and congestive heart failure.

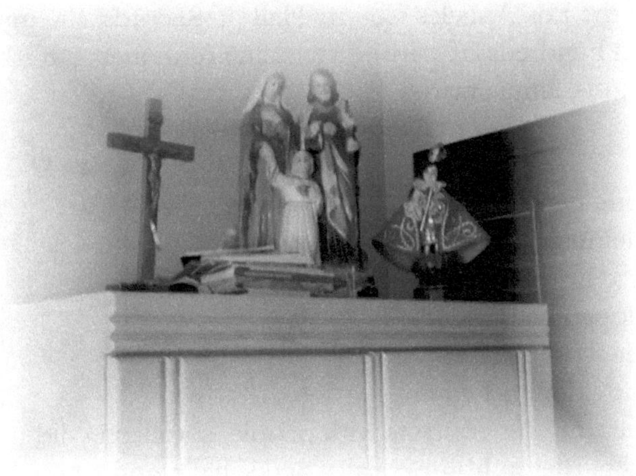

Socializing Amidst Adversity

Even at the sad physical and mental condition that Amelia has been, her eyes still sparkle at the mention of parties with people from her place of work dating back thirteen years. Most of them are retirees themselves who want to indulge in memories around the times they were working together.

She used to be a school teacher before working with the County of Los Angeles Registrar-Recorder/County Clerk's office, which she held for more than twenty years, so socializing is not new to her. In her tenure at the Los Angeles County Hall of Records, she must have attended hundreds of parties, including retirements, birthdays, special occasions, anniversaries, and others.

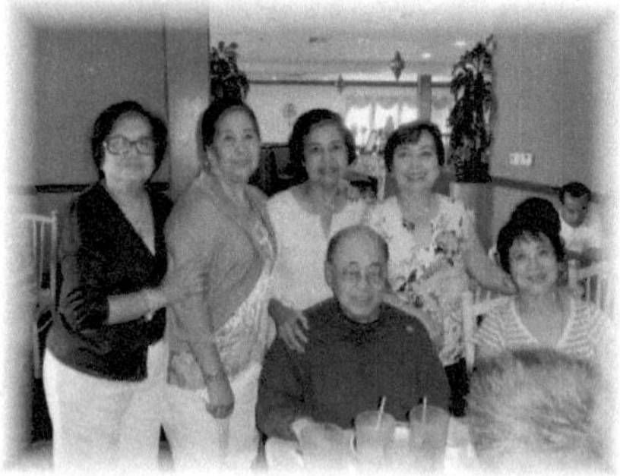

Forced to retire because of strokes, Alzheimer's, diabetes, and congestive heart failure, Amelia developed new friends outside of the workplace. Though slightly diminished in frequency due to fewer contacts with people, socializing did not stop. She had parties at homes, malls, parks, halls, and wherever there are occasions to enjoy and have fun. She was still very active after the first strokes and even with dementia already starting to affect her.

In addition to parties with friends, Amelia initiates gatherings within the family. Through her encouragement, we celebrate birthdays, anniversaries, holidays and other special days when she is aware of them. Although Alzheimer's has, to some extent, taken hold in her brain, she still tends to control the family.

Socializing Amidst Adversity

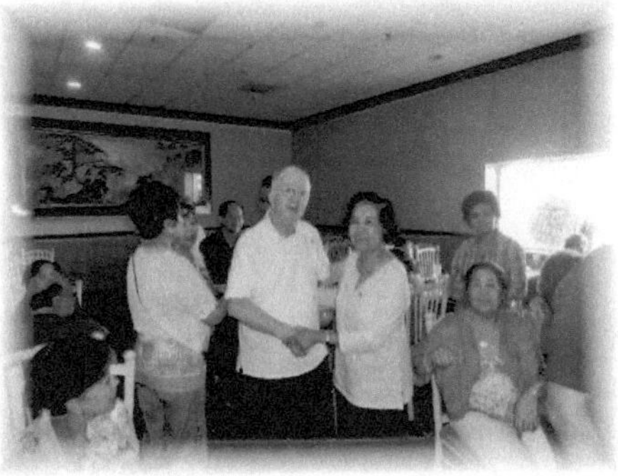

When she can, Amelia loves to attend parties with friends and relatives from our local community of immigrants. Limited only by her taste, she likes to eat native foods while she mingles around. She needs a chaperone and intermediary though, because Alzheimer's has caused her to forget names and faces of even very close relatives.

The difficulty of walking has hindered Amelia's desire and ability to socialize. When she does want to attend parties, I do everything to oblige. Socializing helps her release tension; it helps me too, to a large extent.

She does not miss naming the places in which she had parties previously, including the ones of her own and those of her friends. Strangely, she remembers events that happened many, many years ago.

The desire to socialize is still high in Amelia, discouraged only by her difficulty of dressing up. Strokes, Alzheimer's, diabetes, and congestive heart failure, have a way of spoiling one's spirit, particularly hers. Amelia's case is a living evidence of the ignominy and dishonor the diseases inflict. It is up to my family to let her have as much fun as she can while she still appreciates being alive.

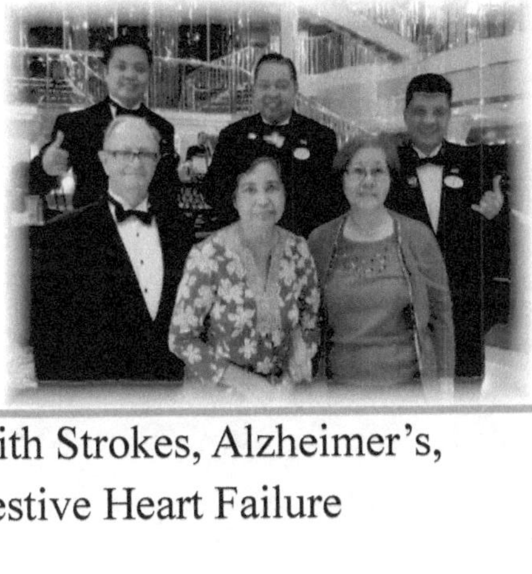

Chapter 4 – Recreational Activities

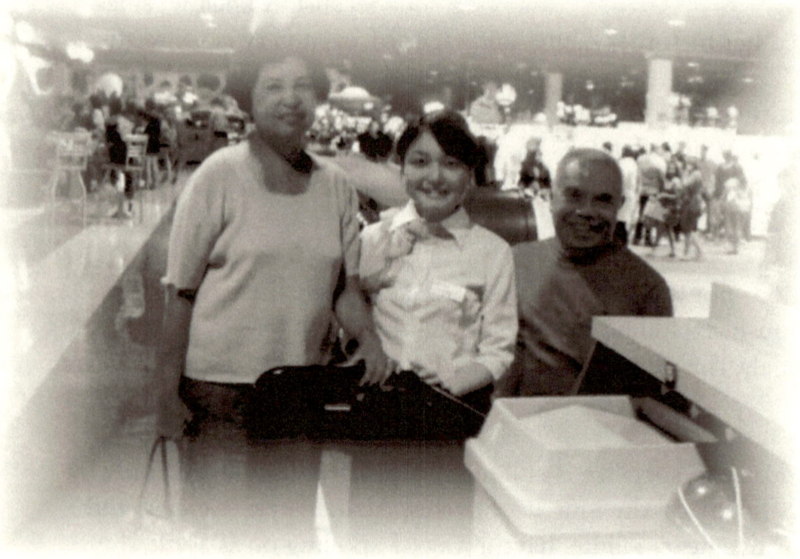

Trip to Solvang, Santa Barbara, California

Located in the beautiful valley of Santa Inez Mountains in Santa Barbara, close to the Vanderburgh Air Force Base, the city of Solvang is a 2-hour drive from Los Angeles towards San Francisco, on Highway 101. The city is east of Highway 101 on Mission Dr. and E. Highway 246.

Founded by immigrants from Denmark, the city has attracted other Scandinavians, helping it grow to what it is now. Its location, though off by a few miles from Highway 101, provides a peripheral destination for travelers who want to explore places between Northern and Southern California. Solvang will certainly grow even more due to its growing popularity as a tourist destination.

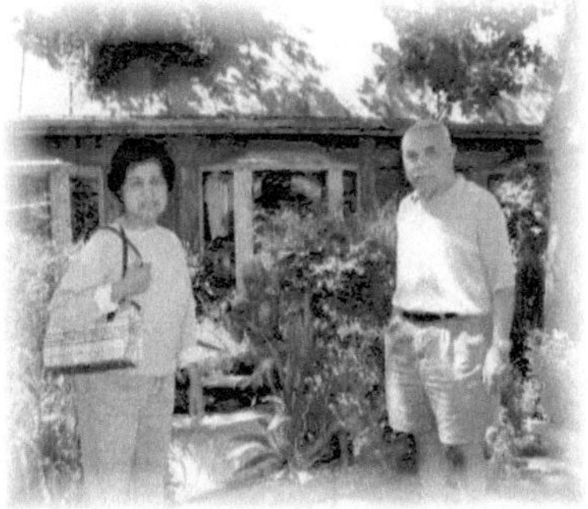

The city is distinct from other California urban cities. With the stores, food, jewelry, furniture, and benches along the streets in Scandinavian designs, one will immediately notice that Solvang has characteristics not shared by other cities in Southern California. The apparels that storekeepers wear, the wares that they carry in their stores, and the mood of transporting tourists within the city, are distinctly Scandinavian.

Like beacons immediately visible from a distance, massive windmills are strategically located, sending notice that the city is a virtual Scandinavian territory in California. Starting at the entrance, the city comes alive with some tourists crisscrossing the streets shopping for souvenirs while some are taking shelters at dining places from the moderately warm weather. Rest benches that offer

Trip to Solvang, Santa Barbara, California

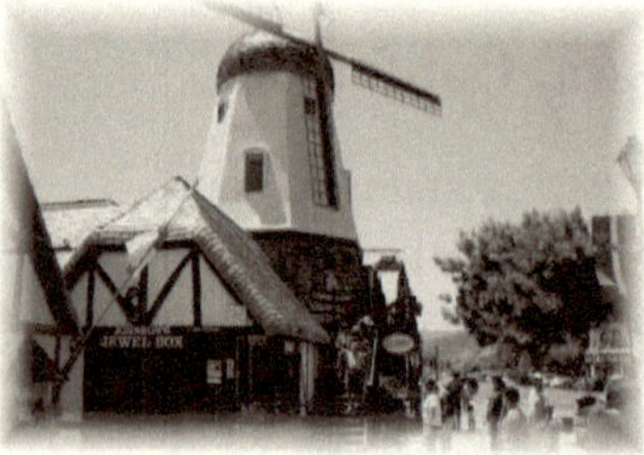

recovery from exhaustion are placed in ideal locations for a quick resumption of the shopping itineraries.

The city is one of the cleanest I have ever been to despite the abundant trees in well-planned areas. As I learned through casual conversations with actual residents, the city is swept during the night to get rid of the leaves that fell the preceding day. By morning the city is completely ridden off the leaves and then regular street maintenance starts. Weather permitting, city cleanup is repeated every day and night.

Less than 30 years old, the city is still very young to make room for growth that is well planned and meeting the needs of discriminating visitors. Most businesses in the city depend on tourism for income. Dependent on tourism as well for their livelihood, the residents do not move very far from the city. For tourists who want to spend longer than a day at Solvang, hotels and inns are available.

Not too far out but outside the city limit, are casinos for tourists who want to dine and gamble at the same time. One should be aware, though, that the town of Solvang is located where there are not many gas filling stations. Before branching out from the main highway, gas must be adequate for the trip out of the city, and if necessary, enough to get back to the main road where gas stations are available with regular frequency.

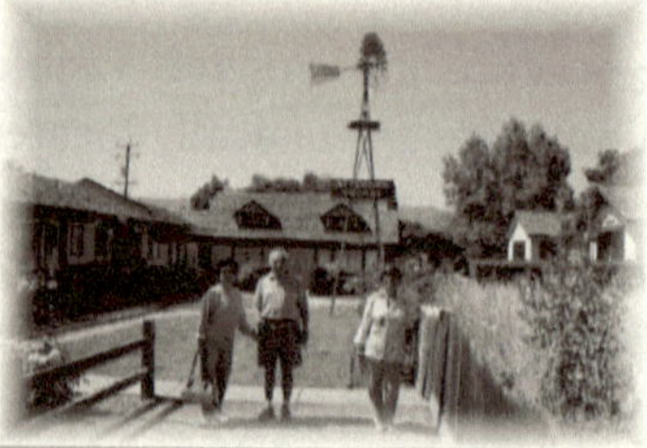

Amelia was delighted with our last visit to the city despite the long drive. Having seen some windmills

Trip to Solvang, Santa Barbara, California

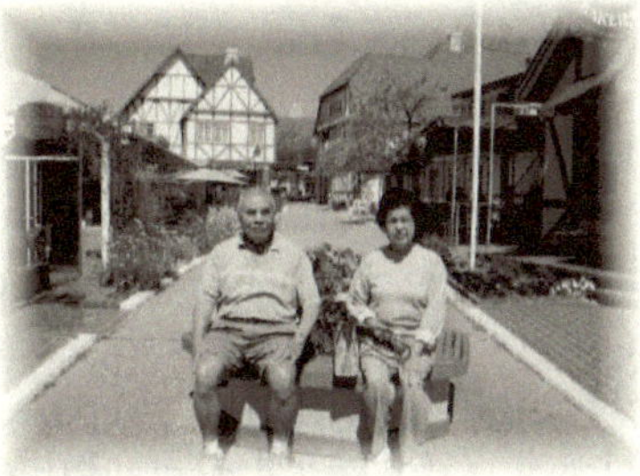

in Holland, she felt like she was touring Europe. The fresh air in the town seemed to invigorate her. Though she was visibly limping, she appeared to be in good spirit and did not look tired. After eating lunch, she even looked better. Solvang is another tourist city Amelia included in her tally of cities she visited notwithstanding her handicap.

We had been to the city a few times before but spaced over a few years. In each visit, the city continues to impress me regarding cleanliness and uniqueness. As long as the city keeps its motif and maintains its unique difference from urban cities, it will always be a tourist destination, and it will be one I will not hesitate to visit again every time I have a chance.

Trip to USS Iowa Battleship, San Pedro, California

It was Veterans Day, and what better day to spend it than with veterans on the battleship USS Iowa! The battleship was on its first public opening after several days of preparation. With the opening day announced on television, I was expecting a big crowd. So hastily cajoling Amelia to prepare to leave for San Pedro where the USS Iowa is docked, I packed the few things I regularly carry around for Amelia, in a pouch. Then very early, off to San Pedro, we went.

We were not early enough, it turned out, and the huge parking lot was almost full when we arrived. Veterans and their families had priority over every parking space including those for the disabled, forcing us to park farther away from the battleship. Vehicles representing the media had the choice parking spaces closer to the temporary grandstand. Hundreds of people were already lining up before the ticket windows opened while a band playing mostly patriotic pieces, entertained them.

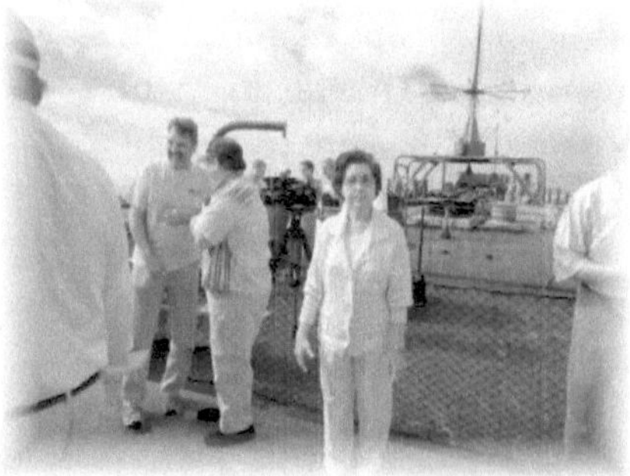

Amelia was discouraged at how far we would be back along the lines forming at the ticket windows, but pleading with her to make the most of our time, we stayed and finally bought our tickets. Then we followed even longer lines to the entrance of the battleship. Again we persevered, and when the entry to the ship opened at the designated time, we just went along with the crowd on the long ramp of about 10- to 15-degree incline. Once

Trip to USS Iowa Battleship, San Pedro, California

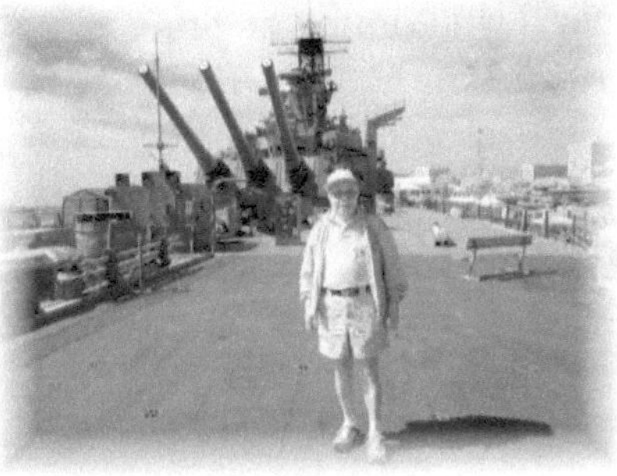

the lines started moving and the crowd kept pushing forward, there was only a limited chance for one to give up and turn back.

Somehow we made it to the open deck where the monster guns are located and where the tour started. The tour was laid out through intricate doors and stairs descending to the lower decks, allowing only one direction of movement towards the exit, and forcing the tourists to appreciate the battleship and its hardware altogether.

On our own, we first checked out as many locations as available to the public on the main deck where we were not obstructing traffic. After taking a few pictures, I decided to tour the battleship without Amelia, owing to the extreme physical demand in negotiating the many almost perpendicular stairs. I left her comfortably seated on a bench shaded by the big guns, assured that I would be back when the tour terminated at the stern end of the battleship.

One of the attractions in the tour of the battleship is the little room that President Roosevelt occupied en route to a treaty in Europe during World War II. For one of the most powerful men in the world during World War II, the room is too small and humble, although it has the amenities and controls consistent with the needs of a commander-in-chief, let alone the President of the United States.

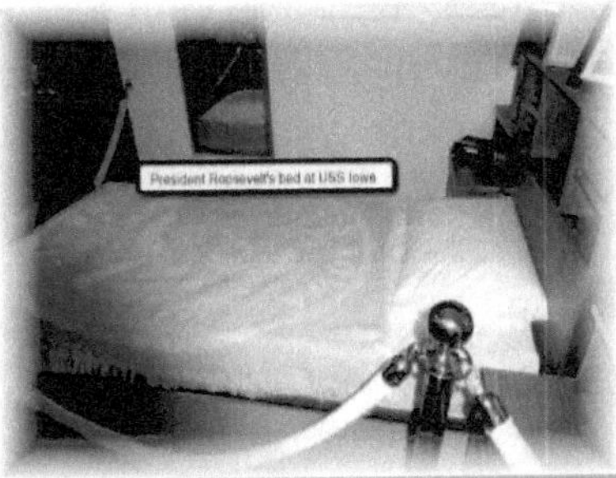

With its big guns, accurate fire control system, speed, and heavy

Trip to USS Iowa Battleship, San Pedro, California

armor, the USS Iowa was the greatest naval ship during its time. It served in World War II, the Korean War, and the Cold War. Her service lasted 20 years in active duty and 50 years in the Reserve Fleet. In 2011 it was awarded to the non-profit organization, the Pacific Battleship Center.

At a top speed of 40 miles per hour, the USS Iowa was already the fastest in its class. In an exercise during the Cold War, the USS Iowa surpassed the rated speed when it reached 43 miles per hour. Already a record-breaker as a battleship, it fired a 16-inch projectile at 26.9 miles in 1989, another record, causing the guns to recoil 47 inches and leading some to believe that the ship moved sideways; the ship did not move at all.

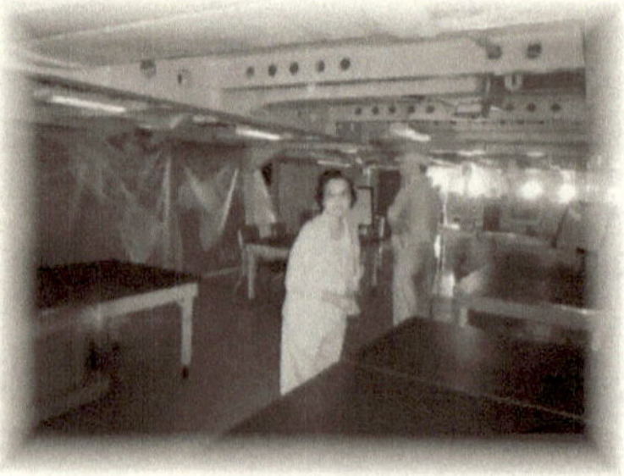

The original cost of building the USS Iowa was $110 million. The same construction, adjusted for inflation, would have cost $1.8 billion if done in 2013. The battleship was constructed with 1,135,000 rivets and 4,209,000 feet or 800 miles of welds. There were 900 various motors, 1,090 telephones, and 5,300 lighting fixtures which required 250 miles of electric cables.

The USS Iowa, although out of service, is properly maintained to keep it in readiness to be put back in service in case of emergency, the kind that involves warlike positioning to wage war if necessary. In the meantime, it is one of the main public attractions at the City of San Pedro in Southern California, for the public to see, admire, and explore. Volunteers handle the various functions held at the battleship.

Trip to USS Iowa Battleship, San Pedro, California

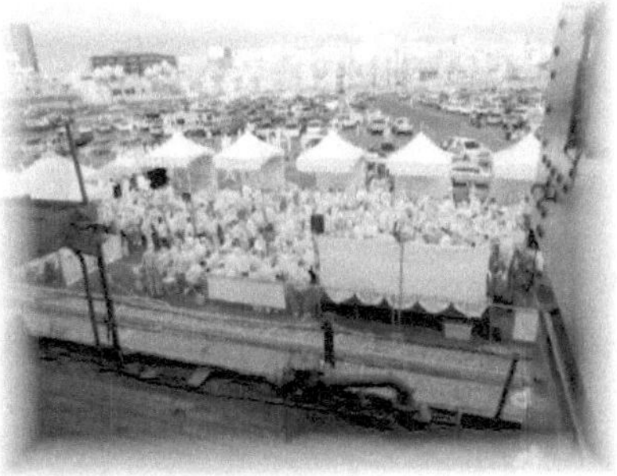

I completed the tour and went back to the tour entrance, to pick up Amelia. She was patiently waiting, hungry, and worried. Observing that Amelia is disabled, the volunteers allowed us to cut through the line and let us out. It took us a while to drive out of the parking lot owing to the hundreds of vehicles coming in and going out. Lest Amelia's hunger syndrome start, we ate at the first available restaurant out of the parking lot.

Fond of military exploits and history, the tour served me well. Other than the disappointment that Amelia was unable to join me in the tour, I considered the visit very successful. From her looks though, I could tell that Amelia did not enjoy the visit.

The battleship certainly reminds people of how mighty the USS Iowa was in its time, not to mention the protective shield that it provided the United States, its territories, and its allies. When in Southern California, particularly close to the Los Angeles Pacific Coast, a visit to the USS Iowa Battleship is one I would recommend to anyone.

Trip to USS Midway Aircraft Carrier, San Diego, California

Trip to USS Midway Aircraft Carrier, San Diego, California

Why a long queue of vehicles was heading towards what, from a distance, appeared to be an aircraft carrier raised our curiosity. That the vehicles were carrying people in civilians clothes instead of in military uniforms, intrigued us even more. I know that usually on regular days, only small fishing boats, museums, and harbor cruise ships dock along Pacific Coast Highway in San Diego. As the aircraft carrier loomed even more, I slowed down and asked what was going on. I found out that the USS Midway was decommissioned several months ago, turned into a museum, and was being opened to the public.

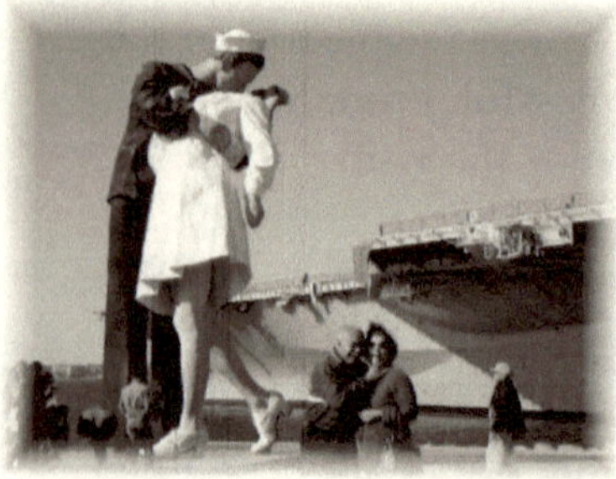

Fond of military history including weapons of war and after convincing our passenger friends, we joined the long queue of vehicles heading towards the USS Midway. I was never in one before, neither was Amelia, and neither were our passenger friends. Except for Amelia who appeared subdued due to her limited movement, we were anxious to tour the massive aircraft carrier.

Able volunteers manned the ticket booths making the purchase of tour tickets effortless. Many of the volunteers served in the USS Midway at some point in their careers with the Navy, so their knowledge of the carrier was an invaluable guide for tourists. I planned on buying food for Amelia, having her sit in one corner at the restaurant area of the carrier while I, together with our passenger friends, proceeded with the tour. Amelia did not want to be left alone, so all four of us joined the tour of the USS Midway.

Having seen its best and worst actions in the Pacific during World War II, the USS Midway was a terror in the eyes of a formidable enemy, particularly Japan, who had an equally impressive array of military hardware. The USS Midway roamed the Pacific like a monster seeking preys for destruction, deterring further aggressive actions by Japan, and proving that aircraft carriers would be dominant mobile bases for carrying the fight to the enemies at a sustained and relentless firepower.

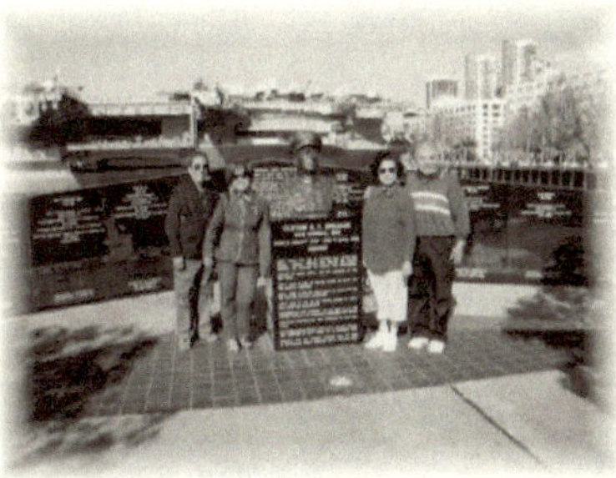

The USS Midway's last action before being decommissioned was in the Mediterranean against the forces of Saddam Hussein. Able to launch a fighter plane every 45 seconds, it had a very impressive and lethal firepower. Besides fighter planes, it handled support aircrafts like helicopters and spy planes. Such was its power that its presence alone led enemies to think first before initiating any provocative actions against the United States and its interests.

Ironically, USS Midway's miles and miles of physically laid out wiring system and the fuel cost to operate it helped in its demise. It had to make way for the modern nuclear powered and electronically sophisticated aircraft carriers like the USS Ronald Reagan, presently anchored across, near the Coronado Island in San Diego. The USS Midway is now a museum, occasionally serving as a venue for sports and ceremonial activities. Its deck is vast enough to handle large events like football and basketball.

Trip to USS Midway Aircraft Carrier, San Diego, California

Thanks to the efforts of numerous volunteers, the aircraft carrier is still maintained as a symbol of the United States power and might.

To my surprise, Amelia was able to negotiate the narrow and almost perpendicular stairs of the aircraft carrier without incident. We descended all the way down to the quarters of the crews and took pictures of exhibits. Some areas of the aircraft carrier where actions used to be initiated, were explained and demonstrated to us, including how aircrafts were launched.

Actual aircrafts were displayed on the aircraft carrier's hangar and deck allowing tourists to frame pictures with them as background. For make-believe pictures, visitors who wanted to appear as fighter pilots had access to the cockpits of some fighter planes and other aircrafts.

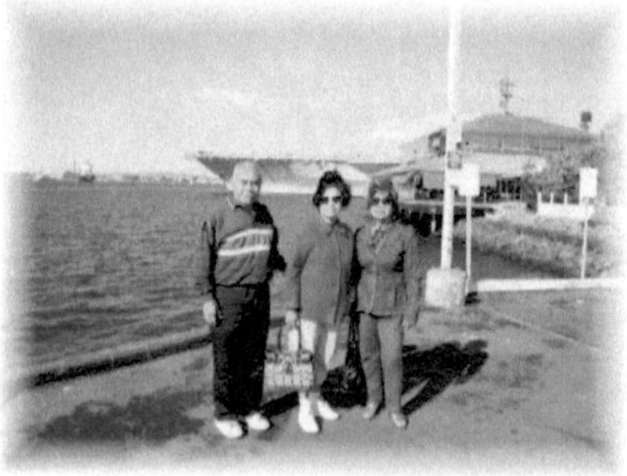

The tour lasted more than two hours. After taking numerous pictures, we had lunch at the aircraft carrier's stern, heading for home thereafter. We were elated that we just toured one of the mightiest aircraft carriers in the world.

Proceeds from the ticket sales contribute to the maintenance of the museum as a symbol of the United States might and pride. The tour which I considered as an act of patriotism to some extent is historical and educational, and I recommend it to anyone interested in military history.

Trip to Grand Canyon, Arizona

On the highway most of the day from Los Angeles, California, to Williams, Arizona, seven of us including a child, settled at a motel, expecting to proceed to our final destination, the Grand Canyon, the following day. A good meal and a couple of cold beers helped us recover from travel fatigue. In the morning we expected to use up more energy to drive another sixty miles to the nearest entrance to the Grand Canyon, not to mention the energy to explore points of interest while in the park.

Already in the park the following morning with tickets on hand and ready to proceed to the viewing area but, motivated by the adventurous spirit in us, we spontaneously decided to leave the South Rim and drive to the North Rim. Having been to the South Rim a couple of times before, I welcomed the change in viewing location.

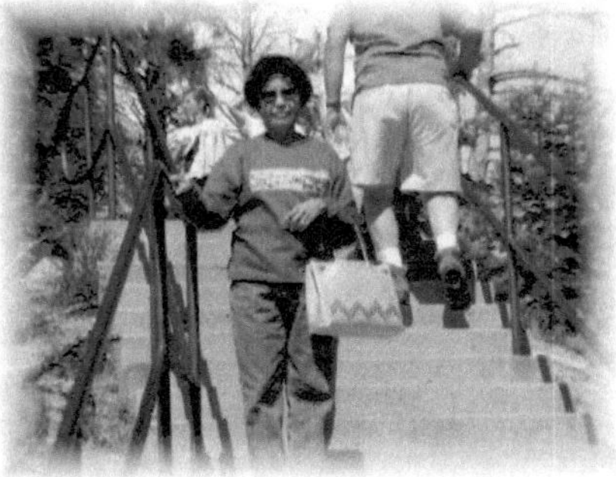

The drive would take us four hours, the same length of time if we had driven from Williams, so we did not lose much time other than the hour of driving to the South Rim. The drive was through stretches of boulders and desert and seemed endless because there were not many vehicles going to and coming from the North Rim.

Along the stretch of boulders and desert, there was only one refueling station, reachable only after four hours of driving. Running out of gas before reaching the gas station, would be very unfortunate and disconcerting. Further, being stranded in the middle of nowhere when the sun is getting down and being overcome by darkness is chilling. There is no satellite signal with which to communicate with someone outside the desert area. Even if there is, one can only imagine how long road assistance would appear. Luckily we were driving a diesel powered newly maintained sports utility vehicle.

We reached the gas station and could have skipped lunch except that it was time for Amelia to eat to avoid triggering her hunger syndrome. I prevailed on stopping to buy some sandwiches. Because it is the only source of fuel and food, the place was so crowded that the wait time was fifteen minutes or longer. Compounding the problem was the fact that seats appeared to be at a premium, even though there were plenty of them.

While the rest of our company ate in the sports utility vehicle, I was forced to eat standing in the yard, which I did not mind for the sake of Amelia. After eating, we drove two to three more hours to reach our coveted destination, the North Rim of the Grand Canyon.

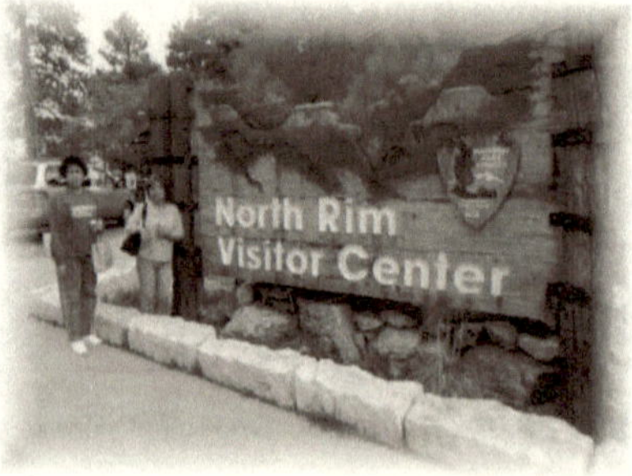

Elevated higher than the South Rim, the North Rim is prettier and has more panoramic views. It is less crowded, perhaps owing to the distance from the nearest city and the fear of isolation in case of emergency along the travel route. Obviously, during holidays, hotels and cottages get good business, but probably not as brisk as in the South Rim.

From the huge glass viewing balcony of the Grand Hotel, one can look across the canyon as far as the eyes can see. Looking down deep into the canyon is limited by the safe viewing distance from the canyon rim. The hotel was where President Roosevelt used to

Trip to Grand Canyon, Arizona

stay when visiting the Grand Canyon. For sale historical memorabilia as well as souvenir items are displayed in the hotel. Due to the different levels of the hotel which limited Amelia's ability to move, we spent most of our time on the balcony than in any other area.

Well-landscaped and shaded by trees to protect visitors from the sun, the North Rim is like a small city, with cottages to accommodate guests who decide to stay longer in the canyon. There are stores other than the Grand Hotel, which are stuffed with souvenirs for sale. With so much walking and exploring of the canyon, weary visitors can indulge in the restaurants, which we did. Concerned with Amelia constantly, I saw that she was feeling good, having eaten enough for the travel back to our hotel at Williams.

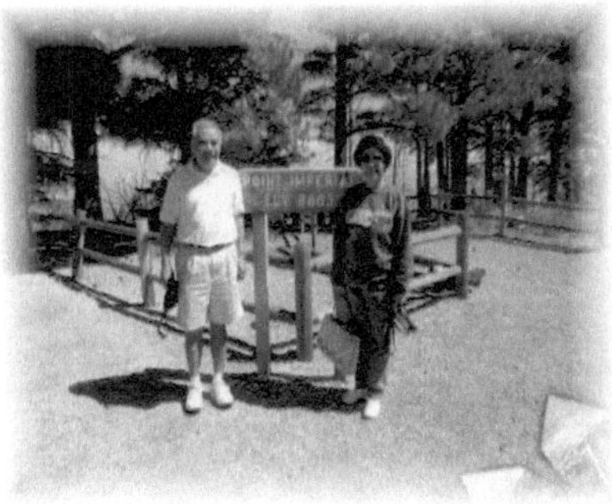

We did not want to be driving at night in the desert area. On the way back while it was still daylight, we had the opportunity to take some beautiful pictures of the wilderness landscape. Our visit to the North Rim was a once in a memorable lifetime experience, unexpected to be repeated due to the concern of having a vehicle breakdown in the middle of the desert. However, I unequivocally recommend the trip to anyone who has the chance to make it safely; the North Rim of the Grand Canyon is just unbelievably awesome.

Bidding Goodbye to USS Endeavor, Inglewood, California

Bidding Goodbye to USS Endeavor, Inglewood, California

Its status as a space ship already well-documented for making twenty-five voyages into space, the shuttle Endeavor was being retired, an occasion dubbed as history-making. The 26th trip was not in space; it was a journey on top of a trailer from the Los Angeles International Airport to the Science Center west of downtown Los Angeles. The 2-mile per hour travel of the shuttle was a far cry from its enormous 17,000-mile per hour speed in space outside the gravitational pull of the earth, on each of the twenty-five voyages. It was a chance, though, for the public to see it firsthand in a close up presentation.

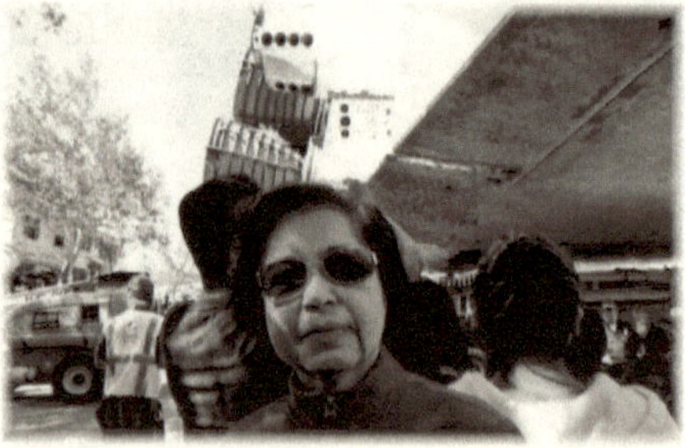

I did not want to miss the opportunity of watching history unfold; the retirement of Endeavor climaxed a lengthy feat of providing a platform for space exploration. The Endeavor is a testament to how much mankind had accomplished in space science. The Endeavor was being retired to its permanent home, the Science Center to allow the people to admire, wonder, and speculate about the accomplishment. Of all its voyages, this last one was the most painstaking, and was one that required careful planning even at its ridiculous slow rate of travel.

Having worked in Inglewood for some years, I thought that this occasion was an opportune time to revisit the city. From the published itinerary, I knew the particular streets in Inglewood where the shuttle would be rolling by from the Los Angeles

Bidding Goodbye to USS Endeavor, Inglewood, California

International Airport to the Science Center, and I figured that if we started early, we could be in a position along the route to have a close-up view of shuttle.

When we arrived at Inglewood, it seemed that the city was having a huge festival. We did not arrive early enough; detour signs were spread out, and the streets that I was familiar with were closed. The city blocks where I used to work were temporarily divided and declared inaccessible. In fact, we were detoured to some areas of Inglewood which I had not been to before.

I decided to take a break from aimlessly driving around to let Amelia eat because she was already tired and starved. I felt that lack of food would soon trigger her hunger syndrome. Having eaten and reconsidered our options, we decided to abandon the idea of witnessing history in the making and just go home.

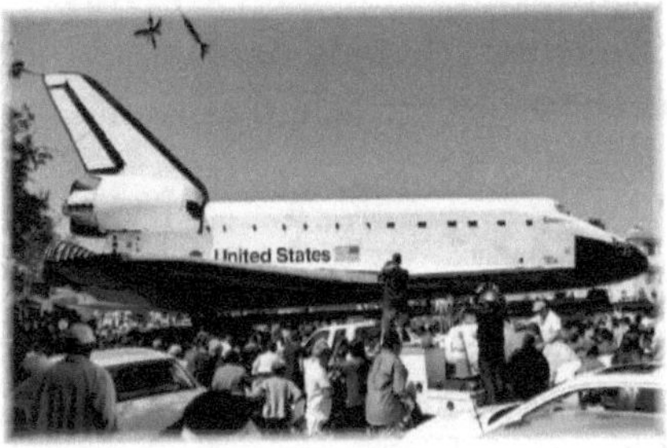

Before we did, however, I checked a residential part of the city which I guessed was along the route of the shuttle. It was being cordoned off too, but we got in time before the barriers were put in place.

It turned out that the shuttle would be rolling by just one block away from where I parked the car. Thousands of people were already lined up along the route; we could hardly find an open space. As the crowd got deeper and deeper, we were being pushed back farther and farther away, denying us our initial vantage view of the street. Everybody appeared to be staking their prized places on the curb.

Bidding Goodbye to USS Endeavor, Inglewood, California

Meanwhile, Amelia was getting tired and unable to remain standing for more than a few minutes at a time. Luckily, a couple unloaded a bench from their truck, and sensing Amelia's predicament and having more than enough space for the two of them, they offered her a seat at the end of the bench. After thanking the couple graciously and with Amelia seated slightly comfortable but appearing uneasy, I walked back to the car to get some crackers and water for her.

It took more than two hours for the shuttle to turn a corner, some five hundred feet from our location. The opportunity of watching the Endeavor being tenderly and carefully towed along narrow streets was a spectacle that would not happen again.

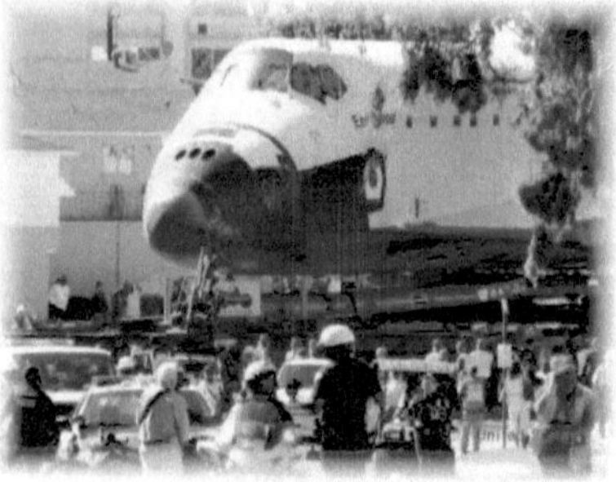

Meticulous mapping of the shuttle's route was a feat of enormous skills that I felt should not be missed. Tree branches were pulled and tied, and overhead lines were restrung so that they did not touch the shuttle. The streets were laid with metal plates to protect the underground utility plumbing. Hundreds and hundreds of barricades were put in place to restrain the people from intruding into the shuttle's path, and hundreds of police officers were patrolling the route to keep the crowd orderly.

We had taken a few pictures of the shuttle before we left for home. Going home was a traffic nightmare as the streams of smaller traffic from the residential areas fed into the humongous central traffic. We had to wait our turn in getting out of the cordoned off

Bidding Goodbye to USS Endeavor, Inglewood, California

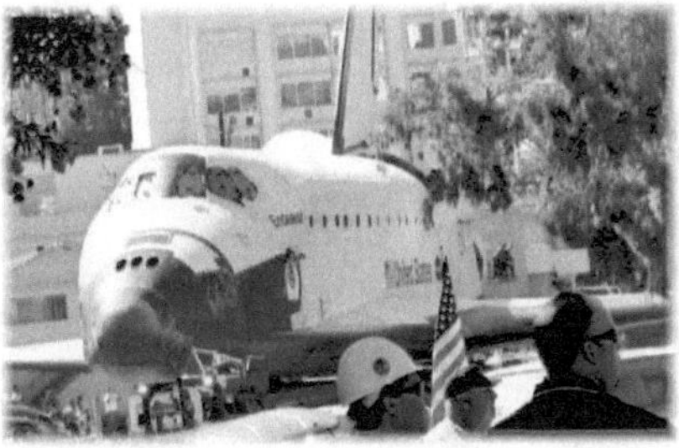

area. There were hundreds and hundreds of cars queued along the narrow residential streets.

The long nine hours of witnessing the Endeavor's last voyage was well worth spending – it was history! Above and beyond other consideration, this was a free spectacle witnessed by the general public regardless of age group. The USS Endeavor was a pioneer and contemporary vehicle in the endeavor to learn more about the space surrounding our planet and beyond.

Trip to the Yosemite National Park, Yosemite, California

The 700,000-acre Yosemite National Park is only a seven-hour drive from our residence in Southern California. Having come from a country of giant trees from thousands of acres of rainforests, I was not very anxious to visit the park, not without strong encouragement. If ever, what would perhaps interest me about the park would be the 3,000-foot high El Capitan, the world famous and well-publicized granite rock popular among rock climbers. So, when our daughter persuaded us to join them on a camping trip to the park, without hesitation, I booked a three-day reservation at one of the lodges in the park, paying a premium for a unit that had the view of the famous Yosemite Waterfall.

Starting at 5:00 AM, we figured that Amelia and I would be joining our daughter's family and eating lunch with them at the park. It had been a while after all, since we had been to Northern California, and I liked driving along the slightly scenic California Highway 99 which offered magnificent views of the vast farmlands.

I did not have to rest from driving, but I did at a rest stop, just to observe and admire the symmetry at which plants, shrubs, and trees were planted on the fields. Until I witnessed firsthand the vast farmlands in California, I did not appreciate the sweat and effort that come with the production of the variety of food that is served at dining tables.

Hoping to eat snacks and add some fuel, we stopped at Fresno after four to five hours of driving, but witnessing a great crowd at the pumps, we drove on. After all, I estimated that the current fuel in the car appeared to be adequate to reach the park. We realized

Trip to the Yosemite National Park, Yosemite, California

later on that the gas station at Fresno was where the last opportunity to add gas before reaching the park, hence the big crowd at the pumps; the next gas station would be inside the park.

We reached the park entrance at the anticipated time. After receiving all the information about the park as we paid the entrance fees, we proceeded to our destination, the rendezvous with our daughter and her family where visitors mingle, rest, and eat. I had a picture in my mind where to go, having consulted the map of the park before continuing with the trip.

Out of confusion, we made a turn too soon on the forked highway. The road appeared to be going up and up, while the number of vehicles on the road became less frequent. From asphalt, the road turned into gravel. We drove in this condition for about 15 minutes, 15 minutes too long on the park's wilderness where there was no satellite signal. We finally turned around and stopped to ask for direction. To my consternation, because of the early turn on the forked highway, we ended up on the wrong road.

As we drove, I noticed that Amelia was showing signs of uneasiness. She was feeling hungry and needing to use a restroom, but with my encouragement and urging, she hanged on. I feared that her glucose level might be dropping; she needed to eat, but we ate our last supply of snacks just before reaching the park entrance. As I was driving, we were watching out for an eating place or a vending machine so that I could feed Amelia; there was none.

We reconnected with the main highway, but by then it was almost 1:00 PM, well past Amelia's meal time. She was starting to shake; her hands were cold, and her face was pale. I was getting desperate; she needed to eat. Luckily, the visitors' area soon loomed ahead.

Trip to the Yosemite National Park, Yosemite, California

We proceeded to a restaurant without stopping at the lodge. I bypassed the customers in front of me to get some food and drinks for Amelia. Observing me frantically caring for Amelia, I guessed the customers understood why I was rude and disrespectful. After drinking water and soda, and eating food, Amelia started to feel comfortable, her facial complexion returning to normal. We spent the rest of the day relaxing in the lodge, viewing the famous Yosemite Waterfall. We did not even care to seek out our daughter and her family.

After our daughter and her family had checked on us the following morning to be sure we made the trip, they went back to their campsite, and we went on to explore points of interest close to the lodge. Our exploration started with a tram ride through a long tunnel to reach a viewing location of the El Capitan and the Half Dome. After the tram ride, we walked to the base of the waterfall, a short distance from the lodge.

The following day we rejoined our daughter and her family to take another tram ride to the Mariposa Grove, where magnificent giant sequoias appeared to be reaching up to the skies in their majestic heights. Due to limited time, we quickly tried to absorb as much information as we could from handouts at the visitors' bureau, about how nature propagates and replenishes the trees. We returned to our lodge, tired and exhausted.

We headed for home the following day, after a spending an hour at the base of the waterfall, while our daughter and her family continued a trip to the San Francisco Bay area. We spent the next two days relaxing and recovering from the rigors of the journey. We considered our trip to Yosemite National Park very exciting and satisfactory. Needless to say, the park is world-famous and is a must-see for anyone having the opportunity to visit it.

Trip to the Yosemite National Park, Yosemite, California

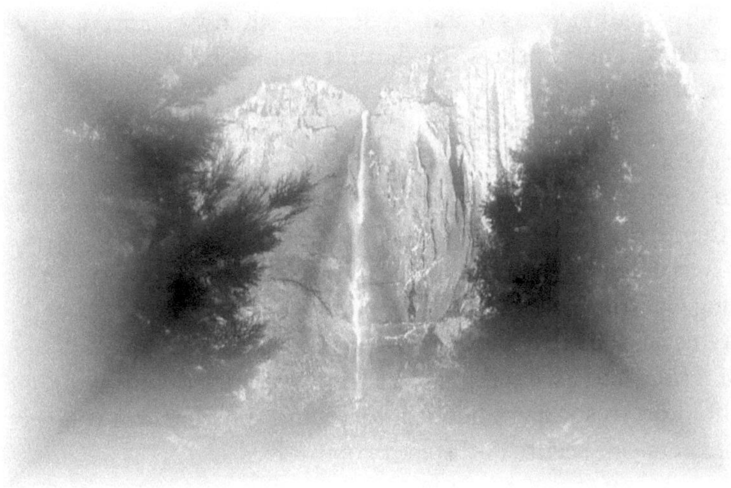

Ascent at PS Aerial Tramway, Palm Springs, California

The Palm Springs Aerial Tramway is a tourist attraction that is only two hours away from the general area where we have been residing for forty-seven years. We know about it, read about it, and have been driving by it several times, and yet, we have been ignoring it until today, Independence Day 2016.

Driving leisurely, we made it to Palm Springs early, beating the traffic, which I anticipated to be above average because of the holiday. The weather was around 95 degrees when we arrived, very comfortable by Palm Springs standard. It would change rapidly as the hours of the day went by.

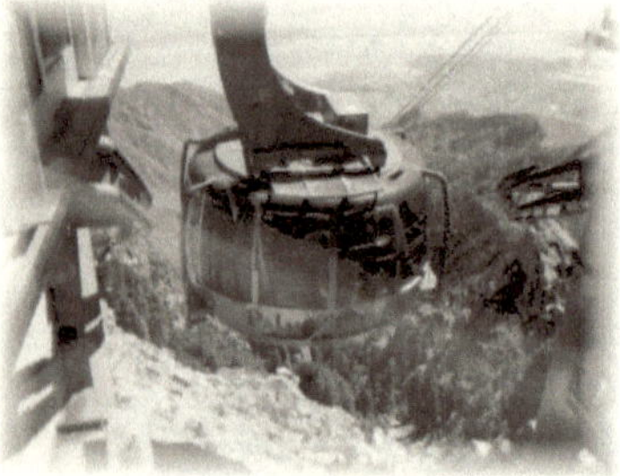

The aerial tram with its rotating platform is the largest of its only kind in the world, making Palm Springs Aerial Tramway an identifying California landmark. Other trams of the same kind are in South Africa and Switzerland. The tram is installed with grab bars to hold on to so that when it lurches and the platform rotates the passengers can secure and steady themselves.

Our tramway ride was scheduled to depart at 10:00 AM, but since we did not have to follow the line to purchase our tickets, having done it online, we were allowed to take the 9:15 AM ride. It was a good start time because we did not expect to be in the area for much longer than two to three hours to avoid the heat while driving towards home.

Ascent at PS Aerial Tramway, Palm Springs, California

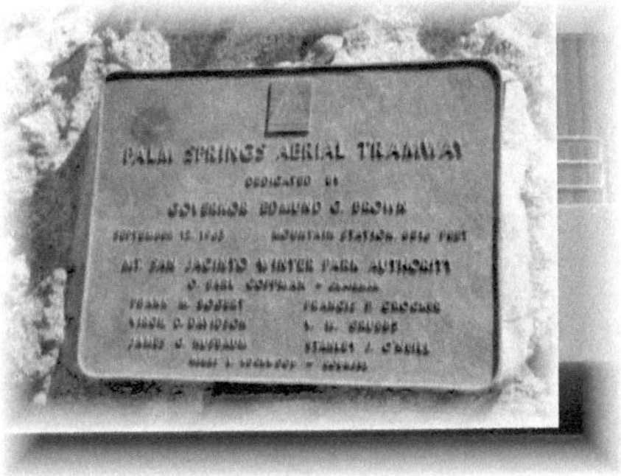

Based on my estimate, the tram traveled at approximately 65- to 75-degree incline on cables strung more than 8,500 feet along the Chino Canyon, up to the San Jacinto Mountain Range, and traversing through eight life zones. About fifteen minutes was all the travel took from the base station to the top, an eternity for some and a joyride for others. Fear of height – there was nothing that can be done about it once the tram started its journey.

Observing Amelia's handicap, a couple of volunteers were kind enough to have her sit at the end of the operator's bench. At the start, Amelia and I were adjacent to each other allowing me to hold her steady, but because of the rotation of the platform, we ended up on its opposite sides while her walker was on another location.

The rotation of the platform allowed the passengers to have a 360-degree view of the valley below and the gorges of green vegetation over which the tram traveled. Interrupted only by the tram's lurching and swinging, the passengers were able to take pictures through thick walls of transparent glass.

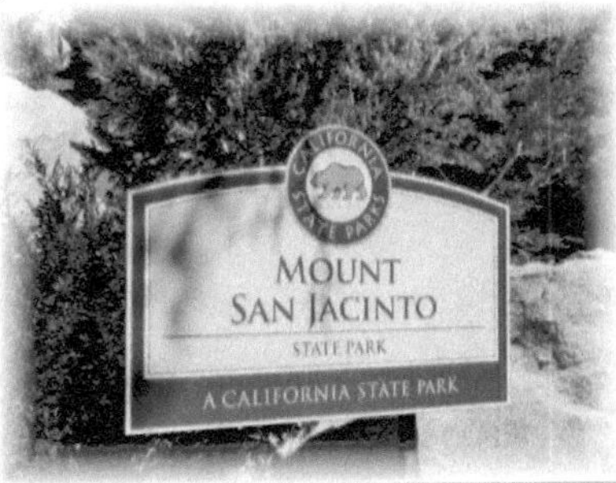

The best location to take pictures was the one next to the walls, but that was where I was most horrified; I felt that the glass would break if I leaned on it to look down. Amelia, on the other hand, was fearless of

Ascent at PS Aerial Tramway, Palm Springs, California

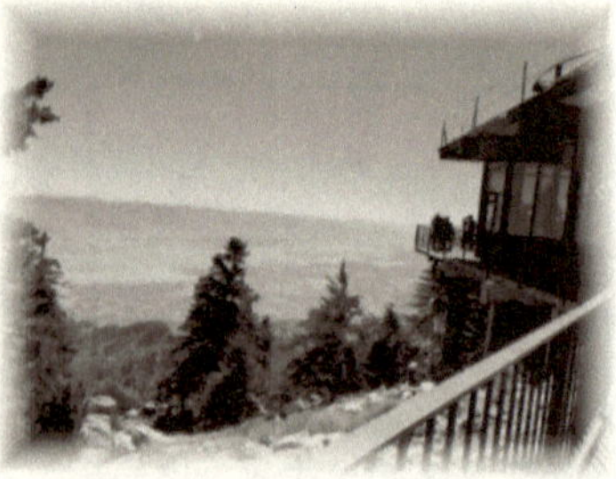

height, be it here in the tram, at the Grand Canyon in Arizona, at Waimea Canyon in Hawaii, or on the 17th deck of a cruise ship.

Our aerial journey ended at the Mountain Station in the San Jacinto Mountain State Park. The east side of the station overlooks the whole valley below while the west side directly faces the pristine forest. The station is equipped with elevators and stairs to all three levels, allowing access to the viewing platform on the third level and the terraces on the first and second levels leading to the hiking trails.

At a theater, a movie was continuously showing the history of the tramway from its conception in 1935 to final construction, the manner of maintaining it, and the facility to supply the stores and restaurants at the station. Souvenir and toy shops carry mementos for sale, to record the visit to the tramway if one so desires.

Even with the naked eyes, on a clear day like the one we had, one can see distant mountain ranges in the horizon hundreds of miles to the north towards Las Vegas. The Salton Sea, more than 50 miles away due Southeast, can be seen clearly. For even more details of the panorama of the region and for use by the visitors, coin operated high-powered telescopes are installed at the east-facing viewing platforms on the third level.

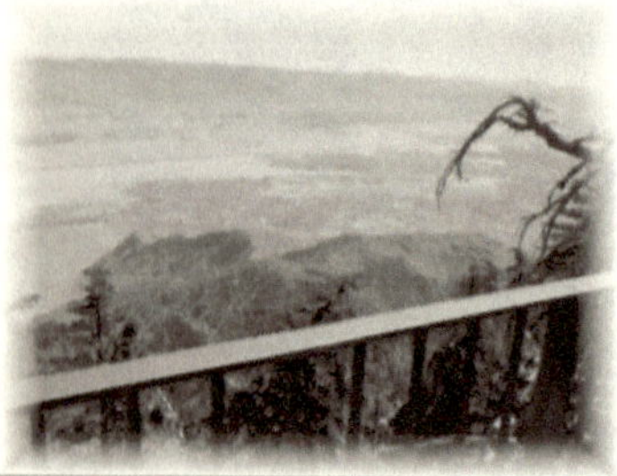

I did not explore the hiking trails because I could not leave Amelia by herself; she tended to get frequently lost on account of Alzheimer's. So we departed after only an hour stay at the station. Returning to the station below, the operator, another couple, and ourselves were the only passengers, compared to more than fifty on the journey up. I did not have to fight for a position to take pictures. It did not matter that the platform was not rotating, I could move freely in the tram.

Before we descended I checked the temperature at the San Jacinto Mountain Range Station - it was cold at 73 degrees - for comparison with the temperature at the valley. The average temperature difference between the two stations is 40 degrees, so it was not surprising that when we departed for home from the base station, the temperature was 115 degrees.

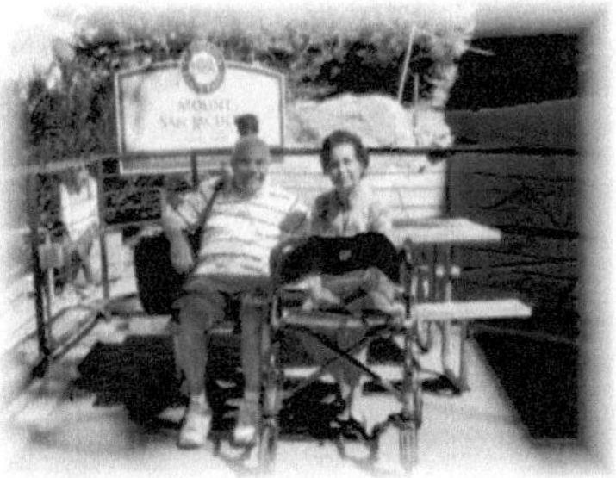

Like the other excursions we had previously, the Palm Springs Aerial Tramway outing was awe-inspiring; it took us to another point of interest in California, particularly in the Palm Springs area. The Palm Springs Aerial Tramway excursion is one I recommend to anyone who has the opportunity to take it. It is not expensive and does not require elaborate planning.

Palm Springs itself and the surrounding cities are world renown for warm weather, making them desirable for winter residence and vacation. Adding to its lure, the valley around Palm Springs is home to some of the finest golf courses in the world where celebrities of different categories and distinguished world leaders make their rounds.

Trip to Historic Julian, San Diego, California

Though not yet due, I scheduled the payment of the tax on a real property we owned in San Diego, California, early, to free myself for other tasks related to Amelia's afflictions. The day I scheduled the payment was also the day when I had to have Amelia walk as part of her therapy. I figured that walking along the pier on a stretch of Pacific Coast Highway in San Diego with a view of the harbor and with the refreshing ocean breeze would be good for her. So we started early for the one and a half hour drive to San Diego, in time for the county tax office to take our payment.

Brochures and handouts about a fair going on in Julian were displayed at the county building. Since Julian is in the general area of Anza Borrego Valley where we owned the property at Indian Head Ranch, Borrego Springs, I decided to drive to Julian to witness the fair.

Driving north on Interstate 5, we passed by Carlsbad to link up with state Highway 78, the road which would lead us all the way to our final destination. It was about 8:30 AM, so we had enough time to reach Julian and tour the town after a short rest. The more than two-hour drive was very lonely with nobody to talk to because Amelia was dozing off due to the effects of medications. With fast driving and missing road signs, it was also confusing with Highway 78 becoming Highway 79 and back to Highway 78 again.

We reached the base of the town, and the road turned into a very steep climb with a deep gorge on our side. I was scared to glimpse down as the road was separated from the rim of the canyon by only a few feet. Amelia, always unaffected by height, just watched the beautiful scenery slipped by as if being swallowed by the deep descent behind. I almost changed my mind and turned back, but the point on the highway for making a U-turn was at about halfway to the town; moreover, the road was so crowded that a hesitation on my part might cause congestion and possibly a traffic mishap. Located more than 3,000 feet above sea level, we finally reached our destination, the town of Julian.

Bumper to bumper traffic started at the edge of the downtown proper; cars were parked at every open space; parking rules were obviously not enforced at the time because some of the vehicles were parked illegally. Unable to find a parking space close to an eating place, I followed the traffic flow to the end of the downtown proper and back, and then crisscrossed the town in different directions. While doing so, in effect we were touring the town.

I drove as far south as the Julian Pioneer Museum, as far north as the American Legion, as far east as Hillside Church, and as far west as the Julian Bookstore. I found plenty of parking spaces, but they were too far out of the downtown proper to be even considered, given Amelia's condition.

Our trip was destined to be a frustration, it seemed, unable to find a parking space where I could push Amelia on the wheelchair to an eating place. My default mission by now was to find a parking space at a location away from the downtown proper to eat and rest for a few minutes before heading for home. But before I did, I wanted to drive on the main street one more time to have a last look of Julian.

As I drove on Main Street, a car pulled off from the curb. I let the cars behind passed, so I could maneuver ours into the tight parking space. As I unloaded Amelia's wheelchair, I noticed the Mom's Pie House sign. I pushed Amelia towards the place and waited fifteen to twenty minutes before I could place an order for what else, apple pie, the pie of which Julian is famous. I knew that a single pie was enough but in case we liked it, I ordered two to avoid waiting a few more minutes to place another order. With hunger gnawing at our stomachs, we finished the pie in no time at all, reserving the other for snack. It was the best apple pie I ever tasted. By then, it was almost 2:00 PM, the time for us to leave for home.

A gentleman helped me load the wheelchair onto the car before I could help Amelia, who was leaning on the half-opened door. Another man caught Amelia in time to prevent her from sliding onto the curb. I thanked both gentlemen and drove off while a car was patiently waiting to park on the space we left behind. We retraced the route coming into town, to head for home.

Descending from Julian, I had to drive on the lane closer to the hillside, making me feel secured away from the deep gorge, but still being extra careful because drivers were haphazardly passing moderately slower traffic like the manner I was driving. I saw to it that Amelia was comfortable; I had to maintain a steady down speed until we reached the level area where Highway 78 turned into Highway 79.

Having driven on Highway 79 a few times going to Borrego Springs, I eased the car into a safe and comfortable speed until we reached Warner Springs when we noticed that the apple pie was melting. We stopped to eat it, but it was already too mushy for consumption. We threw it away even though we felt hungry and thirsty.

I did not want to drive at night on the Cleveland National Forest where drivers appeared to be in so much rush as to over speed on a two-lane highway. I continued driving until we descended into Temecula where we had dinner, time now being close to 5:00 PM. We had plenty of rest before proceeding home for another fifty-five or so miles. The original purpose of paying property tax turned

Trip to Historic Julian, San Diego, California

out to be a 5-county highway undertaking with less than an hour of rest.

Back to the topic about Julian, we witnessed the remnants of the gold rush which made the town famous. Julian, designated as a historical town, meticulously preserves the evidence of the rush to mine the ores from the ground, for younger generations to recapture significant periods in the past. For a bit of history of the gold rush, I recommend a visit to Julian. I relish every moment of our short glimpse of the town.

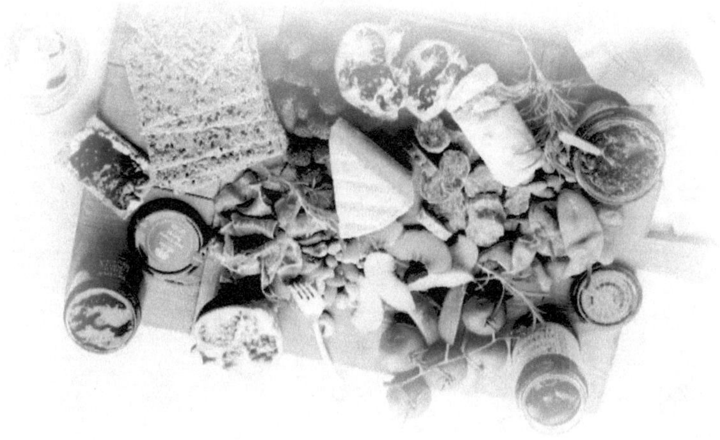

Trip to Historic Julian, San Diego, California

Chapter 5 – Anxious Moments

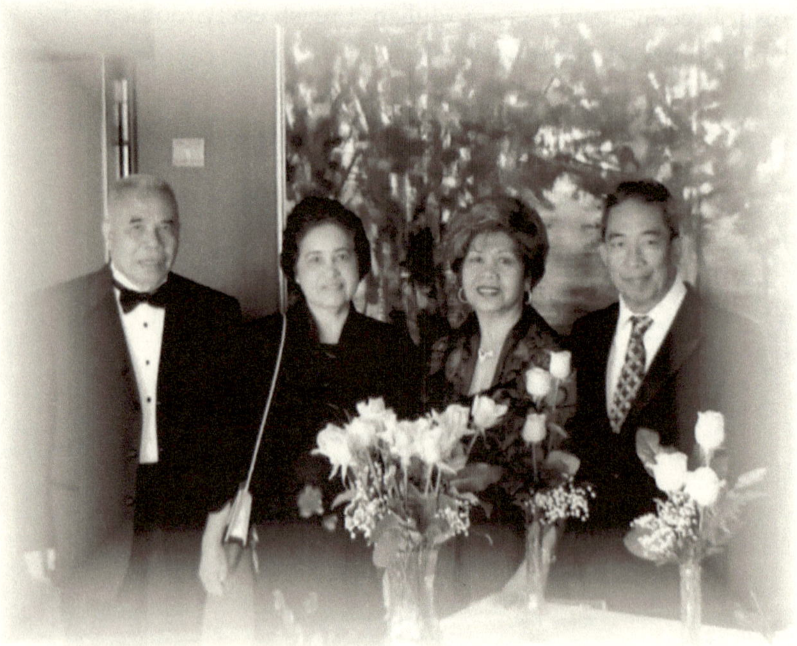

Bad Day at Puente Hills Mall, City of Industry, California

Bad Day at Puente Hills Mall, City of Industry, California

Puente Hills Mall at Rowland Heights, California, is conveniently located for informal meetings; it is only a bus ride for those who do not want to drive their cars. With a small area of its big parking lot designated as park-and-ride, the mall serves as a transfer point for passengers taking public transportation, before proceeding home from work or vice versa. The open space at the center of the mall is a good reference point for giving directions to those unfamiliar with the mall and its surrounding areas, and for arranging different meeting places if necessary. During summer, the mall is also a gathering place of those who want relief from the heat.

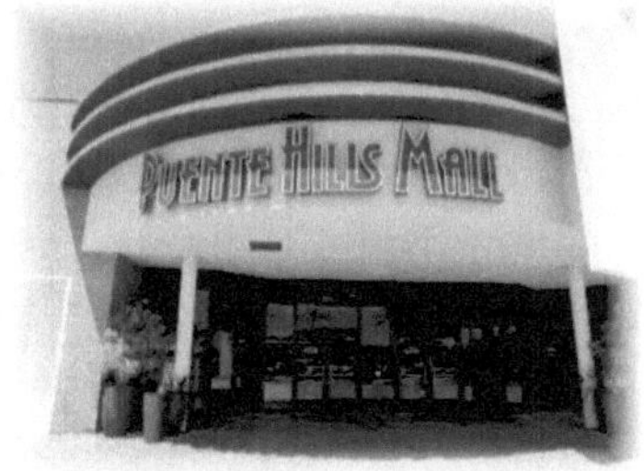

Amelia and her group of more than fifteen retired and semi-retired friends had been meeting at Puente Hills Mall for longer than ten years. The meetings were their way of socializing and making new acquaintances. It was at the mall that information about what was going on in their churches, in their children's schools, in the associations they belong to, and other not-so-private affairs, were exchanged. Each one had each other's telephone number, making coordination of their meetings fast and easy.

It was in one of those meetings that at about 3:00 PM. I drove Amelia to the mall. As a share of the afternoon's snacks, Amelia asked to stop by a bakery to buy some pastries. I did not observe anything unusual with Amelia then; in fact, she was calm and collected during the drive. A few of her friends were already at the

Bad Day at Puente Hills Mall, City of Industry, California

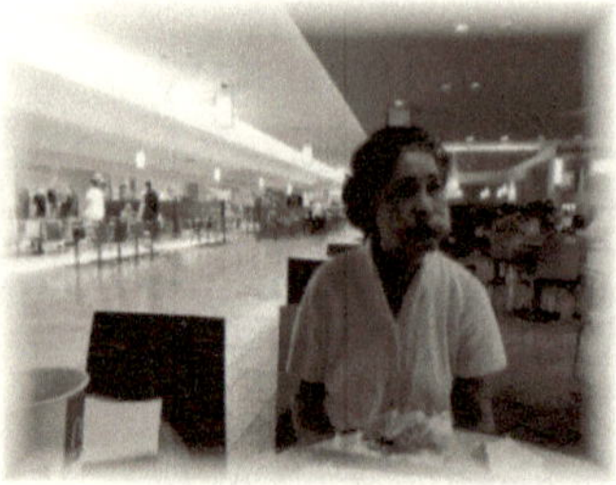

mall, and seeing that they were already staking their usual places, I left Amelia with them.

About an hour later, one of Amelia's friends called and asked me to come to the mall immediately because Amelia had an emergency. It only took me ten to fifteen minutes to get to the mall. Amelia was already on a gurney ready for transportation to the hospital. Before the paramedics drove away, they told me that Amelia's glucose level was dangerously low – about 48, they said. I assumed that was why she was weak and slow to respond to questions.

Advised that following the ambulance in my car was a traffic violation and that the hospital would probably need more information from me about Amelia, I took the time to ask Amelia's friends what exactly happened, before proceeding to the hospital. Her friends described to me that Amelia walked to the restroom appearing dazed. When she did not reappear from the restroom after several minutes, and she did not respond to repeated calls by her name, a friend kicked the restroom door open. Finding Amelia slumping, weak, and appearing ready to pass out, they called the emergency hotline 911.

Amelia was attended to immediately at the emergency ward of the hospital. It took a few hours for Amelia's glucose to elevate to an average level. Even when it was already normal, the hospital did not release her for another hour or two, for further observation. It was past midnight when the hospital

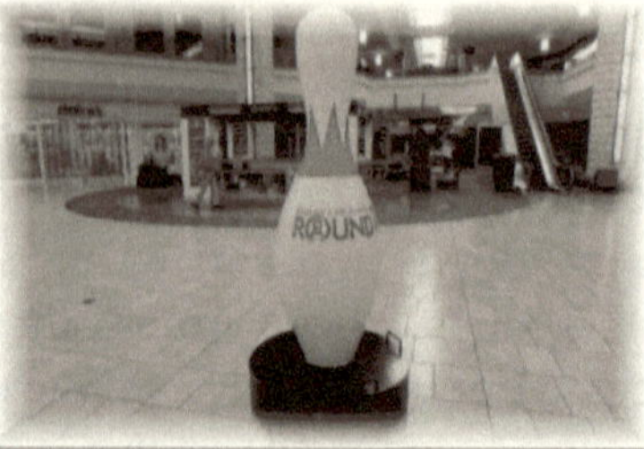

Bad Day at Puente Hills Mall, City of Industry, California

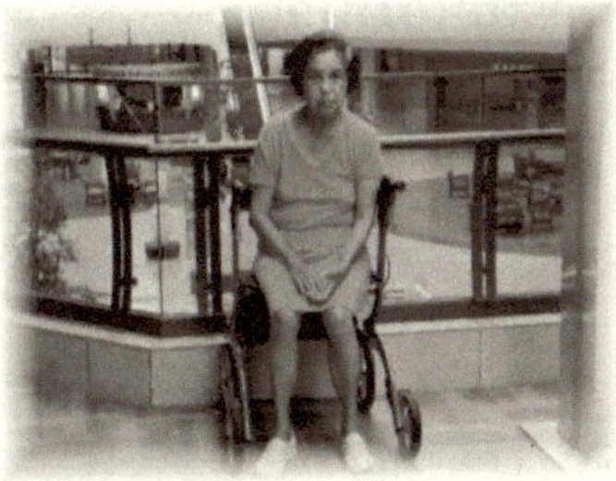

released her with explicit instruction on how to monitor her glucose level, while she was recovering from the incident. Furthermore, she needed to see her personal physician for a follow-up consultation.

Other than what was already in her medical chart, the follow-up consultation with her personal physician did not reveal any new threat to her health. To be sure that Amelia was well, the doctor ordered several tests which returned negative results.

What could have been a tragedy for Amelia was averted by her friends' quick actions, for which we were very thankful. Amelia and her group had, since then, disbanded because some moved to other states and some just simply got tired. We continued going to the mall for a while longer so Amelia could walk around; walking is her way of exercising when she does not want to go to the health club.

Bad Day at Brea Mall, Brea, California

Amelia was shopping for a dress at her favorite store, the Macy's. We agreed that she would go alone and that she would not be gone for more than a few minutes. I positioned myself not far from the store entrance inside the mall where she could easily find me.

After about thirty minutes my cell phone rang. The call was initiated from Amelia's cell phone by one of the store employees, letting me know that she had a confused female individual, asking her to call me. Failing to get enough information from Amelia about whom to call due to incoherence, the employee guessed that I am the emergency contact by looking at Amelia's cell phone.

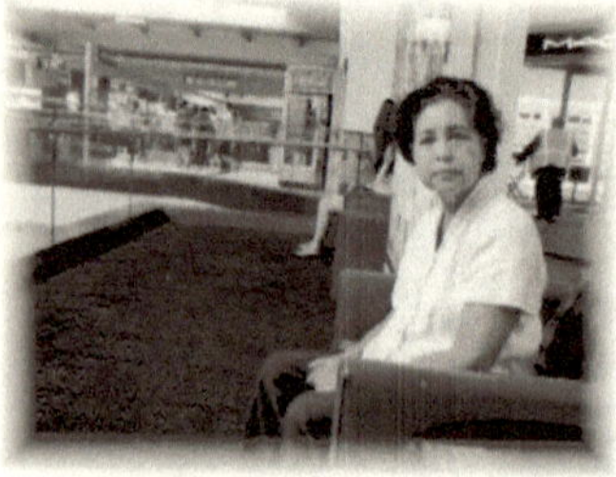

While I was on the second level, the same one where Amelia left me, the store employee did not mention from which store location she was calling. Apparently, the employee handed back Amelia's cell phone which remained unanswered when I called repeatedly.

I searched for Amelia in all the sections of the women's department asking every store employee I encountered, if anyone of them was aware of someone in trouble as described to me on the phone. Not getting an exact answer, I searched for her on the first level, without success. I asked one of the store employees to locate Amelia by announcing her name on the store speaker system. The employee helped me, but after announcing Amelia's name, the telephone was put on hold for what seemed to be an eternity. Time was of the essence; I could not waste any of it.

Bad Day at Brea Mall, Brea, California

Instinctively, I thought that Amelia would stay in the women's department, so there I went again, still no sign of Amelia. With frustration building up, I stepped out of the store and looked down the hallway towards the first level. There was Amelia being attended to by one of the store employees, outside the store. I ran down the stairs and took over assisting Amelia.

Amelia was pale and unable to stand steadily. I concluded that her glucose level had gone down precipitously. Nearby was a candy store with the attendant talking on the telephone. I begged the attendant to please hang up her phone and attend to my request for some candies. While I was talking to her, my eyes were turned towards Amelia, concerned that she might drop to the floor.

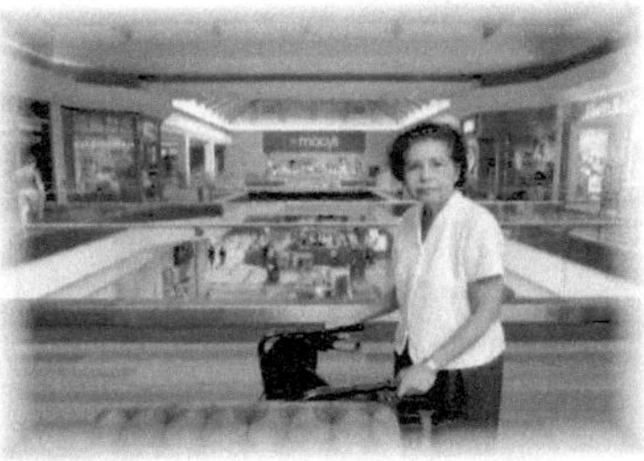

Witnessing the emergency, the attendant obliged, rang a sales transaction, and handed me a bag of mixed candies.

I eased Amelia on a bench and had her chew some candies. She slowly regained composure; she was now able to communicate. When I asked her how she felt, she indicated that she was feeble, thirsty, and needed to drink water or soda. Up to the second level, I hurriedly went to buy soda. In my haste, I did not realize that I handed the store clerk a $100 bill; I was surprised to get back a large amount of change.

I had Amelia slowly drink the soda which helped her to relax more. However, when I asked her to stand up after a few minutes, she appeared to stoop awkwardly and tended to walk sideways. I requested one of Macy's store employees to call 911. Amelia was taken to the hospital where blood and other tests were performed.

Bad Day at Brea Mall, Brea, California

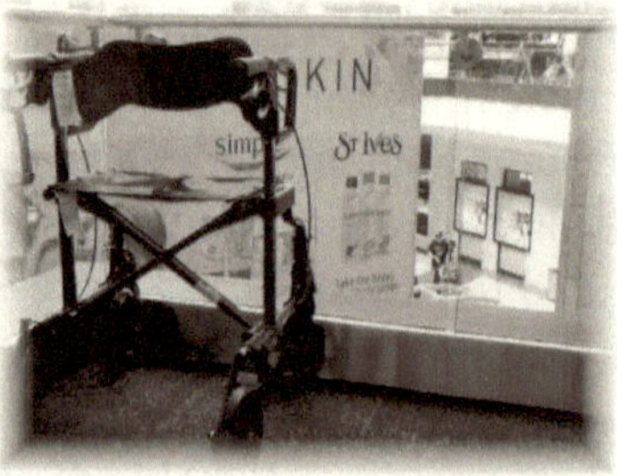

The tests did not reveal any sign of a stroke as I thought she might be having. She stayed in the hospital for more than six hours. When she was finally released from the hospital, she appeared as if nothing happened. The doctor at the hospital told me that perhaps Amelia's glucose level dropped very low, not to mention that she was also dehydrated. Subsequent tests conducted by Amelia's personal physician a few days later returned negative results as well.

As illustrated by Amelia's case, diabetes affects one in various ways not the least of which are general weakness of the body, incoherence, and stuttering.

Bad Day at Fashion Island Mall, Newport Beach, California

Bad Day at Fashion Island Mall, Newport Beach, California

The Fashion Island Shopping Mall located in Newport Beach, California, is one of the premier shopping destinations in Southern California. Widely known department stores include Nordstrom, Bloomingdale's, Neiman Marcus, and Macy's. Equally popular among shoppers are smaller stores spread out in an open-air random but orderly groupings that entice customers to shop while unhurriedly walking around. Excellent restaurants within the main mall area and a short distance away satisfy every customer's discriminating taste. Nearby hotels accommodate customers who intend to stay in the area for an extended period.

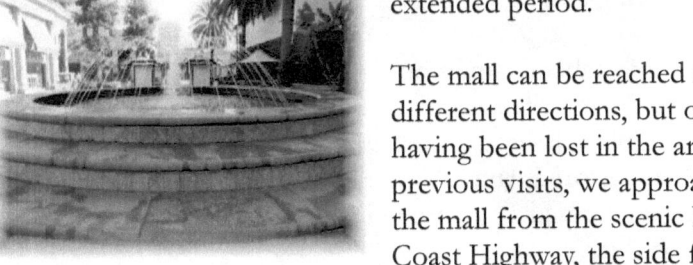

The mall can be reached from different directions, but owing to having been lost in the area in previous visits, we approached the mall from the scenic Pacific Coast Highway, the side facing the Pacific Ocean which blows a constant breeze towards the mall. Bypassing Macy's where we usually use the elevators, Amelia and I decided to use the continuously running escalators from the parking lot level. Amelia appeared to be healthy enough to walk the extra hundred feet farther from where we parked the car.

For a reason we did not know, the escalators turned out to be inoperative at the time. Instead of walking back to Macy's, we climbed the non-operating escalator, one step at a time. Halfway in her climb, Amelia suddenly felt feeble; she could not climb any higher; she could not come down either. Leaning on the side rail of

Bad Day at Fashion Island Mall, Newport Beach, California

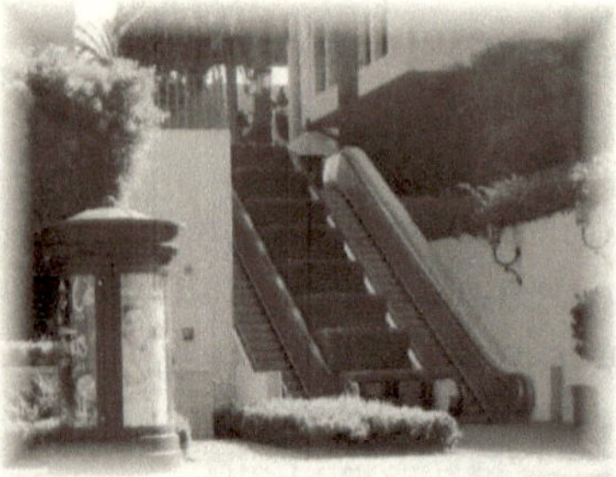

the escalator, she sat down on one of the steps. In the meantime, I was already at the top landing of the escalator, a regretful mistake; I should have stayed behind, watched, and assisted Amelia.

I ran down the steps towards her. With hands as cold as refrigerated water and forehead wet with perspiration, she asked to be left alone to rest. As is usual with her, she declined offers of assistance from passing shoppers. Then for each of the next few steps, I had her rest for a minute. Then I gently held and coaxed her to proceed, finally making all the way to the escalator landing and the mall level where there are benches.

I sat Amelia comfortably down in one of the benches whence I hurriedly shopped for coffee, soda, or food, convinced that her glucose level might be down. I ended up buying ice cream which appeared to have restored Amelia's energy. After resting for some thirty minutes, we decided to go home instead of walking around the mall to shop.

Gently assisting her, we walked towards Macy's where we took the elevator to the parking lot level; the car was still a few hundred feet away. I had her wait on a bench outside the store while I drove the car around to pick her up. In the car and until we reached home, I kept asking her how she was feeling, just to create a conversation to be sure she was coherent. Getting positive responses from her helped me get rid of anxiety and disconcerting feeling.

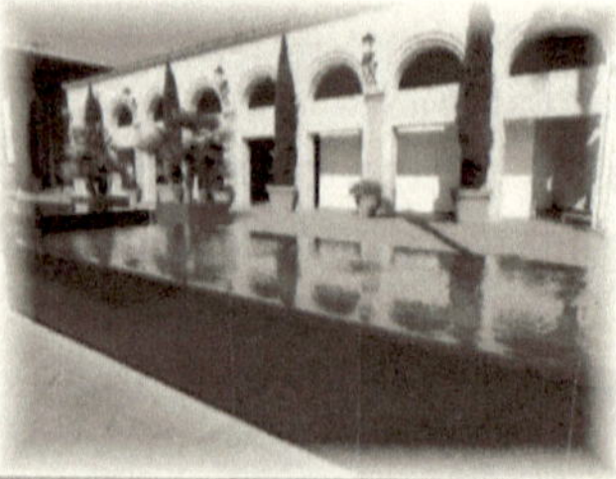

Bad Day at Fashion Island Mall, Newport Beach, California

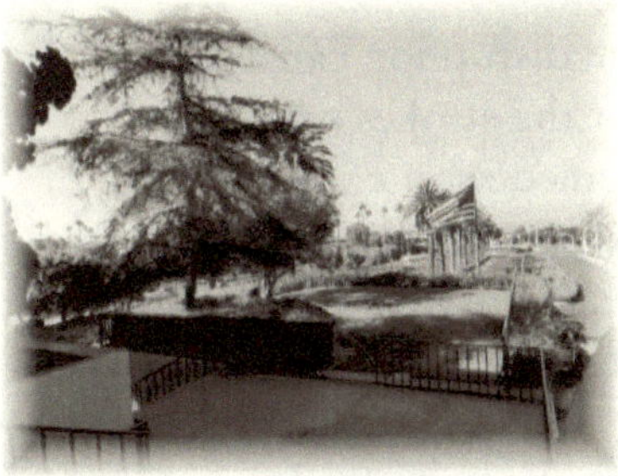

At home, I took readings of her glucose level and blood pressure. Both were within tolerable ranges. Speculating that she needed food and liquid, I gave her both. Four hours later she felt normal again.

As I thought over what could have happened disastrously at the mall, I kept reminding myself that Amelia's condition is so unpredictable that an emergency can occur at any moment. I cannot overemphasize the need to be keenly watchful of Amelia's condition. Caregiving is a personal routine task that requires an unending devotion.

Borrego Springs Incident, San Diego, California

Borrego Springs Incident, San Diego, California

The family had slightly improved from the disruption caused by Amelia's first two strokes. Unsure whether the strokes were a prelude to more severe afflictions, I scheduled asset consolidation as the next order of business. With only our residence to remain fixed, I had to turn a small real estate investment into a liquid resource in case we needed cash for emergencies.

It was an 11-acre lot at Indian Head Ranch, Borrego Springs, in Northern San Diego County. Before I initiated a sale transaction and as a matter of personal satisfaction, I decided to make a last minute observation of the development in the area. Last time I looked, there were some eight or more million-dollar homes widely spread out.

One of the appeals of the subdivision was its huge lots, allowing the residents to build homes distant from each other, at the same time maintaining equestrian trails in each lot. They are second homes in some cases, of people escaping from the harsh winter weather condition elsewhere. Since we had not been visiting the property frequently, I did not care to have the code to open the restraining gate.

Observing some tire tracks on the desert sand around the gate, I repeatedly thumped the tracks with my foot to test if the sand beneath was compacted enough to sustain the weight of the car. The sand appeared compacted, so I maneuvered the car to bypass the gate, following the tire tracks.

As soon as the four tires cleared the asphalt road, the car started to sink in the sand. The more I revved the engine, the deeper the car was sinking; we were stuck. I unloaded the wheelchair, had Amelia settled on it, and pushed it towards the gate where there was a shade from the trees.

After explaining that I was a property owner too, some residents driving by seemed to understand why I was illegally bypassing the gate but probably heaping shame on me. One gentleman offered to help with his 4-wheel drive Rubicon, but his vehicle was not a match for our car because of weight difference.

He offered to drive by a farming warehouse though, to inform the crew of the possible need for a skip loader to pull our car out of the sand. It would be fifteen minutes before I could expect a crew to come.

In the meantime, Amelia was starting to be affected by the heat. She was perspiring in the shade by the gate. She needed to stand and stretch to keep her blood circulating particularly on her right side which was affected by the strokes. I declined offers by some residents to take us to the central area of the town because help was on the way, I was hoping.

Not even fifteen minutes went by when a 2-man crew came, one driving a skip loader and another one in a car. Seeing that Amelia was terribly affected by the heat, the man in the car offered some cold water and sweet unpeeled grapefruits which we accepted. He also offered to have Amelia sit in the air conditioned car which was kept running.

The man on the skip loader tried different lengths of chains between the car and the skip loader. When none seemed to measure up, he improvised a longer chain. I was not sure if he used water or oil, but he soaked a link with liquid. After five or so minutes he eased the link into the hook of the chain. He explained later that the link did not catch earlier because it expanded due to the heat.

Hooking one end of the chain to the chassis of the car and the other end to the skip loader, the man started the skip loader to pull the car forward. In less than two minutes, the car was positioned on the road away from the sand. The car appeared to be alright when I started it. I offered the crew $30.00; they took only $20.00. Amelia was let off the crew's car, and she transferred to ours.

We drove by our property at the ranch; not much change has occurred since we purchased it. Then we proceeded to Rams Hills Country Clubhouse, some fifteen minutes away, because Amelia was not feeling well; she was being overcome by the heat and she needed to drink some liquid. At the clubhouse, I took a measurement of her glucose level; it was normal.

A lady doctor happened to be resting at the clubhouse after her round of golf. After a brief introduction, she felt Amelia's neck and wrist. She then asked to see Amelia's tongue. She told me to give Amelia orange juice and something to chew and have her rest. Amelia would be alright after a few minutes, she said. If Amelia needed further assistance, the doctor could be summoned from the golf course. After an hour and before we left, I asked the clubhouse staff to thank the doctor for me.

I did not want to drive at night in the Cleveland National Forest which we took coming to Borrego Springs. Highway S22 instead would lead us through the more populated Imperial County towards the Salton Sea. Lightning being very visible at the Santa Rosa Mountain Range, I had to be aware though, of flash floods because Highway S22 traverses the Carrizo Badlands in the Anza Borrego State Park.

Borrego Springs Incident, San Diego, California

The name "Carrizo Badlands" appropriately describes the landscape with deep crevices and fissures carved by floods, as if scratched by a giant hand. Highway S22 links with Highway 86 which then links with Interstate 10. At last, we were heading for home driving west on Interstate 10.

I sold the property at Indian Head Ranch, Borrego Springs, at less than break-even, through a local real estate agent, in less than a month. All transactions were done by mail; I did not even meet the real estate agent. The sale freed me from having to think about what I now consider a futile speculative investment, leaving us in possession of just a home as the sole real estate investment.

Garage Fall, Rowland Heights, California

After many years of taking care of Amelia, I have become emotionally hardened and uneasily startled to jump into swift involuntary action. I only react with so much emotion when I feel that she is endangering herself through her senseless actions, because to an enervated person like she is, let alone one who suffered multiple strokes, mishaps lurk everywhere. My fear is that she might get into a serious accident like the one she almost had at home.

Amelia was just learning how to walk again after the third stroke. The therapy she had been going through quickly improved her mobility; her confidence was returning, albeit less profound. Although I was hiding my diminished hope that she will ever walk normally again, I was excited about her rapid improvement. She appeared to test her ability to walk beyond the space designated for her to move around. The challenge though, was that as I relented on my warning to her about overextending her space, she was becoming even more daring.

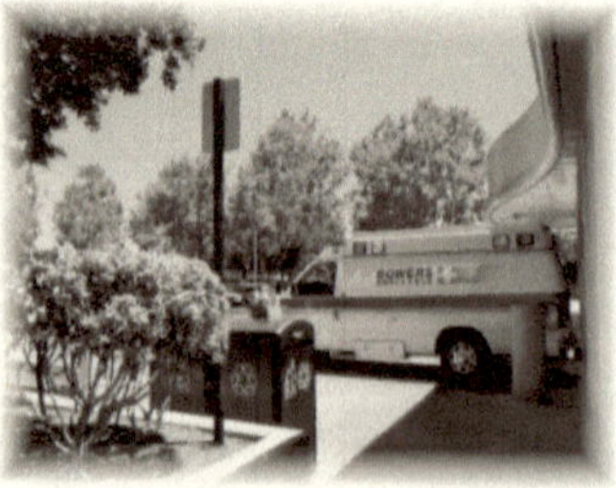

As has been our practice every morning, we eat breakfast at a restaurant ten minutes away from our residence. This day of the incident, I asked Amelia to wait for me in the living room, for my help getting into the car. Not listening to my advice and hearing that I started the car, she headed to join me by going through the garage. When I went to the living room to pick her up by way of the main door, she was gone, to my consternation.

Garage Fall, Rowland Heights, California

I knew she could not be going very fast, and the only way she could have disappeared from the living room was through the garage, so there I went in a hurry. Amelia was on the cement floor, lying on her side, feet straight out along the door, and her head barely touching the steel pipe that protects the water heater. She was moaning and complaining that her right arm was hurting; it was the arm that absorbed the fall. It turned out that she was reaching out to a work table for support with her right hand, but because of injury to her arm from the strokes, the arm was unable to support her weight causing her to fall.

Afraid that I might cause additional harm to her body, I did not raise her up right away; I was contemplating whether to call the emergency number 911. When she answered "no" to my question if she hit her head on the steel pipe, I was slightly relieved. After asking her what other parts of her body were hurting, and satisfied that none were, I determined that the fall did not inflict a serious injury. To be exactly sure though, and still fighting the urge to call 911 I let two or three minutes passed before I raised her up.

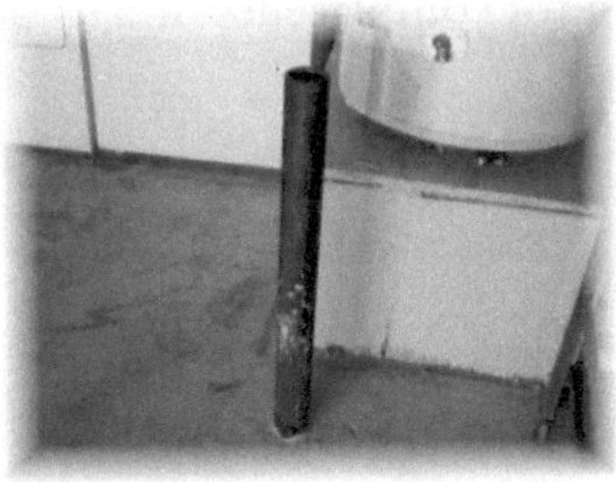

I was roused to anger at her for not following my advice. Suddenly my composure was wearing out, and my mind was swirling at the thought of a potential disaster had she hit her head on the steel pipe. On the other hand, there was nothing that I could do, except to bear in mind that the strokes severely compromised her mental capacity. She was just listening to my rants with a visible facial expression of apology for what she did.

Garage Fall, Rowland Heights, California

We proceeded to eat breakfast. On our way, I convinced her to see her doctor for checkup. When we got home, I called the appointment desk at the hospital and described what happened.

The appointment desk personnel asked me a few questions about Amelia's vital signs to determine whether she needed emergency treatment. When she assessed that nothing seemed to be serious, she set up an appointment for Amelia to see her doctor. The tests performed on Amelia returned negative results; she did not suffer any serious injury from the fall.

A disaster was averted, and luck was with us. With the like of Amelia as a patient, caregiving is a fixed responsibility with no room for complacency and carelessness.

It's in the Mind, Brea, California

Amelia and I had a good lunch at a restaurant. We chose the particular restaurant for its location; it was the closest to the freeway en route to Brea Mall. It was also very convenient for Amelia; she was just released from rehabilitation after the strokes, and I did not want her to spend too much time in motion. The drive to the mall was normal in relation to Amelia's physical and mental conditions. Had there been an indication at all, of discomfort on Amelia's part, I would not have driven her to the mall despite her insistence. I had an idea why she insisted going there, namely, she was going to purchase another purse.

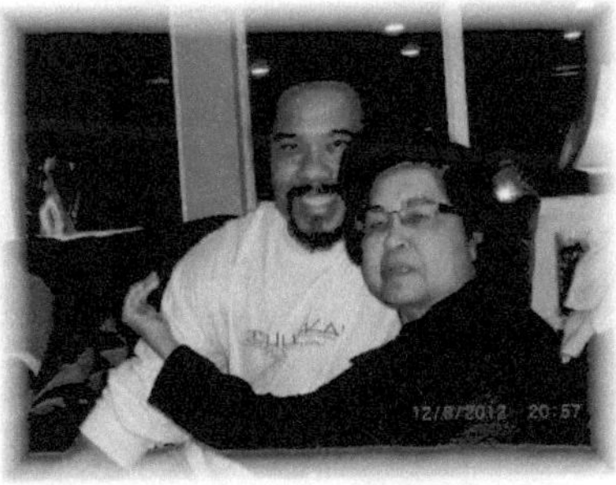

We agreed that I stayed in one particular area of the mall where she could easily find me while she went to the stores to shop. Although I did not want her to go back to the car alone, I reminded her where it was parked anyway. She was fond of a particular brand of purse, so she took a roundabout way to the particular store to mislead me; she did not want me with her to hide the fact that she was at the mall to shop for another purse to add to her collection.

When an hour and a half had gone by without her coming to find me at the agreed location, I decided to look for her at the purse store. Not finding her there, I extended my search to the other stores where she would normally go to shop. She was not in those stores either. Aware of her physical and mental condition, I started to get concerned. Should she decide to find me I stayed at our meeting place a few more minutes, but she did not come.

It's in the Mind, Brea, California

Intuitively I walked to the car, and there she was with our son, shaking and almost in tears. Obviously, she was not able to retrace her way to our meeting place and she got lost. She called our son who drove close to thirty miles to the mall, asking him to pick her up. She was complaining that she was hungry, not having eaten the whole day, and that I abandoned her at the mall. At that time she was still able to use a cellular phone.

I explained to her that before we left for the mall we had a very good lunch, not to mention an early breakfast. As she started to recall, her shaking started to diminish. Finally, she was convinced that we had lunch earlier; her shaking completely stopped. She did not even care for food because she was no longer hungry. Feeling somewhat tired, she abandoned the idea of purchasing another purse; she wanted to go home instead.

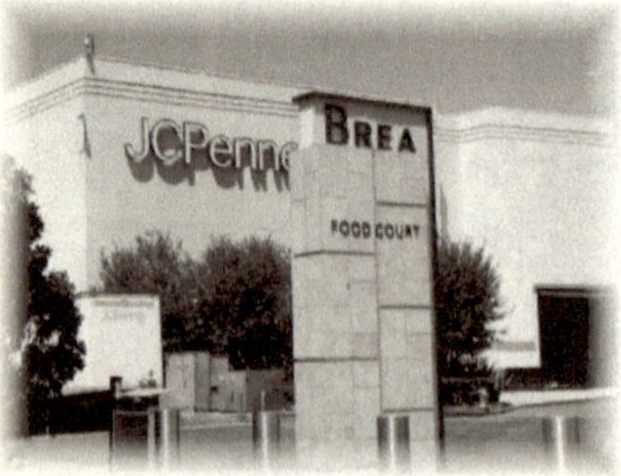

The episode ended well considering Amelia's just-diagnosed ailments. The three of us decided to spend the rest of the day at home and discussed the options for Amelia's continued rehabilitation.

The incident appeared funny, but I was convinced then that her mind was devastated by the massive strokes. I purposely drove by the restaurant where we had lunch to test if she could recall that we had been there earlier. She did mention that we ate there but unspecific as to what day and time. Sadly, Amelia failed to recall the events that happened only hours earlier.

It's in the Mind, Brea, California

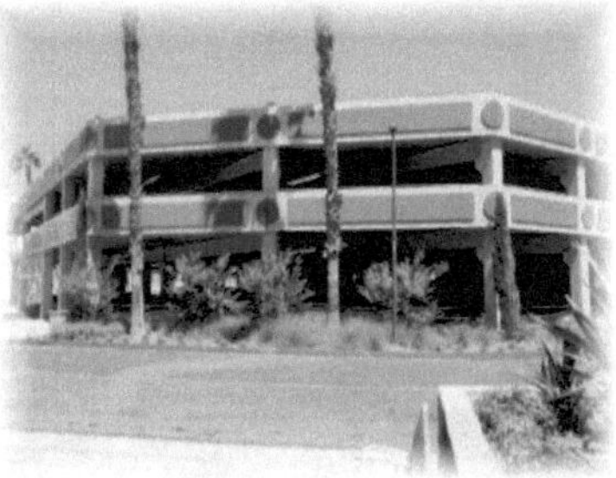

I was told by the doctor that more and more of this type of incidents would be occurring as the effects of the strokes started manifesting. This was just the beginning, and it was already influencing my attitude towards Amelia; she was not perfectly normal anymore. Accordingly, I should be prepared for a major adjustment to cope with her changed behavior.

She laughs whenever I recall the incident to her. Like the doctor's comments, more and more of similar incidents have been happening already. I believe that Alzheimer's has more to do with them than the strokes, although the latter ailment appeared to have triggered the former.

Incident at LA County Hall of Records, Los Angeles, California

At my work at about one 1:00 PM on a warm day, I was eager to leave and exit from a very boring meeting. The receptionist came into the conference room and motioned to me that I had a telephone call. The call was from one of Amelia's friends telling me that Amelia was not feeling well, and that she would be waiting for me in the lobby at her place of work in downtown Los Angeles. That gave me an excuse to leave the meeting.

It only took me thirty minutes of freeway driving from Pasadena where I worked to downtown Los Angeles where Amelia worked. I was happier driving on a warm day on the freeway than watching and listening to a presentation in the meeting. I was looking forward to spending the rest of the day at home.

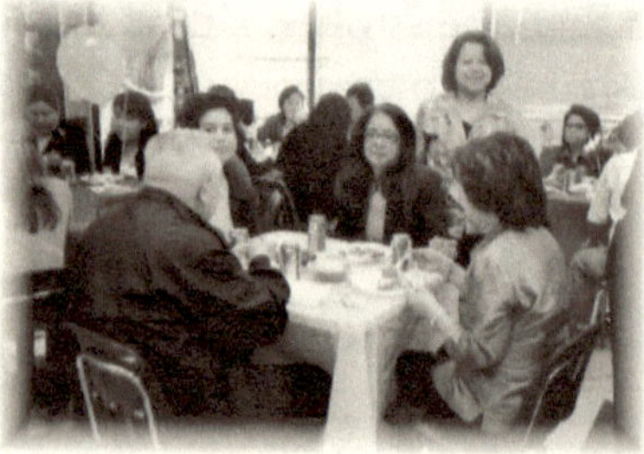

Amelia and few of her friends were already waiting for me in the lobby of the building where she worked. After bidding goodbye for the day to her supervisor, I led her to the car.

While walking, I could tell that she was not usually lively. Once seated, she started to feel weak; her hands were cold, and she was pale. When I lifted her arms and let them go, they just fell back like non-living objects. She was not speaking to me, keeping her eyes closed. I decided then to take her to the hospital instead of home. What a mistake that was, getting her into the car instead of calling the emergency hotline.

Incident at LA County Hall of Records, Los Angeles, California

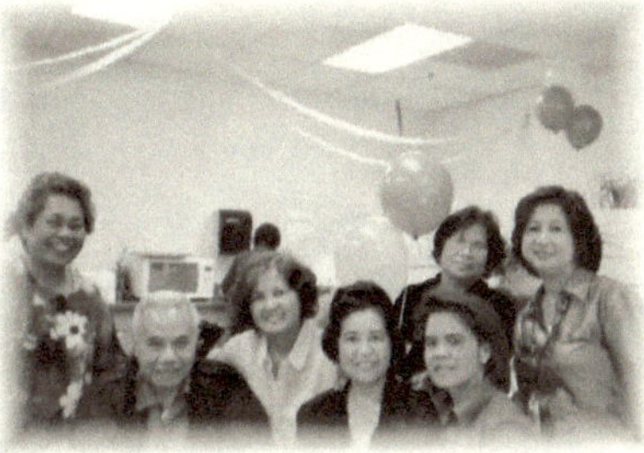

The freeway was like a parking lot because of the amount of traffic; vehicles were moving ever so slowly from what I could tell. What would normally take fifteen to twenty minutes of driving to the hospital of which Amelia is a plan member, was turning out to be an eternity. Even the streets where I would usually take detours were congested with all sorts of vehicles. It was in the middle of the afternoon, and traffic buildup was at its peak.

It probably took me an hour of driving to reach the emergency ward of the hospital. I hurriedly motioned to the personnel at the emergency ward door to immediately help Amelia. They placed her on a gurney and whisked her to the emergency room. The hospital professionals did their emergency routine on Amelia - took her blood pressure, put IV and oxygen on her, so on so forth - before they even did the paper works for checking her in. I was there to assist them later.

After four hours or so, some members of the hospital staff advised me that one of the reasons for Amelia's weakness was the low glucose level. An hour later, they assured me that Amelia was not in real danger anymore; her blood glucose level started to elevate. According to them, had Amelia been unable to reach the hospital in a few more minutes, she could have gone into a coma. They cautioned me against taking a patient in a car; instead, I should call the emergency hotline.

Incident at LA County Hall of Records, Los Angeles, California

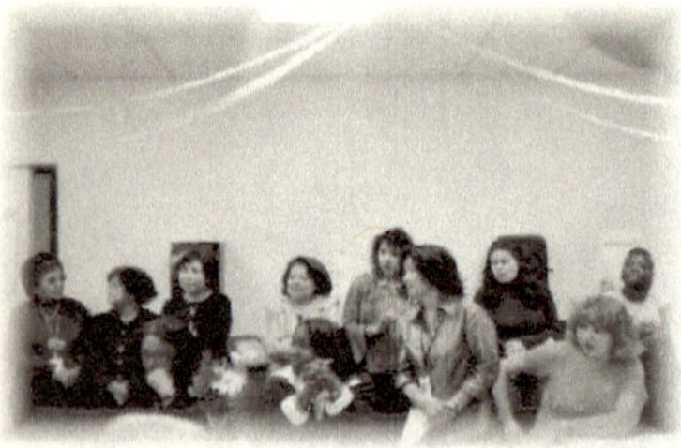

She was released from the hospital after about seven hours from the time of her admission. The day I looked forward to spending at home turned out to be a midnight post emergency disruption.

She had to take a few days off from her work to recuperate. Her glucose level was not fluctuating as erratic as I was told to observe. Although she was recuperating, she was in contact with her friends every day, always eager to go back to work.

The incident was the first that got Amelia sick for having low glucose level. Since then I became more aware and sensitive to any sign of her feeling feeble. As her health was slightly declining and her age advancing, incidents like loss of energy and feeling of general weakness will be occurring more often, the hospital professionals advised me.

When Amelia recovered enough and became fit to go back to work, I did not let her drive for a few more days. She was carpooling with her friends, and when it was her turn to drive, I drove them to work instead. After a month her physical condition had significantly improved.

We were quite relieved and thankful that nothing worst happened to Amelia. Visually, there was no trace of the incident that got her into the hospital. However, we became more aware and wary of her fluctuating glucose level. To control it, the

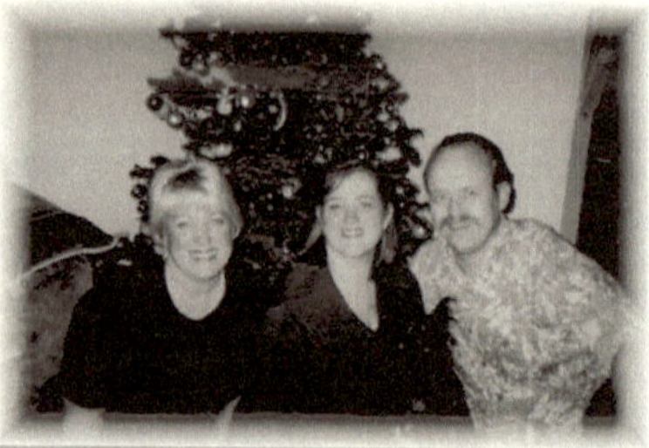

medical staff advised her to adopt a strict dietary regimen and follow a regular exercise routine. Amelia has had no problem following the doctors' instructions.

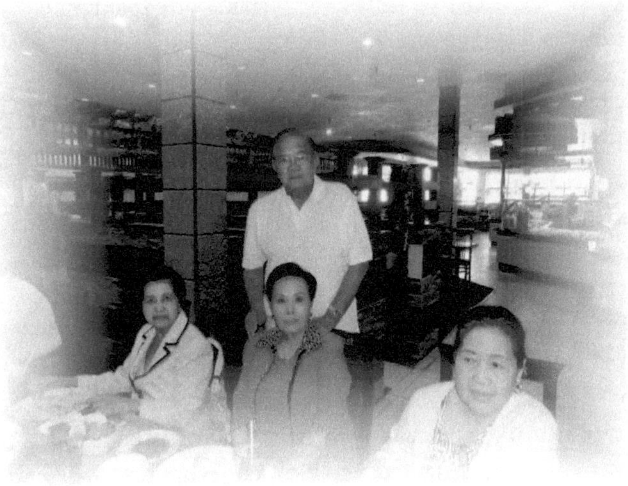

Stepladder Near Fall, Rowland Heights, California

Stepladder Near Fall, Rowland Heights, California

"For the love of God" - these were my words in this particular instance, to describe Amelia's devotion to serve God at her peril. Despite cautionary advices from the medical professionals, children, friends, and relatives, to avoid foolhardy activities which might cause her to fall, she carries them out just the same whenever she has the chance. This particular case always strikes me with horror when I remember it.

The night before we boarded on a cruise along the California coast, an earthquake struck just five miles away from our residence. Damage to our personal properties did not appear to be extensive. In order not to spoil our cruise, I did not even bother to inspect and worry about the broken glass pieces on the floor. The following morning while we were already cruising, another earthquake struck again with our city as the epicenter. The aftershock, I believed, toppled over some of Amelia's religious figurines and crucifixes on her altar. There was nothing we could do from the cruise ship; we just hoped that our house was not severely damaged and that repair works, if there were needed had to wait until the termination of our cruise.

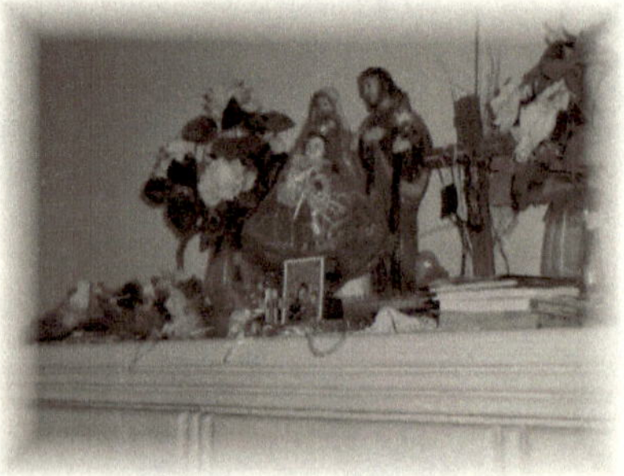

Amelia's altar was atop the 6-foot high chest by design. When she had to rise from and go to, bed to pray she would just look up and face her altar. I did not yet bother to straighten her altar after the earthquakes, explaining to her that an aftershock might topple it all over again. Vehemently insisting that I should fix it and seeing that

Stepladder Near Fall, Rowland Heights, California

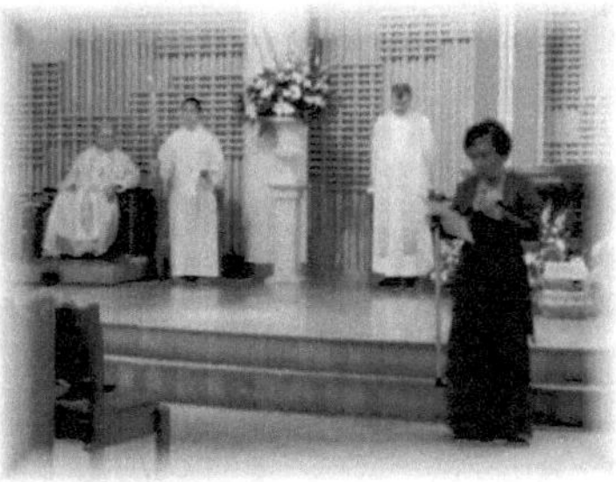

it was not getting done, she waited for a chance to do it herself, while I waited for the frequency of aftershocks to die down.

The aftershocks appeared to have stopped. Then on a day when I was working on my computer, I heard a faint noise coming out of our bedroom. Thinking that the wind was probably causing it, I did not pay much attention to it. Then I heard it again and again. I walked into our bedroom and opened the door.

To my absolute shock and fright, Amelia was on the top step of the stepladder which has no side rails and not-long-enough grab handles, reaching up to her altar, appearing to be hanging rather than leaning on the chest. She was holding onto the top edge of the chest with her stricken and weakened right hand, while she was fixing her altar with the left hand. I did not want to scold, scare, and cause her to misstep and fall while she was off the floor. Gently, I helped her down.

Then my temper, which was all too familiar to her already owing to the constant pressure of caregiving, erupted. I screamed, cursed, and pointedly threatened her with such things as filing a divorce, or leaving her alone in the house, or moving her to a facility for people with disability, and so on so forth. She promised not to do unsafe activities again. So far she was living up to her promise. She had no more access to the stepladder; it was gone out of her sight.

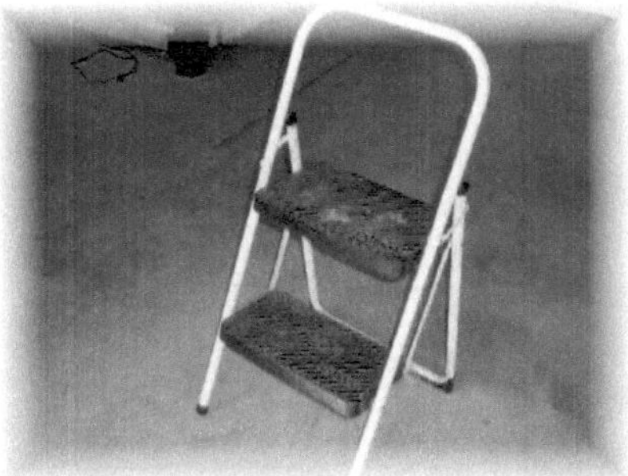

Stepladder Near Fall, Rowland Heights, California

What could have certainly happened was her right arm and leg, severely weakened by massive strokes, would not be able to support her weight causing her to fall. Her head could have hit the edge of the nightstand, the solid hardwood bed frame, or the wooden floor, resulting in real emergency; worst, it could have led to her breaking her neck let alone potential death. Thank God, her attempt to serve Him did not lead to a tragedy.

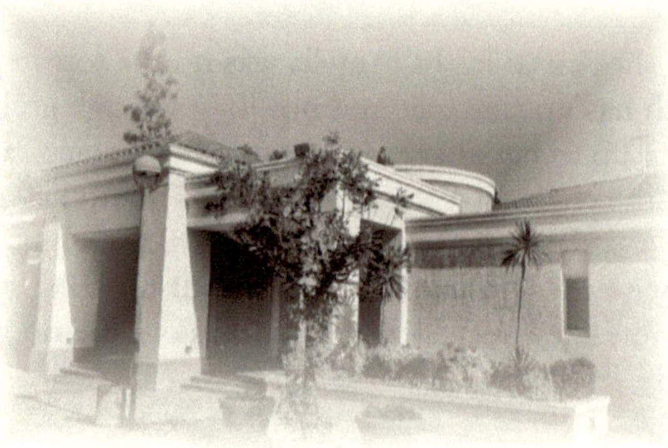

Taco Bell Accident, Rowland Heights, California

After release from a month-long therapy due to two massive strokes, Amelia stayed at home for a few more months to recuperate, returning to work on a part-time basis thereafter.

Her mental capacity having been reduced to a 4th-grade level, Amelia was no longer able to perform her regular duties which were taken over by other personnel during her absence. Workload involving finger dexterity was reassigned to other members of the office staff, her right arm and hand having been severely immobilized by the massive strokes. In short, she was evidently stripped of her duties which she dearly loved. Despite the diminution of her job, she was jubilant that she was still able to associate with her friends in the office. She was driving again.

At first, I did not allow her to drive alone. Either I or one of our children or grandchildren would accompany her as a passenger on short trips. I was hiding my concern about her altered driving skills each time she stepped in the car to drive. She was vehement in her request to be allowed to drive again so she could continue working, free from my constant cautionary reminders. Likewise, her safe driving would be a boon to me for I would be free from taking her back and forth to her office. I had to take care of my separate job also.

With our granddaughter as passenger one day, Amelia drove to the mall to shop. Coming home nervous, our granddaughter reported that during the trip her grandma, at an intersection with stop sign, did not stop, and on another, drove through a red light. Luckily they came home safe, but our granddaughter said that she would never again ride with her grandma as driver. When I confronted Amelia with the report, she said that next time she would be more careful and observant. The "next time" she was referring to, not even a week, came too soon.

I was rearranging our place to make room for Amelia so that she could continue therapy at home. This day when she wanted to go to the gym alone for the first time after the strokes to work out, I was excited about her desire and determination to recover her lost driving skills, after longer than a month without practice.

To hone her skills – I suspected that was precisely why she wanted to go alone. I begged her to drive safely and observe all traffic signals and signs. At the same time I asked her to buy food for lunch from any place that she would not have difficulty parking the vehicle.

She was parking the sports utility vehicle at a Taco Bell parking lot to buy food. I believed that instead of stepping on the brake, she stepped on the gas pedal. The car lurched forward and jumped over the cement barrier, crossed the space between the barrier and a wide grassy island, crossed the island, crossed the drive-through lane, and hit the drive-through window of the food place.

It was the window that stopped the vehicle. Luckily, there were no cars on the drive-through lane despite that the place was always crowded with cars and foot traffic at noon, it being a few blocks close to a high school. Amelia was not injured, no one else was. She still had the presence of mind to sternly tell would-be accident responders not to touch her purse.

The accident cost a $12,000-damage to the vehicle. The food place was closed for several days. I assumed that it must have cost the insurance company a significant amount to have the damages repaired and to compensate the place for the loss of income.

Taco Bell Accident, Rowland Heights, California

Amelia was required to take a neurological test by the Department of Motor Vehicles after the report of the accident was completed. She miserably failed the test that the department seized her driver's license. She was visibly shaken for losing her driver's license which the department replaced with a similar identification card but with no privilege to drive.

I comforted her, telling her that it was better for her to lose her driving privilege than to have one as a potential cause for a serious accident, considering the way she was driving. She assessed herself and finally admitted that she was no longer fit to drive. She never wanted to drive again.

Taco Bell Accident, Rowland Heights, California

Chapter 6 – Vacation Cruises

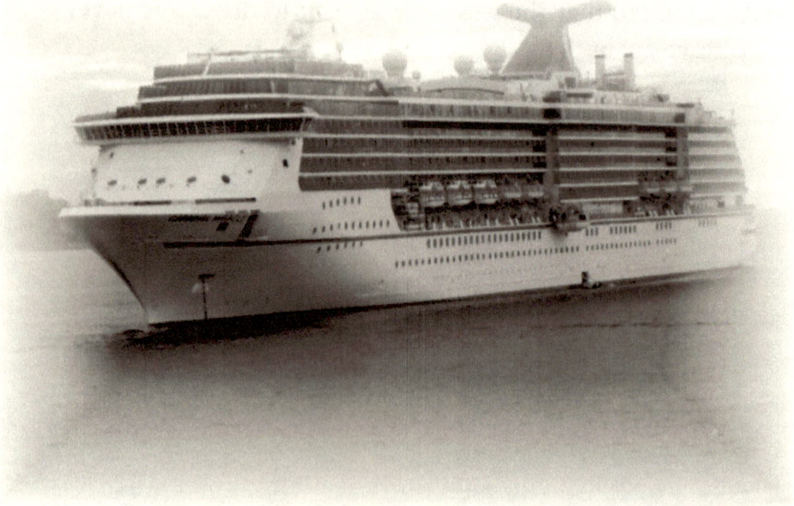

Cruise - Choosing One

My choice of a cruise is determined by Amelia's health and ability to travel, considering her physical and mental condition. A cruise is usually booked a few days, months, or even years, ahead of the sailing date. Price changes may occur in the meantime for early booking discounts, discounts for seniors, family discounts, discounts for men and women in the service, and discounts for certain state residents. As the sailing date gets closer, higher discounts may also be offered for yet unbooked cabins. Upgrades in the cabin selection may also be provided instead of price cuts. Because a cruise is a very expensive form of vacation, I watch for money-saving opportunities.

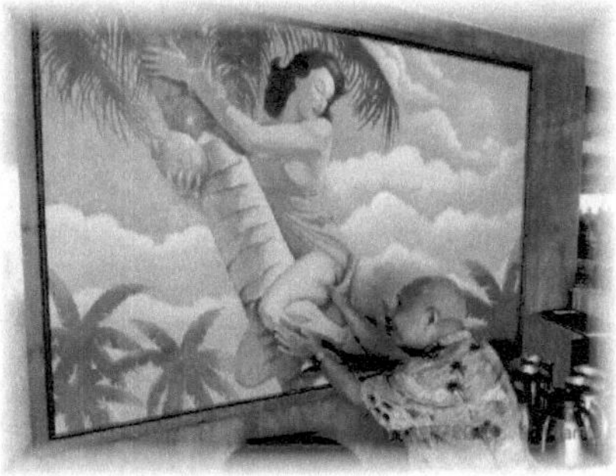

The weather at the embarkation port is crucial in my choice of a cruise vacation. It being unpredictable, avoiding the hurricane months makes more sense with respect to safety and comfort. With hundreds of cruise destinations, the weather is favorable in some ports of embarkation while it is worse in others. In some cases, repositioning of cruise ships due to weather patterns offers more opportunities to save. My choice of destinations is also based on the season.

I do not want to visit a place more than once, so the choice must not be a repeat of a previous visit if it can be avoided. Having determined that the destination is the right one for Amelia, I research the reputation of the ports, regarding peace and order. In a single cruise, one port may be rated very high while another is rated very low. A negative review is an important warning, but I do not drop a port because of it. It is always possible to join a group excursion for safety or to just stay on board the ship for continuous entertainment.

Sometimes cruise lines run more than one ship on the same itinerary but on different schedules. That being the case, I choose the schedule with the newer or recently refurbished ship. Like the newer ships, the refurbished ones are updated to meet the contemporary needs of the cruisers. Refurbishments occur every few years to entice customers making it one of the many approaches the cruise lines advertise their services. At any rate, I feel satisfied in my choice, having explored every possibility.

Not all cabins of the same category on a cruise ship have the same amenities, hence the difference in prices. Because of Amelia's physical condition, I select one among the cabins for the cruisers with disability, if available. Cabin sizes are verifiable from sketches provided by the cruise lines. Among the category of cabins for the handicapped, are selections of locations from which I determine the one that is right for Amelia.

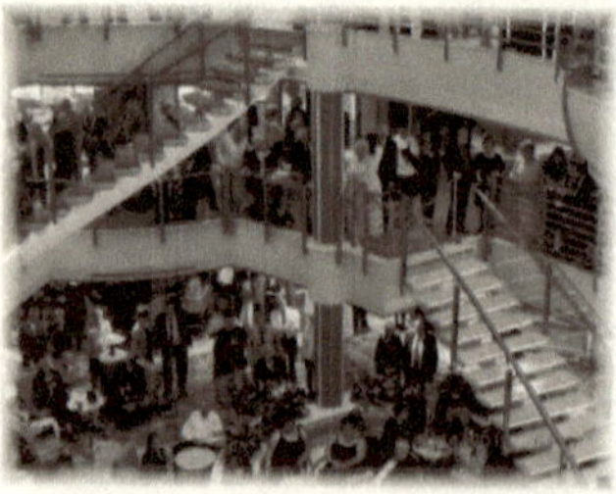

Absent a cabin for the cruisers with disability on a cruise that I really want, I book the regular stateroom cabin. Suites and mini-suites are too expensive. Cabins with balconies may be an option depending on the price. In all cases, I select an available cabin closest to the promenade area.

Most of the time Amelia likes to stay in the promenade area because it is where much of the activities happen. The elevators are accessible at the promenade area, making it easy for her to go to the dining and other decks. Were we to need information, the area is also where we can ask the members of the staff and crew, who

Cruise - Choosing One

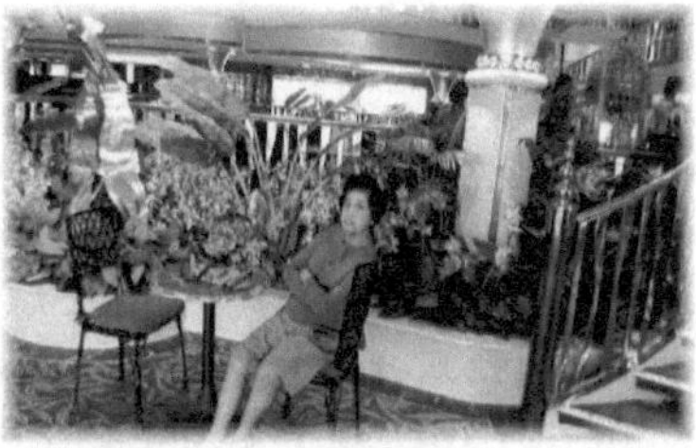

are coming by more frequently. The customer service counter is likely located in the same area. Convenience is a primary criterion in my selection of a cabin.

At this point, I ask the cruise company to hold my choice while I do more research and consult with Amelia. If she agrees with my choice, I complete the booking process, putting the minimum down payment, but reserving the right to make changes until the last permissible date. If she does not agree with the choice, I let the hold on the cabin expire, usually after twenty-four hours.

Cruise - Booking and Preparation

When we started cruising a few years ago when the internet was not yet the popular means for online transactions, I booked every cruise through a travel agent, not knowing that cruise schedules and itineraries were already available online from the cruise lines. We went to Europe, Hawaii, and the Caribbean, with the booking processes exactly identical for most travel agencies. I wanted to do away with the middleman, the travel agent, so I experimented booking a short cruise vacation online, directly with the cruise line. It was successful; I never needed the service of a travel agent again. The required documents for traveling including passports, emergency contacts, discounts taken, and credit card for onboard purchases, are defined by the cruise lines.

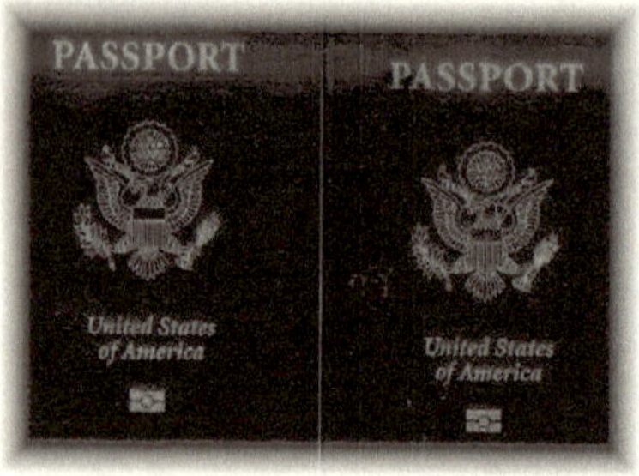

Our passports are valid until 2021, renewable every ten years, so I do not have to check them for expiration dates frequently. I keep ours safe and readily accessible in case an opportunity for short-notice cruise becomes available, offering money-saving discounts. On cruises that sail beyond the United States territory, passengers are required to present their passports at the port of departure and again when they return; I always keep ours available regardless of travel destinations. Except when going on an excursion to a foreign port, I keep our passports in the cabin safe at all times.

Online, I check for schedules of sailings and itineraries, bookmarking the ones that are unlikely to cause physical hardship to Amelia. Since one or more cruise lines may offer similar cruises, I end up bookmarking few with slight variations from different

Cruise - Booking and Preparation

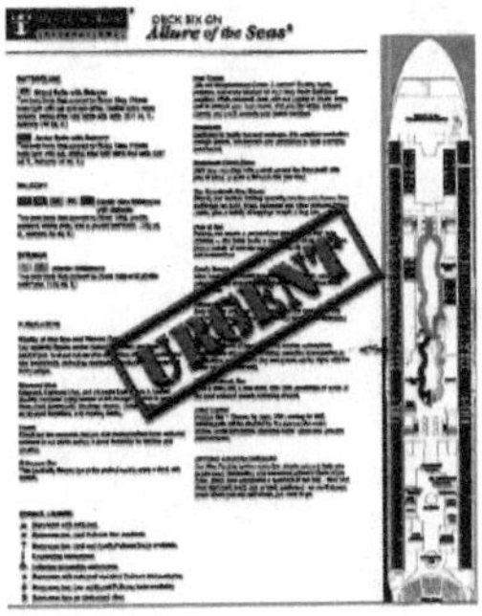

cruise lines. The number of ports visited, level of comfort on the ship, ease of booking, size of the ship, and other aspects of a pleasurable vacation, make up my criterion for bookmarking a particular cruise.

Regularly, I visit my bookmarked cruise for variation in the schedules and itineraries paying particular attention to changes in price. The price may vary depending on the popularity of the cruise. The ship's cabin availability is an indication of how popular the cruise is, possibly causing price movements. I may end up running out of cabins for the price I want, but I do not panic. I can always book one with other cruise lines offering similar cruises, or I can wait for the next sailing date.

When I am satisfied that a particular cruise is one we will enjoy, I pick the cabin that suits us. Not requiring payment to hold a particular cabin, the ship will usually hold the cabin for me for twenty-four hours, while I discuss the plan with Amelia. If the cruise is likely to cause physical hardship to Amelia making it less enjoyable, I abandon the hold and let it expire. Otherwise, I prepare to book it.

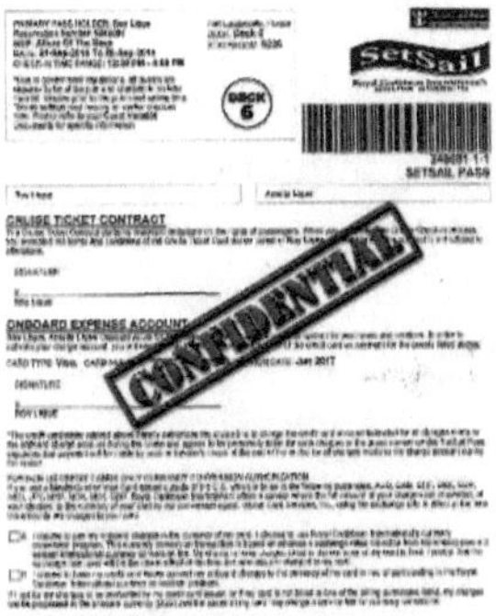

I feel more comfortable booking a cruise online because I do not want to recite any personal information including credit card number to a live person on the telephone. I suppose when entering them online, they go directly to the computer without manual intervention.
Using a credit card that has only enough funds to satisfy the required minimum payment, I proceed with the booking. At

Cruise - Booking and Preparation

this point, the cruise line may require me to create an account, if I do not have one already. Having an account with a cruise line facilitates the transactions for repeat cruises.

Between the booking and sailing dates, I access my account periodically to see what steps are required towards final payment. For later reference in case an issue arises on the booking, I document all communications between the cruise line and me, particularly emails. Towards the final payment date, communications become more detailed with steps to follow. Cruise lines are excellent at explaining what to do to complete the transactions online. If I get stuck with certain items in the instructions, assistance is always available, be it by phone or by emails.

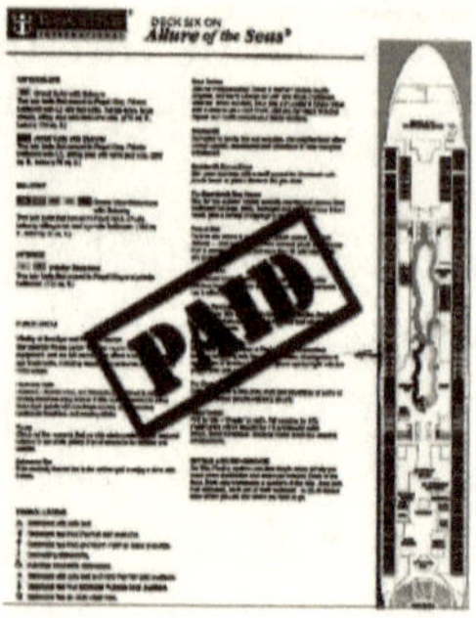

To hasten the check-in procedure at the port, the cruise line may require me to fill in each passenger's information online, including passport number, emergency contacts, discounts taken, and credit card which will be used to charge onboard purchases. With the few cruises we already enjoyed, I never had an issue with filling in the information online.

Having done all of the preceding requirements, I wait for the luggage tags to arrive if the cruise line sends them by mail; otherwise, I obtain them at the port. Twenty-four hours before boarding, I finally prepare to sail and check in - again, online.

Cruise - Why It Is Good for Amelia

Any of the four bodily disorders: strokes, Alzheimer's, diabetes, and congestive heart failure can, in its mildest variety, render one miserable and pathetic; in its severe form, it can cause death. A single stroke, not to mention multiple, causes mild to complete incapacity or death. Loss of memory and dignity is the distinctly distressing characteristic of Alzheimer's which leads one to a life of misery before ending in death. Causing death as well in the long run is diabetes which slowly gnaws into one's well-being, weakening the body and spirit. Most lethal of them all is congestive heart failure especially with no option for surgery, as is the case with Amelia.

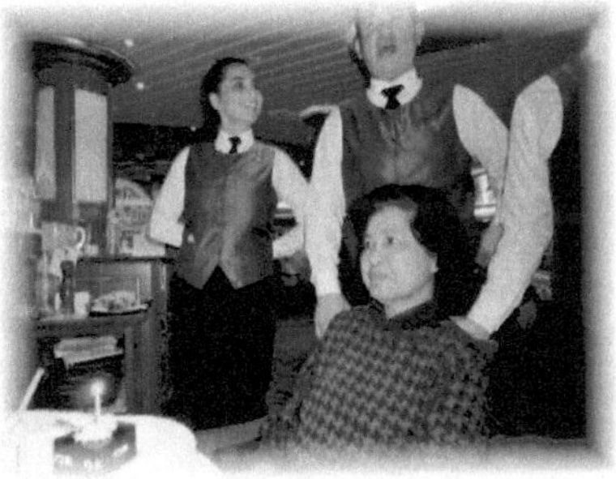

The pernicious aggregation of aforesaid bodily disorders is what Amelia has. Her movement is very limited, and her speech is slurred causing her to be misunderstood. When not closely watched, her glucose level exceeds or recedes beyond the standard levels causing her to come close to passing out. Her physical and mental conditions restrain her activities; she is all but slowly degenerating and dying. With all the restraints caused by the diseases, when asked if she still enjoys life, her response is always positive and would like to continue enjoying it with gusto and aplomb. Her first joyful taste of traveling makes her long for more. It is, in her opinion, the only way she will enjoy the remaining days of her life.

Ocean cruising is the mode of travel that Amelia and I like because I feel that she is safe on the cruise ship. Considering that Alzheimer's causes one to wander around aimlessly, it can not

Cruise - Why It Is Good for Amelia

happen to Amelia for she has nowhere to go beyond the confines of the ship. The ship has eyes virtually everywhere except in the private areas, watching the passengers and their activities. By observing the onboard rules of the ship, rarely can an accident or injury happen without someone witnessing it.

Each cruise ship has a complete medical facility required to treat medical emergencies, and staffed with qualified medical professionals. Confined in the floating ship, the medical staff has nowhere to go either, making the members available twenty-four hours each day during the cruise. A call to the emergency telephone number is all it takes to summon help in case of an emergency. Should a medical emergency occur that cannot be thoroughly

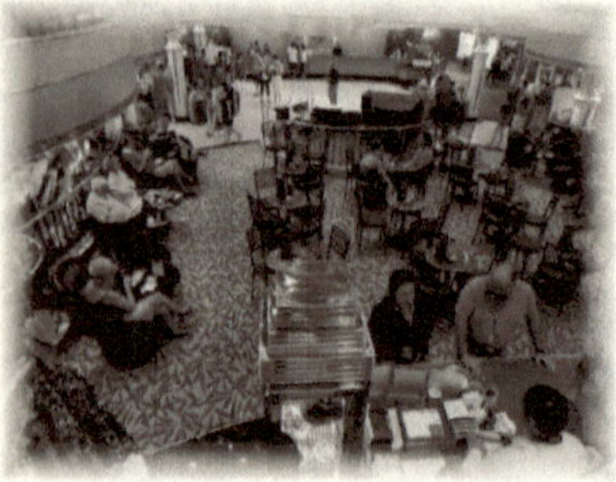

treated on board the ship, the staff can arrange for patient treatment at the next port of anchorage. Needless to say with Amelia's condition, access to a medical facility is of paramount importance when we travel. Having availed of a ship's medical facility a number of times previously, I relate this account from experience.

Food on the cruise ship is virtually unlimited. Since it is a habit of Amelia to sometimes long for food at the middle of the night owing to her medical condition, the availability of food is a desirable aspect of cruising as well. It only takes an elevator ride to locate an open place to eat. Food can also be ordered from and delivered to the cabin. Rush hour dining is in itself a spectacle to behold and enjoy especially on a huge cruise ship with as many as 6,000 cruisers.

Cruise - Why It Is Good for Amelia

The bars, in addition to the dining places, carry most kinds of juices that might be needed to treat simple emergencies such as those arising from enjoying the unlimited food to excess.. In a number of times, I had to do so to help regulate Amelia's glucose level.

Like the food, entertainment on a cruise ship is limitless. In every hour various forms of activities go on: trivia questions, bingo, photography, bowling, casino (when allowed), dance lessons, rock climbing, swimming, movies, performances by the ship's crew - just to mention a few. The ship also maintains salons, sauna, gymnasiums, libraries, computer rooms, and other amenities. Some of them are for fees while some are free. Guests can come and go as they please.

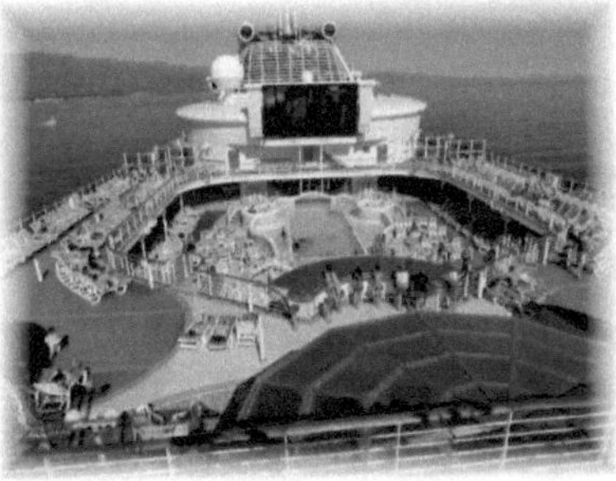

Visiting unfamiliar places by way of excursions from the cruise ship is another aspect of cruising which Amelia and I like. For fees, excursions can be booked at the same time as the cruise itself. Likewise, they can be booked on board the ship allowing one to clarify some doubts about a particular excursion in person. In either booking instance, I have to select the ones that suit Amelia, owing to her physical condition.

These features of ocean cruising are just a few of the benefits we enjoy onboard the cruise ship. For $150.00 per day, I will not hesitate to book a good cruise vacation because it is fun and safe and which I know, Amelia will enjoy.

Cruise - Choosing an Excursion

Contributing to the local economy by way of revenues from the sale of services and merchandise, excursions are a big part of the cruise industry. The coveted currencies carried by tourists need a place to roost apart from the cruise ship. To the delight of cruisers, improved services result from competition for the tourists' patronage, among local operators.

Tourism being their mainstay, some cruise lines, ports, and towns, directly promote certain attractions within their jurisdictions; when they cannot, excursions are subcontracted to local providers.

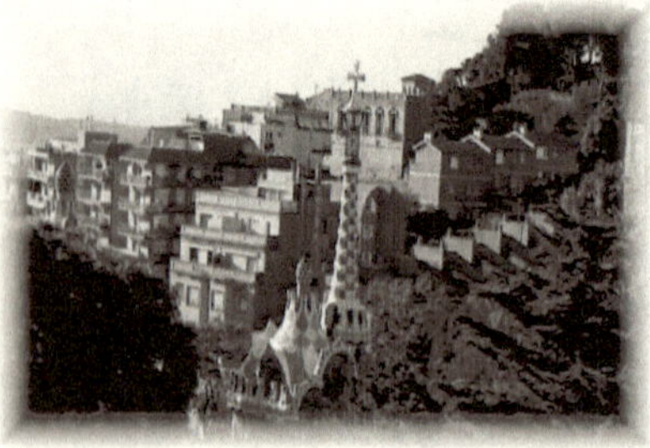

Similar to an afterthought, excursions are a way of exploring places unreachable by other means on short notices. Cruisers only need to make the proper selection from several that are offered by the cruise line, consistent - as is the case with Amelia - with their endurance capability.

What I do next after booking the cruise online is find a suitable excursion from a particular port. Once I register an account with the cruise line, its website becomes accessible for details about the cruise, including the list of excursions. Some websites are harder to navigate than others, in which case I call the cruise line for instructions to obtain the list. Cruise line employees are all but very helpful to talk with online, a subtle way of promoting the company's image.

Cruise - Choosing an Excursion

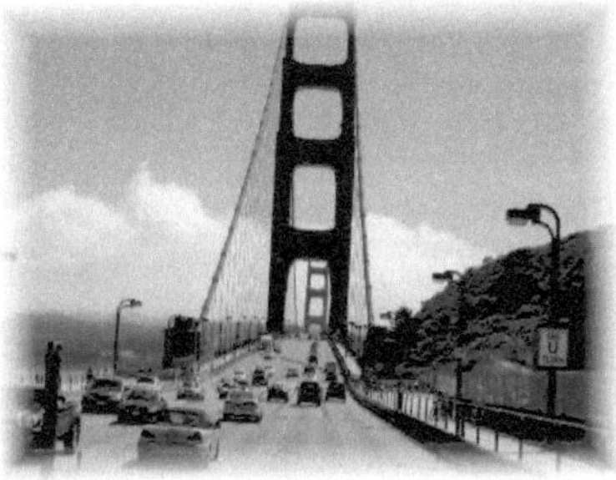

With the goal of finding an excursion that does not require a distant walk I mark the possible excursion that Amelia is capable of taking. Regarding physical exertion, not all excursions are the same even though they are headed to the same identical locations. Thus, I pay attention to the appropriate cautionary signs and icons.

At this stage of my search, I want to find out if the tour bus is equipped for seating passengers with disability, and whether it is air conditioned or not. Absent these criteria, I rate down the excursion from mediocre to undesirable.

Initially, I may come up with few possible destinations, each destination tagged with the corresponding price. Prices may vary depending on departure times, the length of the tour, the degree of service, and the tour operators. With these details on hand, I mark my list for confirmation later, on board the ship. If I get the excursion schedule from a live person on the telephone, I take the name and phone number and record them too.

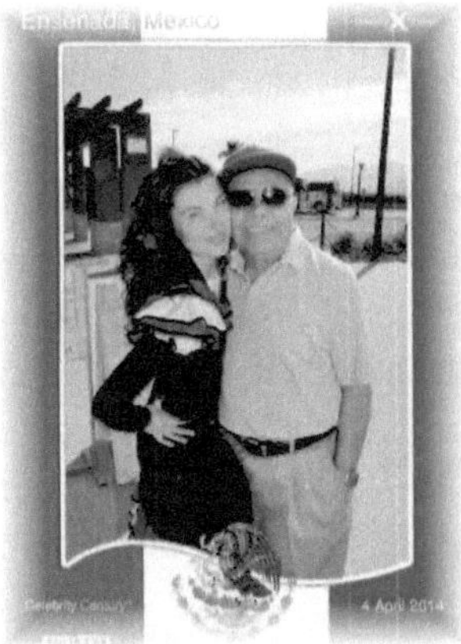

Without booking any of the possible excursions that I find consistent with Amelia's physical condition, I review the list as often as I can think of new unclear points, with the goal of including every detail that can be used during confirmation and booking. Once satisfied with the list, I keep it with my cruise documentations.

Cruise - Choosing an Excursion

Early on board the ship, I confirm my list of possible excursions with the staff assigned to handle them. Armed with the notes that I have written earlier, I make certain that nothing is left out to compromise the excitement and thrill of the excursion that I will ultimately book.

At this point, I add another excursion criterion, namely, the distance from the ship to the tour bus and back. Often this criterion is not known until the passenger is on board the ship. If it involves a long walk or is not wheelchair accessible, I abandon the excursion. I repeat the same confirmation process on every item on the list.

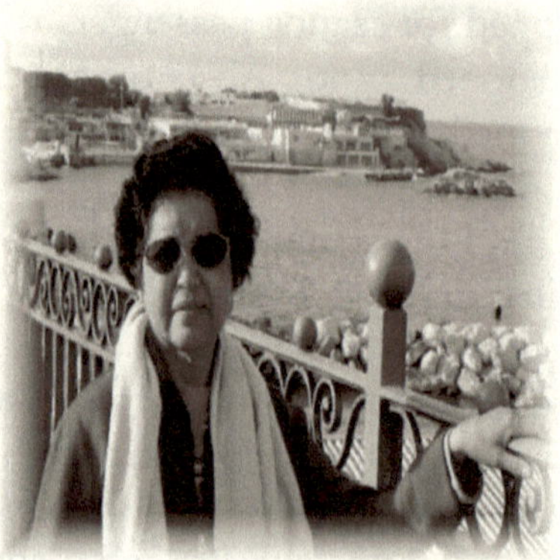

Regarding physical exertion, excursions are marked as easy, moderate, strenuous, wheelchair accessible or something to that effect. Immediately my choice is clear - one with easy walking. Excursions are also identified with what clothes and shoes to wear, and if protection from the element is necessary. With enough experience behind us, I always see to it that we are provided with these essentials even if they are not clearly mentioned.

When everything checks out with Amelia's ability to take on an excursion, I book it before it closes. I am now ready for the next excursion on the list to fill each day of our cruise. Usually, we try to go on one each day we are at a particular port. But if I am not able to come up with an appropriate selection, we just stay on board the ship and enjoy the endless entertainments.

Cruise - What Amelia Likes and Dislikes

Amelia likes some aspects of a cruise vacation more than others. They are not present in all cruises. The following is a list of some of the things she likes:

- Comedies
- Musicals
- Formal nights
- Local entertainers
- Clean sheets
- Excursions
- Window shopping
- Karaoke
- Acrobats
- Pastries
- View of ocean
- Parade of waiters
- Photography
- No food worries at home
- Food
- Deck side conversation
- Magic
- On board entertainers
- Dance exhibitions
- Sightseeing
- Open deck exercise
- Open Wii
- Sanctuaries
- Fruits
- Crew talents
- Flower arrangements
- Talking with crews
- No house cleaning

The following are some of the things she dislikes:

- Bingo
- Movies
- Steps/stairs
- Computer room
- Story telling
- Golf contest
- Basketball
- Card games
- Bars
- Casino
- Trivia games
- Libraries
- Crocheting
- Shuffle boards
- Baseball
- Painting
- Backgammon
- Alcoholic beverages

Cruise - What Amelia Likes and Dislikes

- Embarkation procedures — Disembarkation procedures
- Document preparation — Customs processing

She likes to lazily spend a few hours at the food deck, drinking coffee and munching on a variety of pastries and fruits. It is at the food deck that we occasionally meet new friends and watch the waves and the ever so few creatures that pop up from the ocean.

Amelia particularly likes to spend some time on the open deck beside the pool because it is there where we usually listen to a band playing loud music, watch some tournaments, and participate in light gymnastics.

The list of activities on a cruise vacation is endless; one only needs to make a choice from the daily newsletters.

Cruise – Food on the Cruise Ship

When food is the subject of discussion, the cruise is synonymous with excess. At the mention of a cruise, the first thing that comes to mind for some people including some who have not been to one, is food. Often minor flaws in the cruise ship's features like age and size of the ship are overlooked in favor of good quality food. As some reviews reveal, different cruise lines - in fact, different ships belonging to the same cruise line - have different ratings for food and service. A great number of passengers rate a cruise by the food they eat.

Themed according to the itinerary of the cruise, the type of food being served is aligned with the characteristic of the region. For example, a Hawaiian cruise will always include Hawaiian fruits such as pineapples and bananas as part of their servings, while an Italian cruise will have Italian specialties naturally, such as pizza.

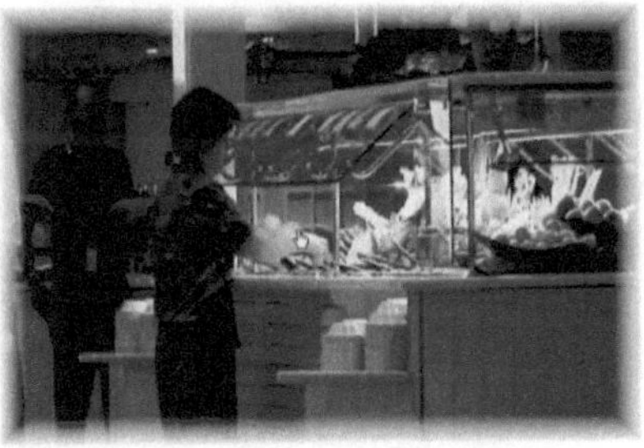

On a regular dining hour when the cruisers converge on the food deck, many trays of food parade through the counters. On a huge ship, the food deck may be split into two, one opening on an earlier time, immediately followed as it closes, by the opening of the other. Irrespective of the time and opened dining area, food is always served to excess.

I can easily count no less than fifty different servings on a regular dining hour - breakfast, lunch, or dinner - just on the open food deck. Separate stands may be stuffed with yet various types of food for the taking.

Cruise – Food on the Cruise Ship

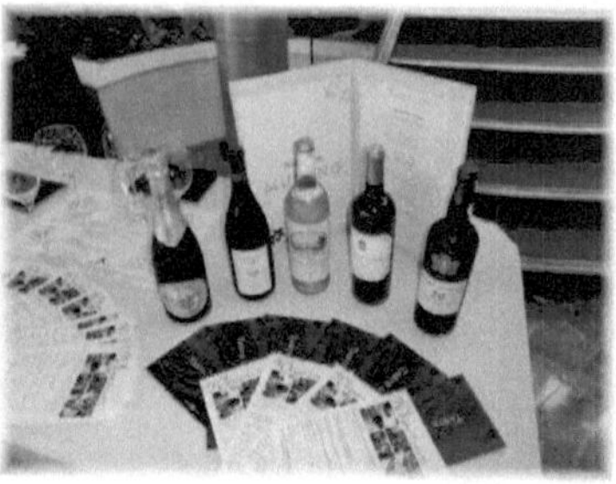

In more formal seating, cruisers are assigned seats in the few restaurants apart from the open food deck, serving yet another type of food. Also, bars may serve food, wine, and alcoholic beverage, up to the wee hours of the following day. If a particular type of food is missing, one can always inquire if it can be specially ordered.

As soon as the main eating places are cleared of the clutter from the previous dining, they are prepared again for the next scheduled seating when yet another appropriate type of food may be served. In the meantime, cruisers walk around, stopping here and there for pastries, coffee, fruits, desserts and other nourishments. While letting the just-eaten food settle in, perhaps a demonstration of how to prepare a certain type of food is performed as entertainment. The output from the event is given away to the crowd, as yet another type of food.

The promenade deck is where most activities are performed to keep the cruisers from being bored. Very likely, food and beverage are served there too. Some may prefer to spend time in a quiet corner of the ship, picking up some pastries to munch and coffee to drink, while reading, resting or dozing. In every place where cruisers gather, food and drinks are likely to be nearby.

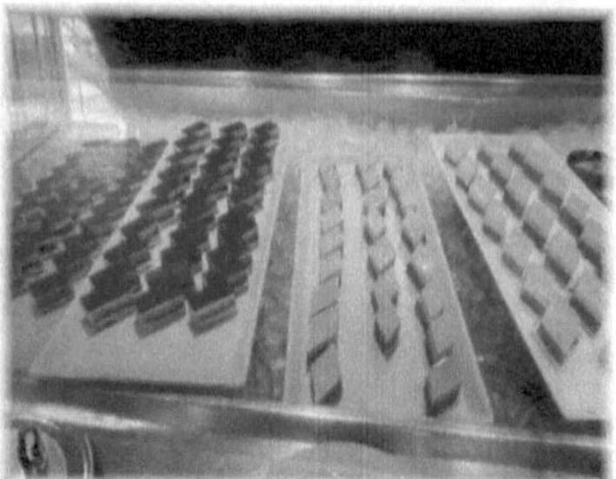

For certain cruisers who especially love wine, wine tasting is always a treat on board the cruise ship. It is advertised when it happens; all one has to do is look at the schedules in the newsletters. Apart from the bars, wine and alcoholic beverage

Cruise – Food on the Cruise Ship

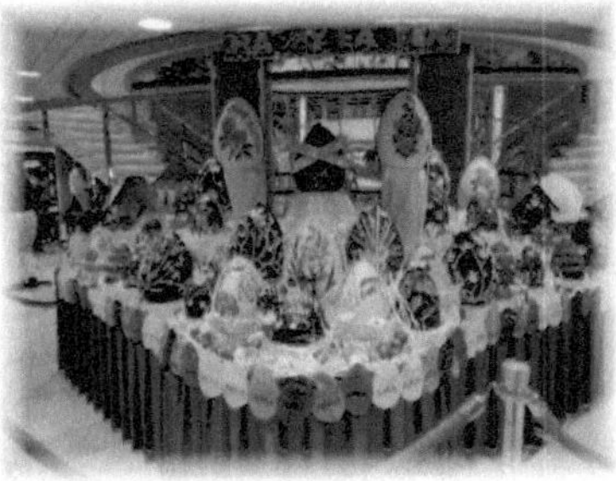

can be ordered from most locations of the ship.

On food safety and with thousands of servings each day, here and there might be a slight flaw in the food that may disappoint a cruiser. All one has to do is report it and get another serving; the servers are always ready to help the cruisers.

Hand sanitation is required before entry to the dining areas, and inappropriate attires are not allowed. There is always a place open 24/7 where one can get food and enjoy to excess, keeping in mind, as a fair warning, that it is easier to gain than to lose weight. It is true that with uncontrolled appetite, one will certainly gain enough pounds to worry about after disembarkation.

Cruise - Packing for One

Usually, packing for a trip is an easy task. It is when certain limitations, restrictions, and requirements are imposed that it becomes slightly difficult.

The first thing I consider is whether direct embarkation is all it takes to start cruising. If it is, there are not too many restrictions on packing regarding luggage size and contents as long as they pass through the x-ray machines when they are checked in. Direct embarkation is when we board the cruise ship immediately after the initial and only check-in. I tend to use an oversized luggage to minimize the number of luggage I have to pull along when checking in and out. Amelia is unable to help me in this regard because of her disability.

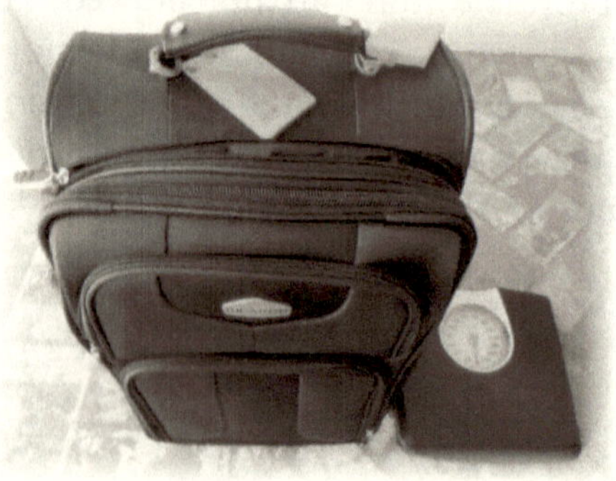

When the travel plan involves an airline flight, then I have to consider: luggage size, luggage weight, and luggage contents. Also, I have to consider the carry-on luggage size and its contents. My primary goal is to travel light because I have to take care of Amelia and our luggage at the same time.

Staying with the luggage size, weight, and contents limitation, I have to provide for the following:

- Optional formal attires for Amelia and me. On a 7-day cruise, there are at least two formal nights when we participate in these options. On a 15-day cruise, there are at least four or five of these formal nights. We had these

Cruise - Packing for One

nights a few times before, so we can choose to ignore them unless we want to have souvenir pictures of the cruise; pictures are very costly, though,

- On board casual attire for dining, swimming, sunbathing, semi-formal dining, etc.,
- Excursion attire - shoes, umbrellas, coats, caps, etc.,
- Most important of all is enough supply of Amelia's personal items.

I have to keep in mind that cruise ships have Laundromats and laundry services. If packing gets even trickier as to exceed the size and content limits of the pieces of luggage, I can use the services just to keep within the limitations.

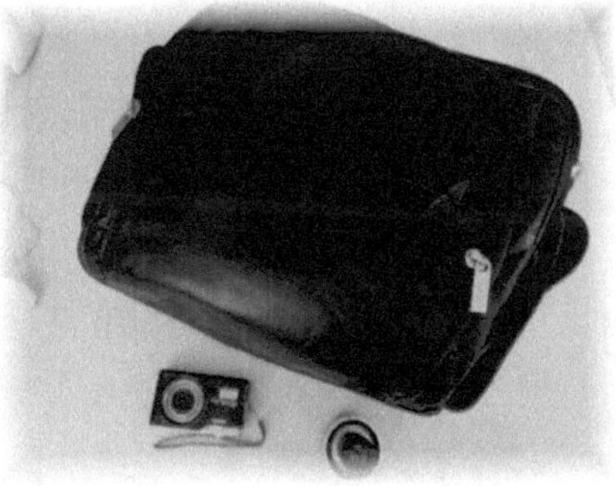

Many items are not allowed on the plane. I have to be certain they are not in any of our luggage. The hand-carried luggage contains my photographic equipment and Amelia's personal items like medications, brushes, combs, and possibly certain allowable types of juice. If I am not sure what is and what is not allowed on the plane, I check with the airlines.

After a few travels and with enough experience, the task of packing becomes somewhat easy and efficient. When it is a cruise that Amelia and I like, nothing will deter us from proceeding with it, not even the most uneasy task of packing.

Cruise – Pre-Embarkation Checklist

Booking a cruise is not complete until final embarkation. To be sure that we are ready to travel, I maintain a checklist that I review few days before the flight or sailing date.

- Travel Documentations
    - Passports, Cruise Ticket Contract, Expense Account Documents, Tags, Cruise Summary, Booking Confirmation, Air Transportation Booking, Wine and Dine Packages, Excursions Documentations and Contracts
- House
    - Sprinkler system, appliances, home protection, pool water/pump
- Mail hold by the post office. 3 days before departure I have the post office hold our mail for the duration of the cruise
- Bills due while on vacation. Online banking helps in this regard
- Photographic equipment. I carry two cameras to be sure I have one always ready in case one stops functioning
- Children notification. I always let them know of our departure and arrival dates.
- Hotel booking at port of departure. I book a 1-day hotel stay near the airport to avoid rushing in the morning of travel

Cruise – Pre-Embarkation Checklist

- Travel clothes appropriate for travel day. Depends on weather forecast for the day of departure
- Currency. Enough for travel cash expenses. This is needed to pay miscellaneous port services and other miscellaneous items
- Insurance if desired. I maintain enough travel insurance coverage even if we are not traveling
- Extra tags, pens, rubber bands, writing pads. They come in handy when in a rush
- Fit for travel certification for Amelia if necessary. Only as precaution if Amelia does not seem able to travel.

Allure of the Seas Experience

Embarkation

Cruise Vacation on The Allure of the Seas. The bus from the hotel dropped us off at the entrance of the processing building. Noticing that Amelia was using a walker, we were immediately led to the lines of passengers with disabilities. We traveled light from the hotel because our pieces of luggage, identified by cabin tags, were loaded separately.

Boarding The Allure of the Seas followed similar procedures employed in the other cruises we had been through before. However, the enormous task of processing documents for all passengers within four hours was short of mind-boggling, considering that there were more than six thousand five hundred of them. Evidently, the crews' training has been paying off; the target departure time has seldom been missed, I learned from conversations with some members of the crew.

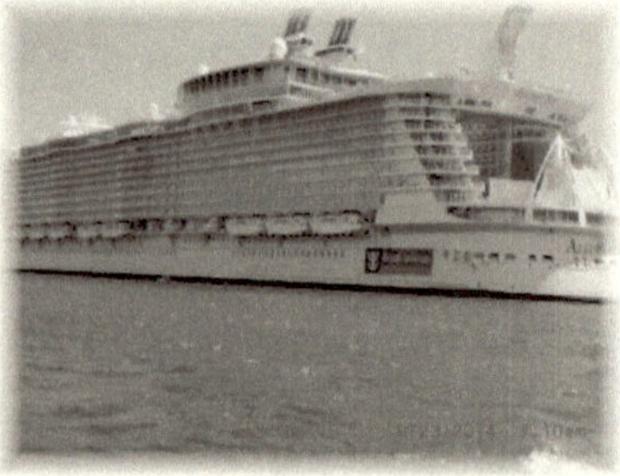

The first step in the boarding process was securing SeaPass cards. I already filled in all the required information online. After verification of identities through our passports and providing the credit card we would be using for on board purchases, we were issued the cards.

Each time that a long queue would form at a particular window, it was cut by leading the rear passengers to less crowded windows. When one had to be referred to a crew member with a special processing skill, all one had to do was follow the color jacketed member being pointed to yonder. Apparently, each team member's rank in the hierarchy of responsibility was identified by the color of the jacket. I have never seen such full utilization of color coded jackets than during the embarkation, and disembarkation after the cruise.

After securing our SeaPass cards, we were transported by elevator to a waiting area for passengers with disabilities. Thence, Amelia was supposed to be wheeled to the final destination deck 5. Since there were few passengers with disabilities ahead of us, Amelia prodded me not to wait for the wheelchairs to come. She was ready to undertake the journey through the 5- 10-degree incline of a zigzagging path with her walker, each turn running approximately 30-50 feet. She was right the wheelchairs did not come in quick succession.

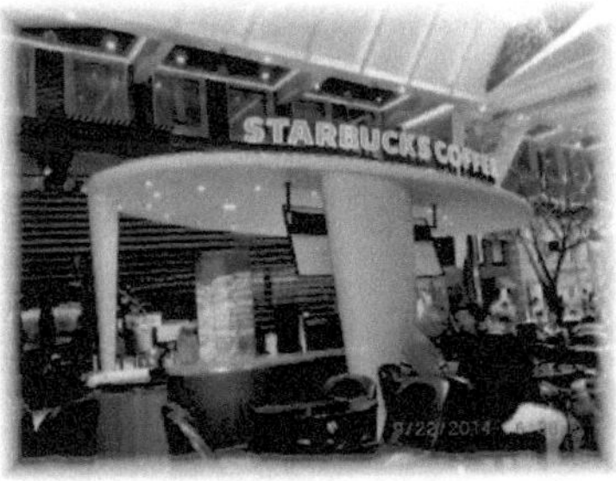

The last leg of the zigzagging path was the most difficult one for Amelia, she being very tired by then. With me slightly pushing and encouraging her more, we made the entire way to deck 5 in about fifteen minutes.
Deck 5 was used as an assembly area for passengers while the cabins were being made.

In the meantime, food and drinks were served at the Promenade Cafe. The band was playing like a great festivity was going on, at the Rising Tide Bar. After the announcement that there was more food at the Windjammer on the 16th deck, the passengers made their way there, clearing deck 5 for more boarding passengers.

Allure of the Seas Experience

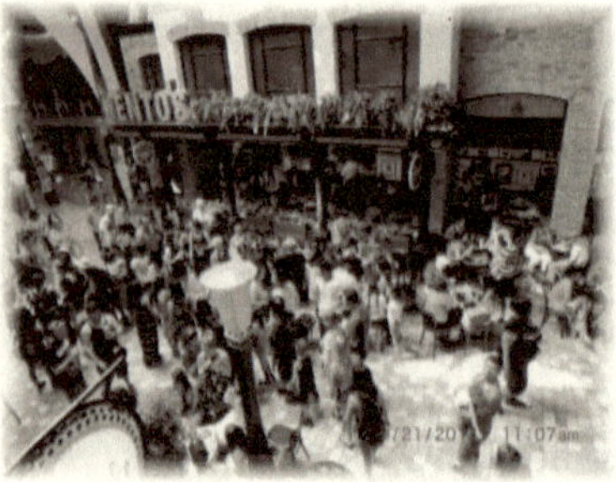

Before long, we were allowed to proceed to our cabin where our pieces of luggage were already deposited at the door. With the boarding process out of the way, we rested a few hours before venturing out to marvel at the size of the monster ship.

We were finally on board the biggest and grandest cruise ship ever built at the time; I have been following its progress since its initial construction. Our cruise vacation was ready to start on board The Allure of the Seas.

Allure of the Seas Experience

Stateroom

Cruise Vacation on The Allure of the Seas. Ours was a 182-square foot Superior Ocean View Stateroom with a 53 square feet balcony that yielded us a 180-degree panoramic view of the Caribbean sky and ocean. The balcony was accessible through a floor-to-ceiling sliding glass door which could be securely locked from inside. Allowing privacy, thick fiber glasses separated our balcony from the adjacent ones. Completing the balcony setup were a table, an upright chair, and two reclining sunbathing chairs.

We had two twin beds converted into a queen to make up for our sleeping comfort. The stateroom had considerable closet spaces to hold our clothes and to keep them from wrinkling. To accommodate Amelia with her disability, a private bathroom with shower, handrails, and proper drainage made up the essential features of the stateroom; they were all that I expected when I booked the cruise. The table in the living area had ample desk drawers and a vanity to hold Amelia's personal articles. A sofa arranged to face the ocean, and a center table provided additional restful convenience.

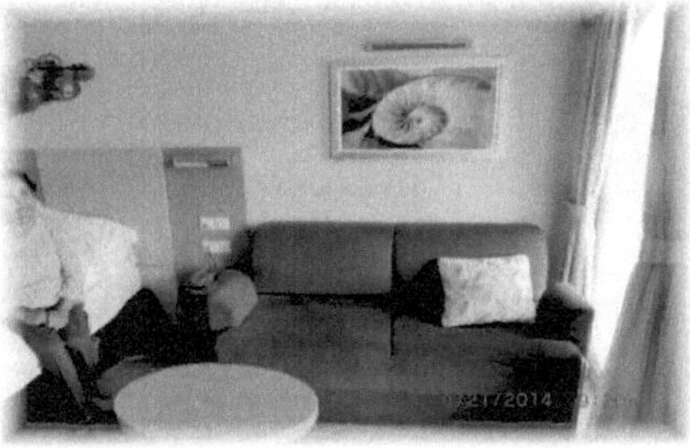

The flat screen television set was big enough for comfortable viewing while sitting on the sofa or getting ready to sleep. For communication, the stateroom had an internet access, direct-dial telephone, and radio. To control the climate inside, it had its separate thermostat to set and adjust the air conditioning unit. As in all cruises, a safe was built-in where our travel documents, some jewelry, and camera equipment were safely locked.

Allure of the Seas Experience

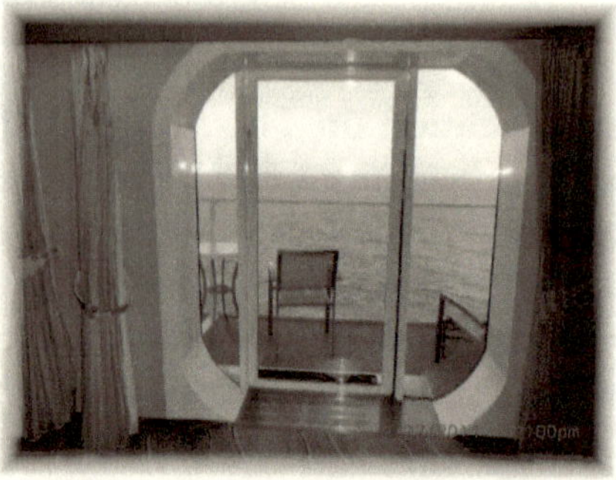

In case hunger awakened us at night and we felt tired to go to the dining areas, the stateroom had a mini bar to sustain us until breakfast the following morning; the 24-hour room service was also available.

With the setup in place, I could hardly wait for the time to sleep at night with the floating clouds seen through the glass door and to listen to the waves from an always moving platform, The Allure of the Seas. Having lived in a country of thousand islands some sixty years ago, I longed for the nostalgic experience.

Night came, but unable to readily sleep in the cabin room, I stepped out into the balcony and tried sleeping there. However, the heat and humidity drove me back after merely a few minutes. Sleepiness finally overcame us, and we soundly slept, with the drapes drawn open, until morning in time to get ready for the first full day of exploration of The Allure of the Seas.

Allure of the Seas Experience

Great Vacation!

Cruise Vacation on The Allure of the Seas. On the dullest day, day 1, of the 7-day cruise vacation, approximately 91 on board fun activities were available for enjoyment. Day 6 had the same number of activities but it also had 40 shore excursions. Day 2 and Day 7 had 151 and 171 on board fun activities respectively; both had zero shore excursions. Day 3, Day 4, and Day 7 had a combined total of 371 on board fun activities and 70 shore excursions.

A grand total of 875 on board fun activities and 110 shore excursions was what choices we had for enjoyment on the cruise vacation with The Allure of the Seas. Of course, staying inside the stateroom and watching the Caribbean ocean and sky floating by was in itself a mini vacation. Had we chosen to indulge, food was available 24/7, in the restaurants or as delivered to the cabin.

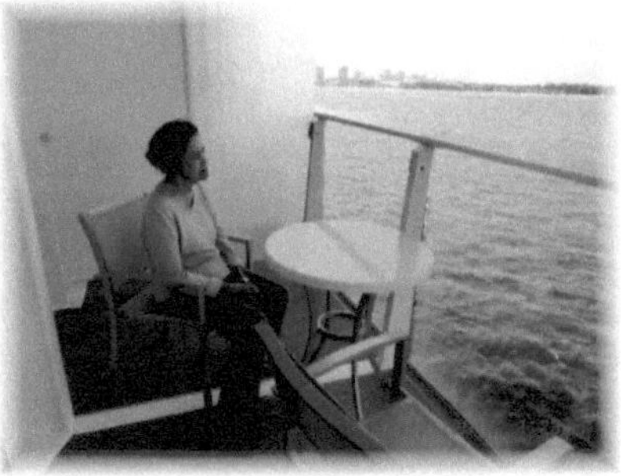

I called the Royal Promenade as the "cross deck" for it was where most cruisers transitioned between the upper and lower decks. Grand sales, parades, and most other spectacles happened on the promenade deck.

Offering free food, the Promenade Cafe was the ideal location for enjoying the ongoing activities, meeting new friends, and listening to the ongoing music. Most other places on the ship offered similar activities as in the Royal Promenade, but in a quieter and subdued environment depending on the theme of the location. Like on the Royal Promenade, we spent significant hours at Central Park.

Allure of the Seas Experience

Day of the Cruise	Approximate Number of Fun - On Board Activities	Approximate Number of Shore Excursions
Day 1	91	0
Day 2	151	0
Day 3	110	23
Day 4	112	40
Day 5	171	0
Day 6	91	40
Day 7	149	7

Chapter 7 – Destination Alaska

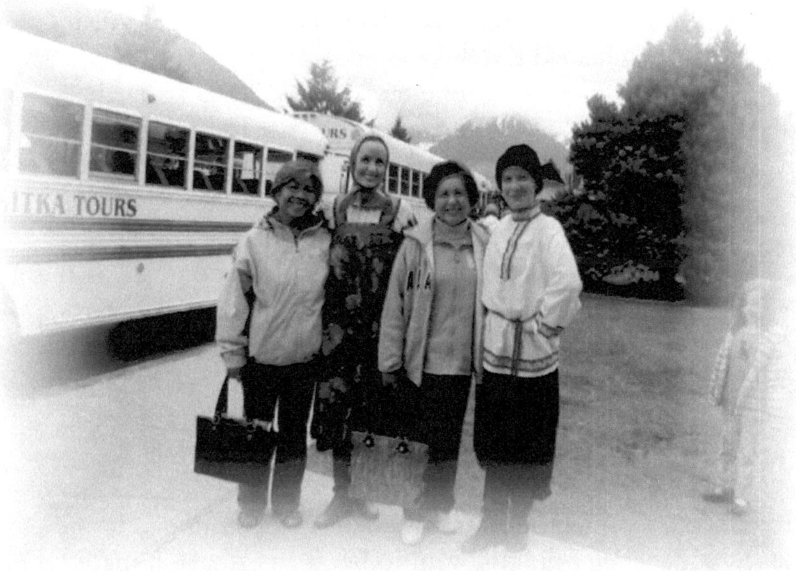

At Ketchikan, Alaska

Our first taste of the Alaskan weather was at Ketchikan. It was not winter, but we had to scramble for warm clothing at the local stores. One store, I could tell, was selling clothes more than souvenirs to tourists from the cruise ships - there were three of them.

Ketchikan was the first stop on our Alaskan cruise towards the north. It was a fishing town that grew with the Alaskan gold rush. Timber and fishing helped Ketchikan's economy so much that at one time, it was Alaska's fourth largest city. Few large fishing boats were docked at what appeared to be a marina on the far end of the pier. Replacing timber and fisheries, tourism is now one of the biggest contributors to the town's economy. I was surprised to see the huge cruise ships able to dock just a few hundred feet from the main seaside boulevard.

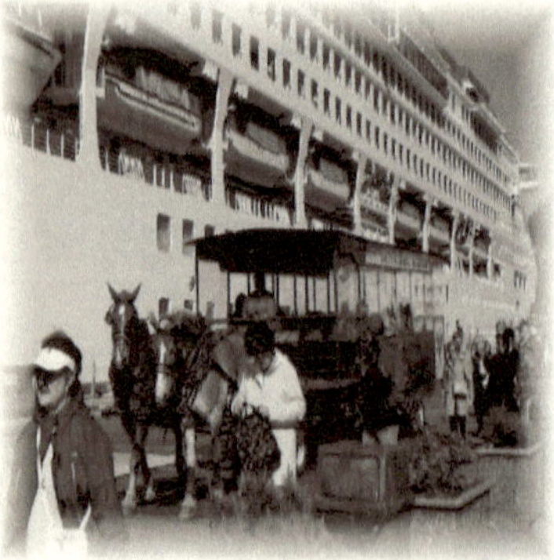

Due to the cold weather, our visit to the town was confined to the central shopping area. I did not want to book an excursion that would start with light physical exertion and later required too much walking, owing to Amelia's physical condition. There were few attractive and historical places to explore outside the town, we were told, but Amelia was not ready for the cold weather. She even regretted to have left the comfort of the ship and come down to walk on the windy boulevard.

Our only opportunity to memorialize our visit of the town this time was to watch the lumberjack show which had been

At Ketchikan, Alaska

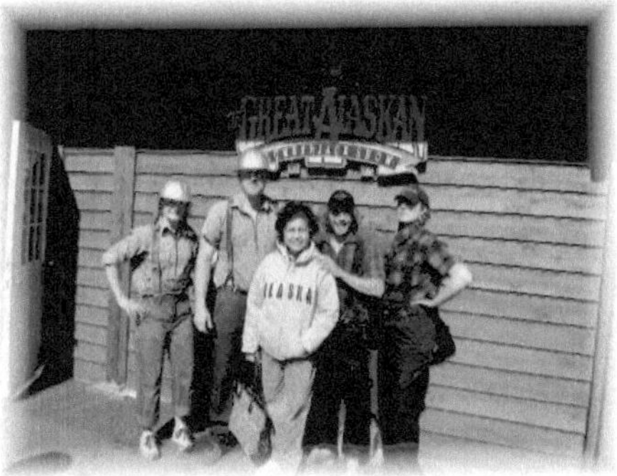

performing few blocks away from where we shopped for warm clothes. I purchased the tickets for the show from the same store. Even with the tickets on hand, Amelia would not go to the show without first having coffee. She would rather forfeit the ticket, go back to the ship, and miss the show altogether, than not having coffee to help her fend off the cold weather. So, I got her a cup of coffee from a stand two blocks away.

We walked to the site of the lumberjack show with Amelia walking close behind anybody - not only me - to shield herself from the cold wind. I thought that was funny watching someone unaware of who was following very close behind. At the bleachers area, Amelia chose the most secluded seat but best shielded from the wind.

The lumberjack show was performed by people from all over the country whose passion involves logs, lumber, and timber. Log rolling, timber cutting, and many other skills were displayed at the show. Comedians also helped in entertaining the crowd who were, by then, pressing to each other in their groups because of the cold wind.

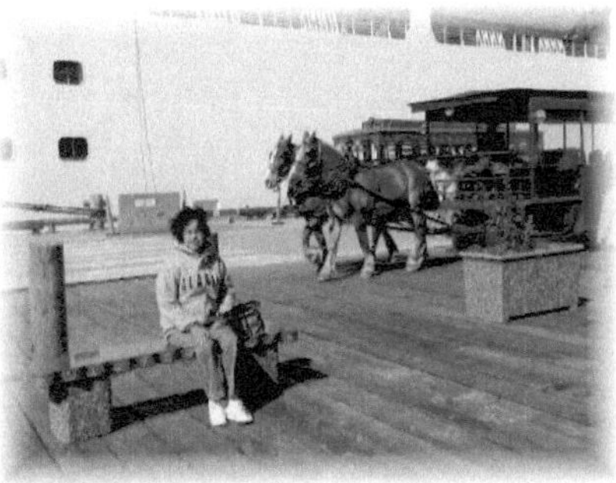

It was a fun show, different from shows that have been presented in the more urban cities and towns. We hurriedly walked back to the ship with Amelia performing her creeping act again. At the comfort of the ship, we had all the coffee and food to relieve us from the cold weather outside. We spent the rest of the day resting and relaxing, waiting for the night entertainments.

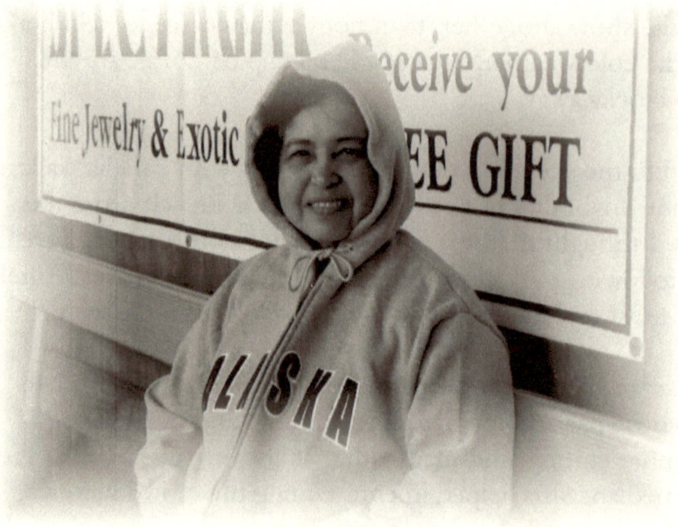

At Sitka, Alaska

Sitka was the last stop of our 10-day cruise to Alaska before heading back to San Francisco. Because of the shallow water at the port, tourists were tendered to the island. A short paraphrased history of the island in my words follows:

The Russians arrived in Sitka in 1799. The native Indians, knowing that they would be subjected to the rules of the Russians, attacked and killed almost all of the Russians and the native collaborators. But the Russians did not give up, coming back five years later, and attacked the natives. The attack raged on for more than a week and finally ended when the Russians overwhelmed the natives and won the battle. After that, the occupation of Sitka by the Russians started.

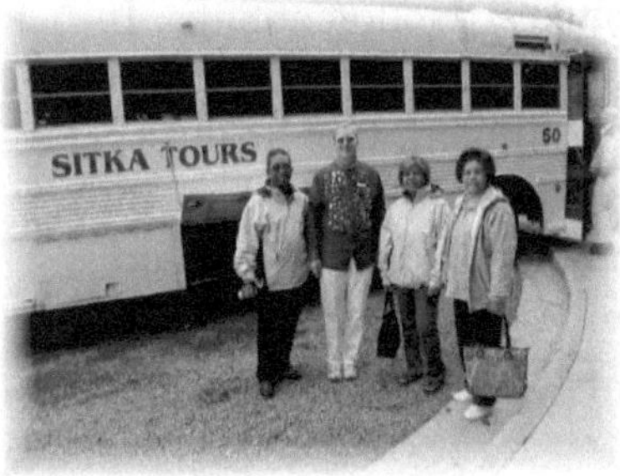

The Russian Orthodox Church clergy came and established residence at Sitka. Subsequently, the homes of the natives were converted to fortress-like structures in anticipation of another attack by the natives. All the successes and failures in battles were documented by the natives in totem poles which are, to this day, are proudly standing as tourist attractions.

With the Russians settling in the island, the fur trade started, and the Russians became the most successful fur traders in the world. When the sea otter population - the source of furs - nearly vanished altogether, the Russians lost interest in the area. They sold Alaska to the United States for $7,200,000. Clinging to their heritage, many residents of Sitka still like to be identified with the Russians.

At Sitka, Alaska

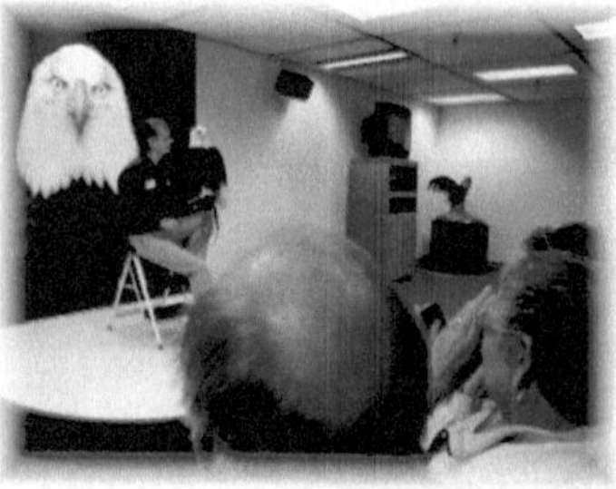

St. Michael's Cathedral located at the center of the town is full of relics, but taking pictures of them was not allowed. With three huge cruise ships anchored in the harbor, the cathedral enjoyed a crowded day at the time of our visit. The Cathedral has a miraculous history according to the Islanders. When the Cathedral burned down some years ago, one person unhooked the enormous and heavy chandelier and saved it. After the Cathedral had been rebuilt, it took five to six people, using a semi-heavy equipment to hang the chandelier back.

The Alaska Raptor Center is the most visited attraction at Sitka. It is where birds particularly eagles, are treated for injuries. Treatment includes flight training in a controlled environment. One such environment is a structure where the birds cannot see and hear the visitors, even when the visitors are not inhibited from talking, and are watching the birds from just a few feet way. Injured birds come from as far as the United States mainland, it being the only center of its kind in the world.

There are enough tourist attractions on the island besides the Raptor Center. Entertainers still perform Russian dances in halls overcrowded with tourists. As we came to the island, three other cruise ships were anchored ahead of us, an indication of the island's popularity.

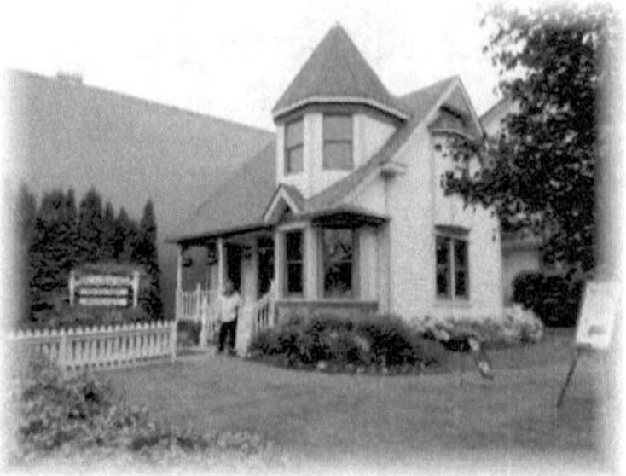

Volunteers mostly perform the services in the town. Our tour bus driver serves as a minister, policeman, and firefighter; he just donned the uniform appropriate for the occasion. Volunteers

At Sitka, Alaska

appear for training in critical services like firefighting and police work even though presence is optional. Some of the services are financed by donations from tourists, explanation for the warm welcome of cruise ships coming into the harbor.

I struck a conversation with a storekeeper. He said that some of the items in his inventory were coming from Russia, making me wonder how he could possibly do so legally in a retail business in Alaska. Because of some quirks in the United States code, he further said, he could sell some merchandise in his store cheaper than those sold in the mainland. Without showing my disagreement as to whom he is selling to, we left the store for another to buy some souvenirs.

Up to this time, Amelia did not have any problem at all touring the island. I was surprised that she could keep up with me when I was in a hurry exploring some places close to our route. Apparently, she was enjoying the shore excursion.

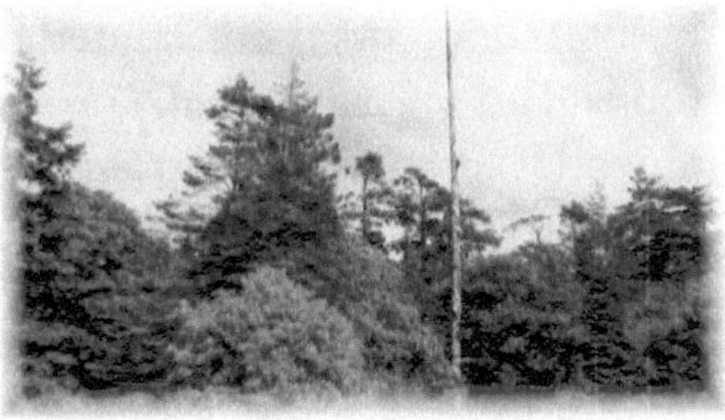

We visited a museum close to the harbor. The museum displays photographs and artifacts about the natives', Russian, and American histories. Huge totem poles are across the museum depicting the historical events that occurred in the island.

It was at this location that hunger syndrome made its presence known to Amelia; she needed to drink liquid. Dennis, a friend who was with us, and I had to run a quarter of a mile to get soda from a vending machine; no food or drink was available at the museum. Amelia significantly improved after drinking the liquid.

At Sitka, Alaska

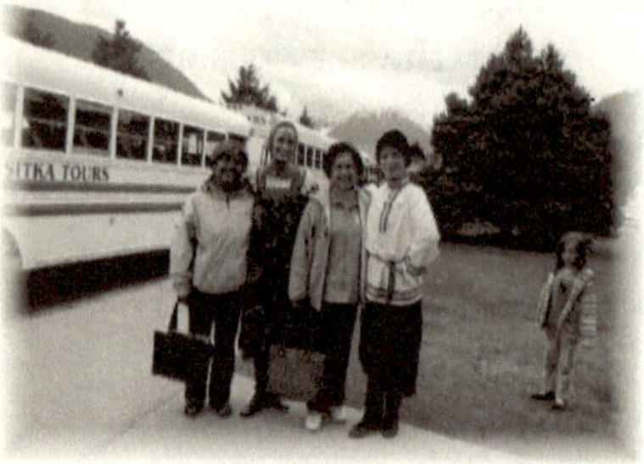

For a certain amount of donation, we watched the presentation of Russian dances at a huge entertainment hall. Seated at the rear of the hall, we could only glimpse at the performances because visitors in front of us were intermittently standing to applaud and appreciate the event. Nevertheless, Amelia liked it; she waited for the performers to come out and had her pictures taken with them.

We took the bus to the pier area from where we were tendered back to the cruise ship. We ate dinner at the ship and waited for the nightly entertainments. I considered our visit to the island of Sitka, educational and informational, and I would not hesitate to recommend it to anyone, as a tour destination.

Fond of history, I was always intrigued by how the United States came into possession of Alaska. With wars erupting now and then for control of geographic territories, the United States acquired Alaska at a bargain without fighting a war.

At Tracy Arm, Alaska

Our cruise package included Inside Passage which meant passage through Tracy Arm. Amelia liked this part of the cruise because we did not have to get off the ship, but we had to endure the cold weather and strong wind on the deck, to appreciate the passage. Deferring to the glass-enclosed dining rooms of the ship, Amelia did not have to join us on the deck, enjoying the trip as well with a slightly obscured view.

Tracy Arm is only one of two or three passages by cruise ship to the Alaskan north, I believe. Navigating the passage allows the visitors the chance to view the ever so tiny interior part of the huge state of Alaska, hence its popularity. But there are some inherent hazards involved in the navigation of the passage.

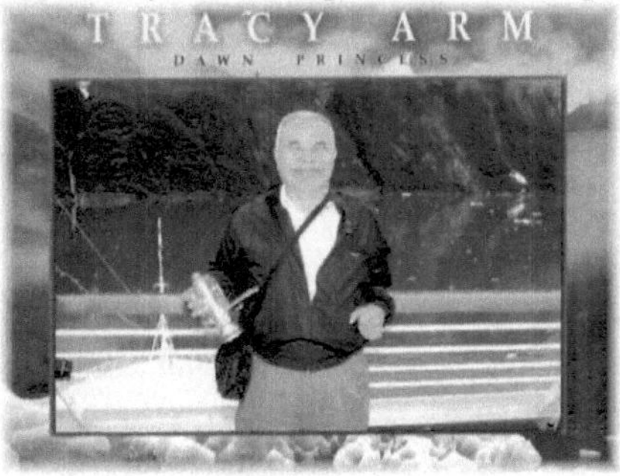

Only a specially trained pilot was allowed to navigate our cruise ship through the passage. The original pilot relinquished control of the ship at a designated point in the passage. With the cruise ship not reducing speed - slowed to about 5 knots per hour - the specially trained pilot caught up with it in a speedboat and stepped up the cruise ship in a casual manner. That feat alone was a delight to watch.

At three to five knots per hour, the pilot tenderly piloted the ship while avoiding treacherous glaciers. Small as they seemed, the ship was careful to avoid them as they are ten times bigger in size below the surface of the water than they are above. That is how dangerous glaciers are; it was glaciers that sank the Titanic.

At Tracy Arm, Alaska

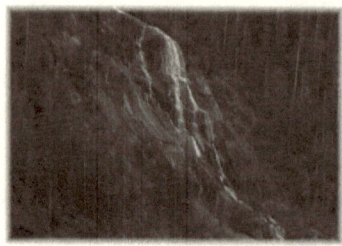

At some points in the passage, it is so narrow that it allows only a few hundred feet of clearance on each side of the ship. There are only certain locations in the passage in which a ship can make a U-turn should it decide to go back in the opposite direction, for whatever reason.

The passage is very narrow as it is very deep, about 1,000 feet in some locations, allowing the cruise ship to get close to the banks. Mostly granite, the cliffs along the banks are not prone to collapse to endanger the ship and its passengers, further allowing the passengers to appreciate the nature of the passage in particular, and the state of Alaska in general.

The coast guards were very active at Tracy Arm as smaller boats were also plying the crowded passage. Their presence ensured that distance from the cruise ship was safely maintained. Not only used by ships and boats, the passage was also a strip of water where hydroplanes were landing and taking off. We even witnessed people paddling their boats along the banks.

The passage area is uninhabited by humans because of the weather condition and the very steep cliffs and mountains capped by snow. During our journey, passengers were alerted by the ship's lookout crew, for some mountain goats and bears. We had our cameras ready, but disappointingly, we did not see any. As if to make up for the missing goats or bears, high up in the skies were bald eagles effortlessly flying in the wind.

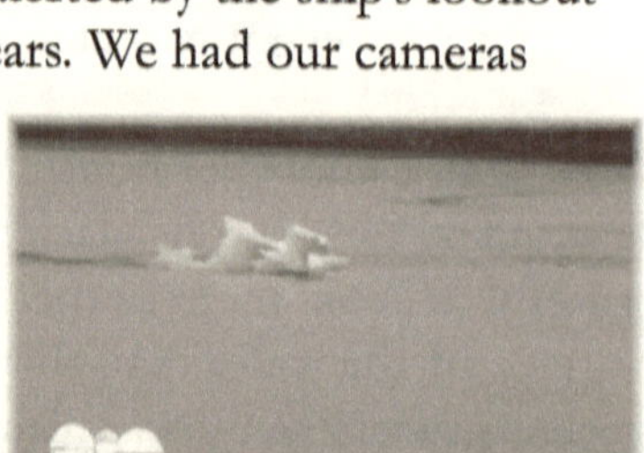

At Tracy Arm, Alaska

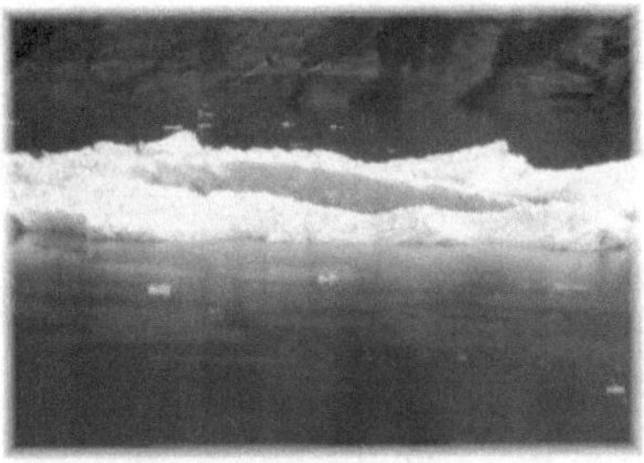

Except for the voices, almost down to murmurs, of the cruisers, there were moments during the very slow passage when one could make out everybody's comment about the calm and placid water. As the ship maneuvered to avoid glaciers, recollections of the Titanic tragedy were whispered unconsciously by some cruisers.

Such was the serene, peaceful, and unagitated motion of the cruise ship through Tracy Arm. The slow passage took us to Juneau by morning, which was another stop in our cruise package. The journey is one I recommend without reservation to anybody who plans on cruising.

At Juneau, Alaska

Our trip to Juneau from Ketchikan along Tracy Arm was more exciting than the few ones we had before in the open ocean, affording us the luxury of seeing land and lush forests on both sides of the ship. Few bald eagles were flying up in the sky; hydroplanes were landing and taking off; and, the coast guards were keeping a close watch on the few boats that were sailing along with the cruise ship. There are some homes and buildings along the route which, we were told, are usually buried in snow during winter.

We found ourselves waking up at Juneau in the morning with the two other cruise ships sailing ahead of us already docked calmly. I was surprised to see the three huge ships docked so close to each other, almost end to end, and just next to the main highway, thanks to the skills of the specially trained pilots.

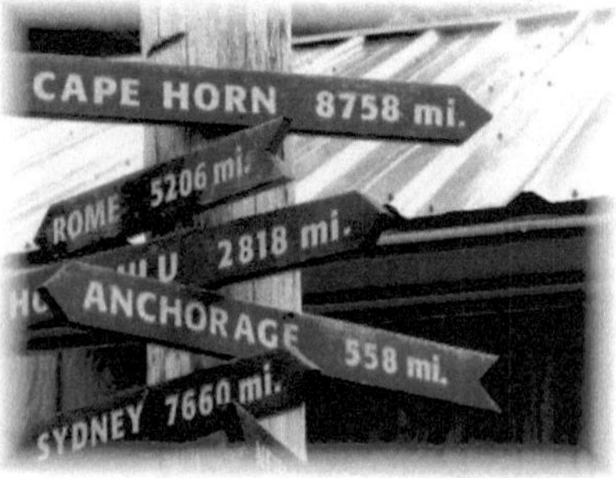
CAPE HORN 8758 mi.
ROME 5206 mi.
2818 mi.
ANCHORAGE 558 mi.
SYDNEY 7660 mi.

Juneau itself is not large in terms of population - just more than 25,000. When Juneau became the capital city of Alaska, it was the biggest city in the north and south Americas, and the second largest in the world, with respect to area of administration; the largest one is in Sweden, I learned. As the capital city of Alaska, Juneau was transformed from a mining town to a city of governance whence administration of the whole state emanates.

The city, we were told, was built from the dirt that came out of the mines in the process of ore extraction during the Alaskan gold rush. It has been constructed very close to the mountains, in fact, so close that the tour bus we were in was being driven along the mountain on one side and close to the few levels of the government building on the other. One can step into the bus from the mountainside and step out of it into the office buildings using the bus as a transition step, according to our tour guide.

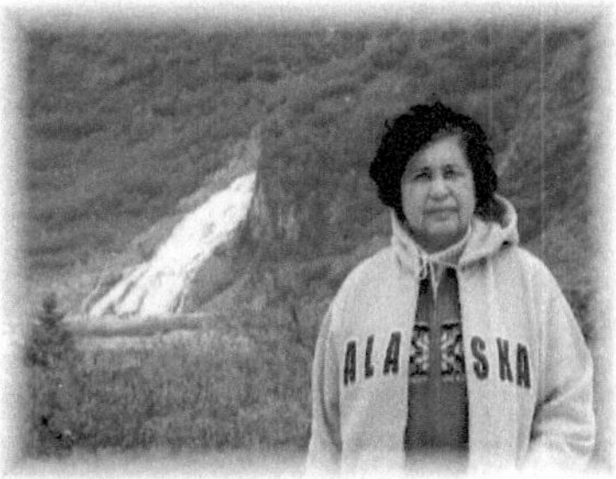

Our visit to Juneau was climaxed by the visit to the Mendenhall Glacier Park. Along the way to the park, we visited a garden planted with the different vegetations present in Alaska including a model garden of the Alaskan tundra. While probing for answers about the tundra and the plants from the garden keepers, we took the last opportunity to rest and eat before proceeding to the park.

During the last few years, the glacier at Mendenhall Glacier Park has receded more than 150 feet, and the recession is still continuing. It is not conclusively decided whether global warming or something else is causing the glacier to recede. Trapped for thousands of years, light causes the glacier to display different shades of blue. The glacier allows the tourists to compose beautiful pictures by shooting at various angles with it as background.

In addition to the main glacier, there are large chunks of icebergs barely moving in the yellowish water leading from Mendenhall Glacier. They are attractions as well, allowing the tourists to take pictures in close encounter, from motionless platforms to wit, the flat land in level with the water and the bridge above the water.

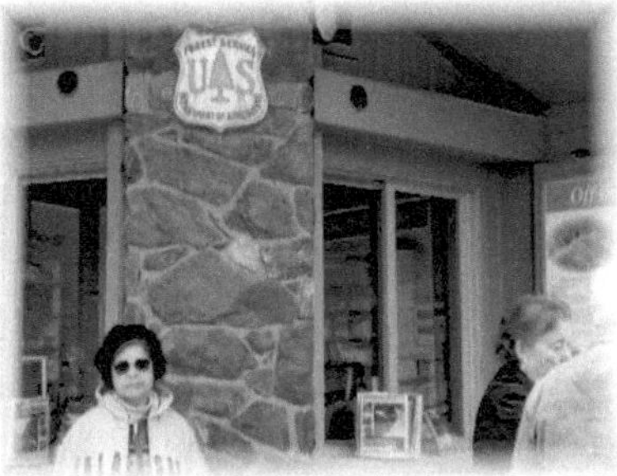

Weather permitting, the glacier is visited by thousands of tourists. A visitors' bureau is immediately conspicuous in the area, and plenty of parking spaces for visitors coming by buses and cars are available. Maintained by the Unites States Park Department, Mendenhall Glacier Park is clean and safe; park rangers ensure that their presence is visible to maintain order and enforce park rules and regulations.

On the way back to the city, our tour guide alerted us to few nesting bald eagles. They were not in any way, perturbed by the hundreds of tourists gawking at them. More eagles were majestically flying overhead as if to announce to the tourists that they are America, the bald eagle being the United States official symbol.

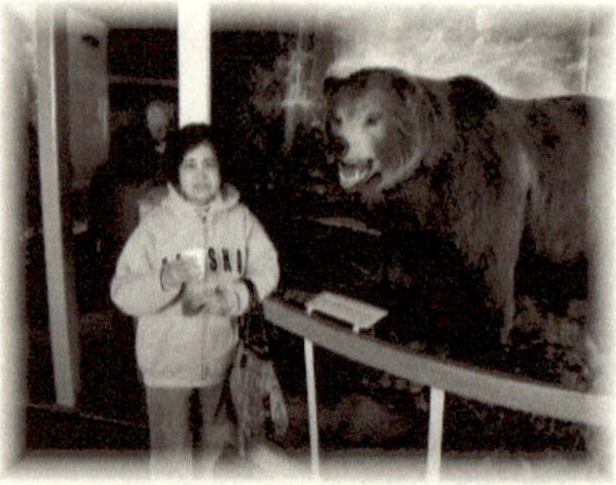

We stopped by the museum where a lengthy history of Alaska is in graphic display. Close by is a spawning pond for salmon, which helps in the propagation of the species and its continuous supply at the dining tables. To ensure that hunger did not overcome Amelia, we ate at the restaurant nearby, allowing her to rest after the exhausting shore excursion to the Mendenhall Glacier Park.

Soon afterward the bus took us back to the ship in time for dinner and the night time shows and other entertainments.

At Juneau, Alaska

Chapter 8 – Destination California

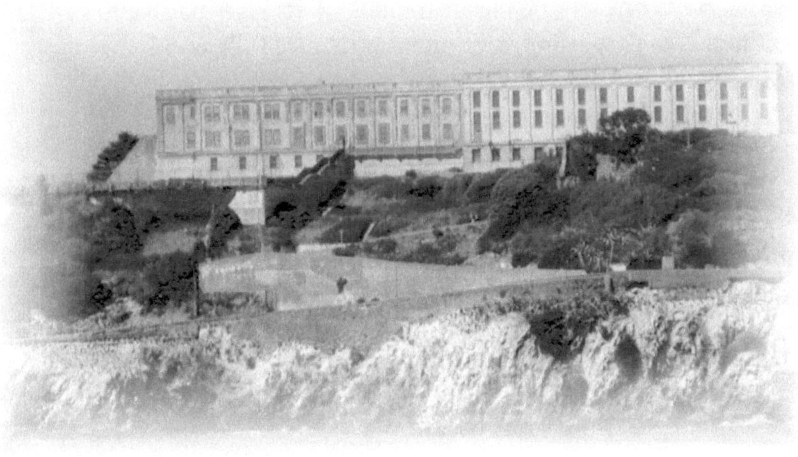

At Santa Barbara, California

At Santa Barbara, California

Santa Barbara, California, was the third stop on our cruise itinerary along the Pacific Northwest. Vying for a share of the revenue from the lucrative tourism industry, the city has been in a vigorous campaign to lure tourists to come. Hospitality groups in makeshift tents handed brochures, newsletters, and other cards promoting the city as a tourist destination. As the groups welcomed the visitors, they took the opportunity to point out the white sandy shores which the city is known for.

Santa Barbara is one of the cleanest cities of its size that we have ever visited. Not surprising, it counts on many Hollywood celebrities choosing to establish permanent and vacation residences in the city. As a matter of fact, the trolley that takes the tourists around the city has a designed route that meanders through the district of the most famous residents. Montecito District, home of some of the wealthiest celebrities in America, boasts of some of the most expensive homes in the United States.

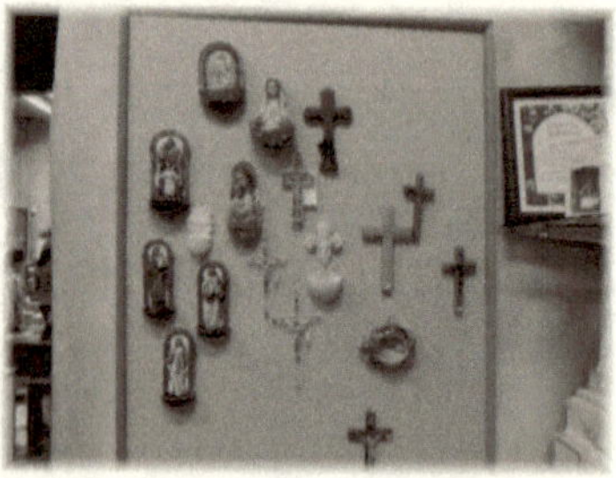

One of the city's proudest possessions is its city hall. Featured in movies and shows, it has brought the city to a new height of popularity. The trolley drove around it twice to allow the tourists to view it at different angles. Mesmerized by the building, some visitors gave up the trolley ride completely and walked to it with cameras clicking. Obviously, they were tourists with interest in architecture or in showing off back home that they had been to the City of Santa Barbara. Other trolleys would take them back to the shoreline.

At Santa Barbara, California

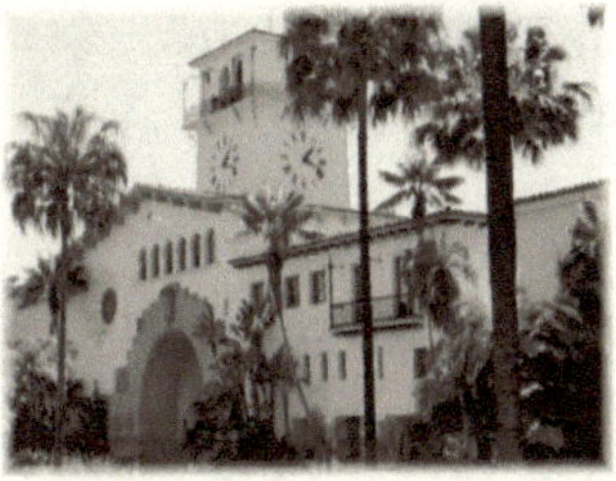

The huge shopping center at State Street was just gathering a crowd as our trolley pulled into an open space in the parking lot. It was noon time, and sensing that Amelia might be having hunger syndrome, I bought some food to fend off a condition that makes her shake, and causes her glucose level to drop. I was relieved that she did not have the uncontrollable attack; she was only tired and starved.

After fifteen minutes, we resumed the tour, this time around the clustered homes with sandstones. Another interesting tourist attraction, sandstones were what the natives used to build walls, fences, and decorative additions to their homes. Mostly confined to the old homes now, they look awesome and unique as they are beautiful. No longer available in commercial quantity, sandstones are now considered specialty products

As we toured the city, the trolley driver provided commentaries about the city. According to him, the city code does not allow homes to be built taller than the palm trees. The requirement inhibits overbuilding and ensures that residents have a glimpse of the beautiful beaches and ocean.

It was not at all surprising that the move to include beach volleyball in the Olympic Games started in the Santa Barbara beaches because of their beauty, span from the water's edge, and quality. Santa Barbara's most crowded attraction, however, was the Santa Barbara Mission. Part of the mission was destroyed by an earthquake in 1929 but was restored and made to

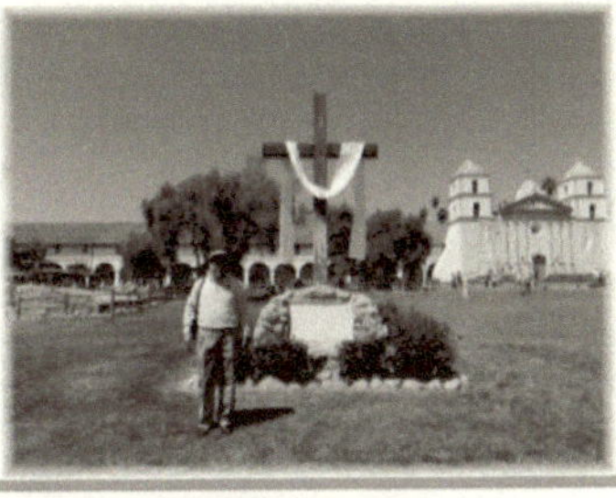

At Santa Barbara, California

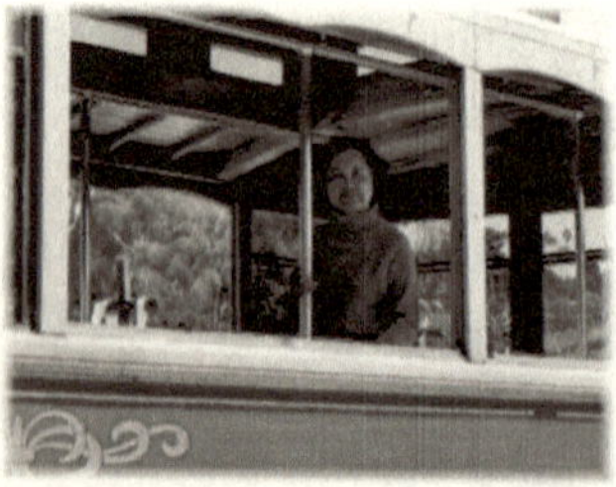

look like the original, using modern building techniques.

Due to the uneven landscape around the mission and the long walk, Amelia did not get off the trolley. She was very disappointed to have missed the mission, for every time that she comes close to a church she likes to get in to say a short prayer. The 15-minute stop was not long enough for tourists to have a complete impression of the relics inside the mission.

The tour of the city lasted about two hours. Heading back towards the pier area on a different route, the trolley drove by more residences of famous celebrities of various categories. Lagoons and banyan trees were pointed out as notable landmarks.

Lacking a pier to accommodate a huge cruise ship, cruisers were only able to get on and off the ship by tenders. We did not have to wait long for ours because as the last check-in time to be on board approached, more tenders were dispatched to pick up the tourists from the shore. We spent the rest of the day resting and relaxing, waiting for the night time entertainments

At Santa Catalina Island, California

At Santa Catalina Island, California

Santa Catalina Island is only 30 miles from the nearest coast in Southern California. The island was formerly owned by Mr. Wrigley, the owner of the famous Wrigley's chewing gum until it was turned over to the Santa Catalina Conservancy.

If Mr. Wrigley administered the island with stiff regulations to maintain the island's flora, the Conservancy pursues his policy even more stringently. Vegetation and wildlife are controlled. The number of rats, snakes, eagles, buffaloes (limited to 500) so on so forth, is monitored to maintain a natural balance in the island.

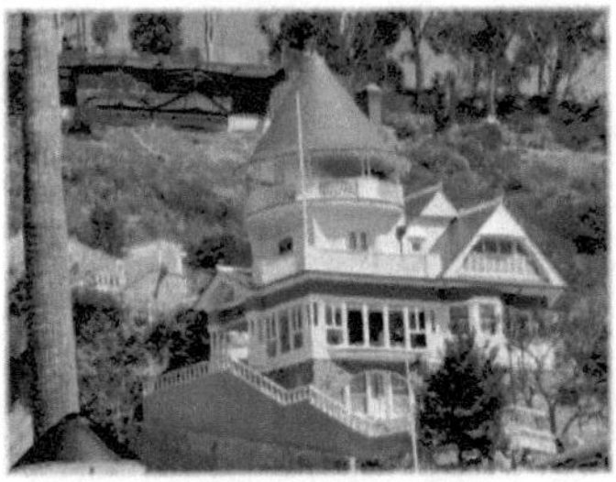

The Santa Catalina Island is reachable more often by smaller boats than by cruise ships. Most visitors to the island use the smaller boat mode of transportation from ports along the California coast, San Pedro being the closest one.

Avalon is the major port in the Santa Catalina Island and the first visitors' destination for exploring other areas of the island. Growth in the island being controlled, Avalon is not a big city. A major expansion is practically non-existent, and if one exists, construction cost is prohibitively very high. On certain holidays and spring breaks, the island is very crowded, and cost of commodities rises as demand increases.

Our cruise ship dropped anchor out in the ocean outside Avalon's harbor which is way too small to accommodate a huge ship, and where only pleasure boats are docked most of the time. We were tendered to the island from the cruise ship, but instead of dropping the tourists at the main dock, for whatever reason the tenders were

At Santa Catalina Island, California

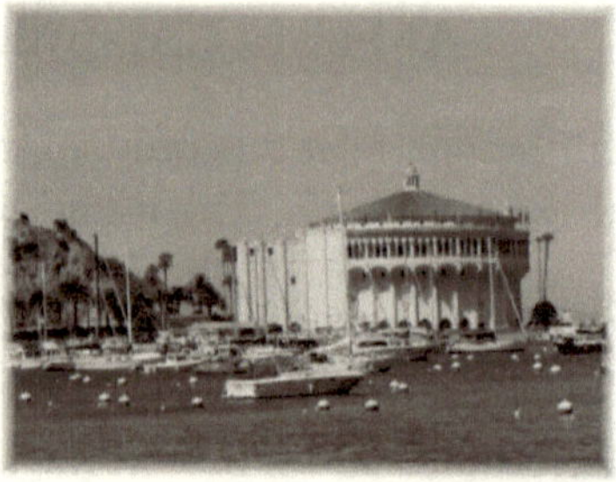

diverted to the smaller platforms. It was low tide when we approached the island, so the ramp was steeper and longer, and not favorable to Amelia; I had to stay behind and help her navigate the ramp.

The assembly point of our excursion was on the main dock requiring us to walk a quarter of a mile to reach it. With Amelia laboriously covering the distance, we made it to the assembly point nevertheless, and we were off to our excursion. Our destination was the airport, a trip that would put our cameras into service to include in our shots the vivid panorama of the island.

Initially, the road to the airport is narrow, winding, and dangerously close to the cliffs. Careful not to disturb the island's landscape, the road is left sparsely paved helping the island look rustic and bucolic. With different kinds of vegetations native to the island dotting the roadside, the road provided us sights of grazing buffaloes and flocks of other wildlife. Past the water supply source of the island, the sight of the airport's tower finally loomed ahead.

It was almost lunch time when we arrived at the airport, and Amelia was eager to eat, lest hunger syndrome would make its presence known. Luckily, a well-stuffed restaurant is maintained at the airport, so I did not lose time ordering food to relieve Amelia of hunger immediately. After spending an hour perusing the displays and mosaics at the airport, we headed back to Avalon.

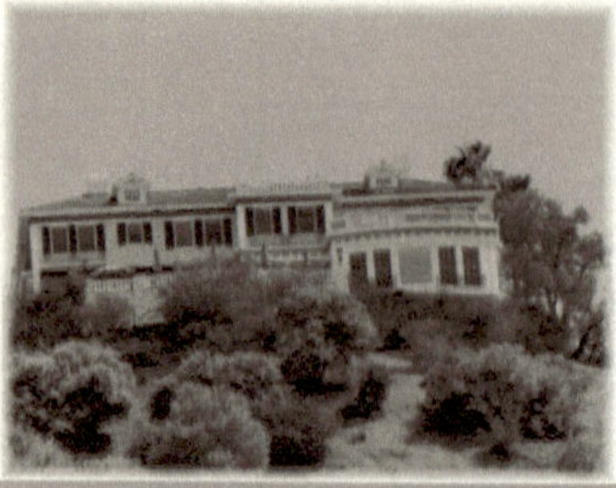

At Santa Catalina Island, California

Back at Avalon, more than a handful of landmarks and structures are worth noting, but the Casino and the Wrigley Mansion are the eye-catching ones that are most photographed by tourists. For most tourists, and because of its distance and difficult access, the Wrigley Mansion is sufficed to be pointed out from the pier area.

The last part of our tour was the fish sighting from the glass bottom boat. For $5.00, the fish feed could be purchased and dropped into the ocean to lure the fish beneath the transparent glass bottom of the boat where they could be photographed. We did well with attracting the fish except, that the competition for space on the boat squeezed Amelia and me, making us feel uncomfortable.

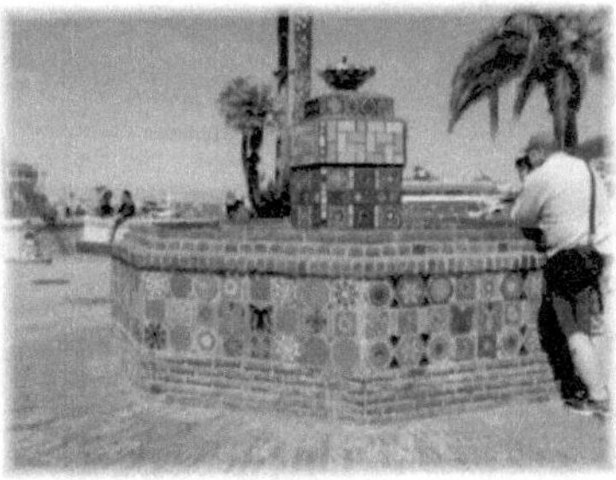

We were tendered back to the ship with aching bodies due to the rough ride to and from the airport, finishing the day resting and relaxing on the cruise ship. The Santa Catalina Island offers an experience of ocean travel, town exploration, and land excursion without the expensive preparation associated with a big cruise vacation. I would recommend spending some time on the island to anyone who wants to use some moments to escape the busy hours and days in the major cities.

At Alcatraz, California

At Alcatraz, California

On a previous cruise from San Francisco to Alaska, I was disappointed for failing to book an excursion to Alcatraz prison because tickets were sold out. On this subsequent cruise, the tour tickets were sold out again before I could read the announcements in the newsletters. But this time I was determined not to be denied the opportunity to visit the island prison, our cruise ship already being so close to the island and the company that ferries tourists to Alcatraz being only two piers away.

I walked to the company and purchased tickets for Amelia and me. The trip to Alcatraz was for the next day, but that was all right because the cruise ship was staying all night in San Francisco. The problem was that the weather forecast indicated a gloomy morning, and rain was expected. Amelia had problems with both, she having a stroke ten months earlier.

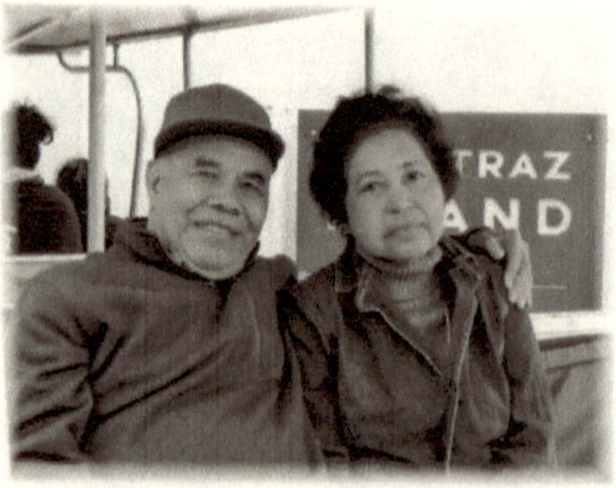

The lines of tourists going to Alcatraz Island were unbelievably long for a rainy sailing. Amelia could remain standing for only a few minutes at a time, but because of her physical condition, she and I were pre-boarded, the term the members of the staff used to process tourists with walkers and on wheelchairs, ahead of everyone else.

On the island and again because of Amelia's disability, we were let on a tram going uphill to the main prison building while other passengers were still waiting in line to disembark. A sense of guilt crept upon me, but other tourists with the same condition as Amelia's were treated favorably as well.

At Alcatraz, California

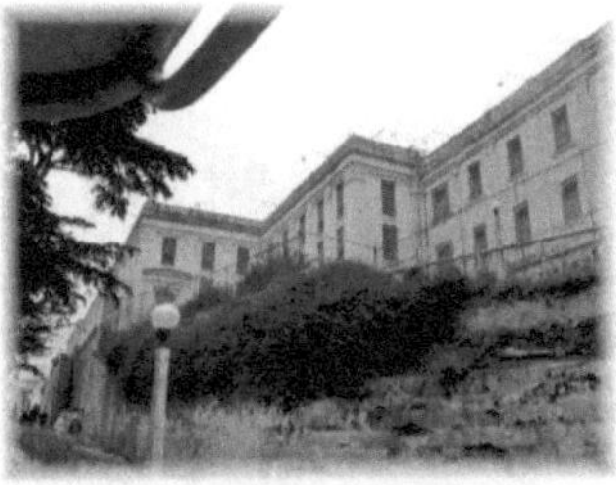

Alcatraz housed the most hardened criminals of their times, among them being Al Capone and Robert Stroud, whose lives were featured in movies, the latter in "Birdman of Alcatraz," and the former in few films relating to gangster culture in America. The island prison itself is featured in the movie "The Rock" with famous actors doing some of their best performances. Equally brutal and ruthless, other inmates including the narrators of the tour left their impressions on the island prison as well.

Although several attempts were made to escape from the prison, not a single one was successful despite some unverified tales about escapees surviving the conditions around the island. The water around the island is very chilly that a would-be escapee will be overcome by hypothermia before he gets close to the mainland.

Because of high operating costs, the island prison was abandoned; it is now managed as a park and is a very popular destination for tourists. As infamous as the island prison was, there are some elements of romance, adventure, and hero worship associated with Alcatraz. While waiting to sail for the island, we sat across two men from Switzerland who purposely extended their business trip for two days just to visit the prison, for Alcatraz is also a name and place featured in magazines and other publications in their country.

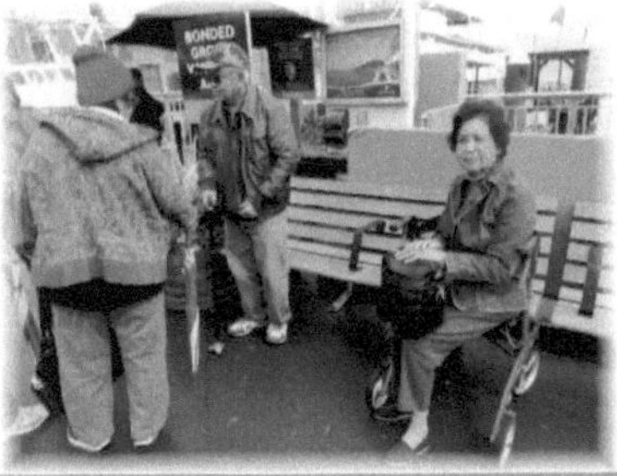

Coming back to the cruise ship, I was surprised to see Amelia briskly walking with her walker, to escape the rain. I was concerned that visibly shivering and with cold hands and chattering teeth, she might not make it to the ship

At Alcatraz, California

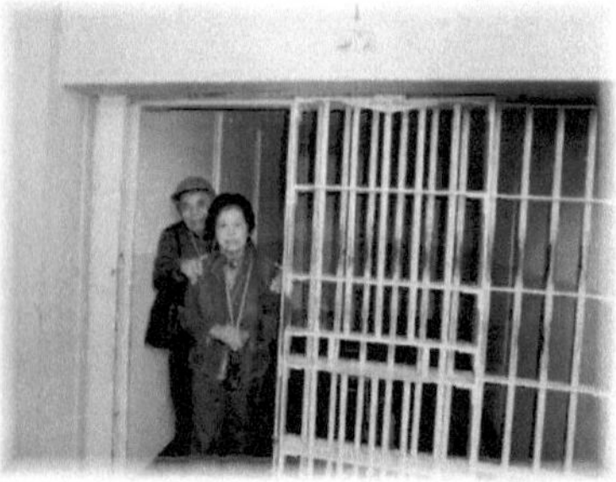

without some type of emergency. We got back to the ship all right where I immediately gave her hot soup and coffee to ease her discomfort.

We rested and relaxed the rest of the day waiting for the ship to depart from San Francisco and for the nightly entertainments. I considered the tour of Alcatraz, the island prison, to be one of the most memorable excursions we ever had.

When in the San Francisco Bay Area, one must not miss the Island of Alcatraz for its historical, educational, and turbulent cultural impact on the American way of life that existed in the early 19th century.

At Napa Valley Wineries, California

While actively employed, wine tasting was never an occasion I would like to go to because wine was never an essential part of my diet. Occasionally wine tasting was a secondary social function to break the monotony of confinement in the office, especially during seminars and conferences. Now that I am retired I seem to appreciate any activity that takes me away from being bored.

Our preferred excursion during this portion of the cruise was to the Muir Woods, but it was fully booked before we could get our reservations in. It turned out to be a good miss because it was raining to be out in the woods after all, and Amelia would have a problem walking in the rain. Our backup excursion, wine tasting, turned out to be handy.

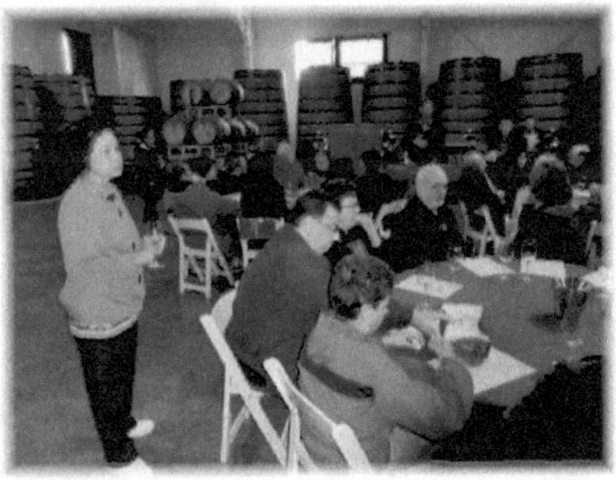

Never been to a wine tasting from real grapes before, a trip to Napa and Sonoma counties was what I looked forward to with interest and light excitement. It would be our first time to be in those counties after all, giving me a chance to compare grape wine with sugar cane wine. We tasted wine from real sugar cane in Barbados, the Caribbean, previously.

It was a two-hour drive from San Francisco to the first winery, the Cline winery. We made it late to the wine tasting room because Amelia, with her physical disability, was avoiding humps and uneven pavements, occasionally following roundabout paths. Visitors including some from other excursions were seated on long benches, and already tasting wines. Even though more benches were brought in to accommodate a stream of arriving guests, we found ourselves sitting in the outskirts of the crowd.

At Napa Valley Wineries, California

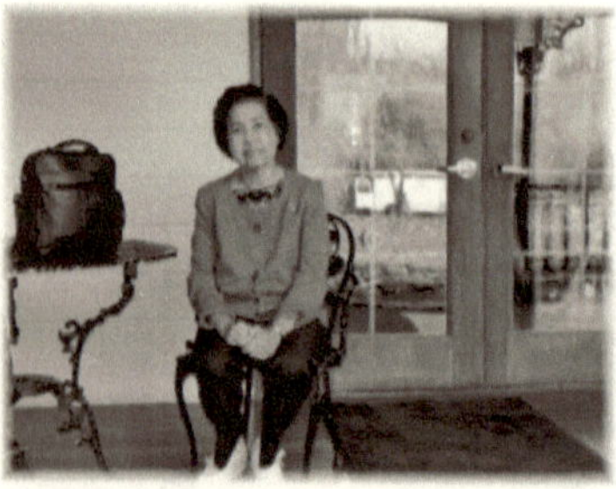

Barrels and barrels of wine were evident in the wine tasting room. I was surprised at some guests' ability to identify different kinds of wine. Showing absolute approval by nodding their heads, some wine tasters derived pleasures from even the most acrid (I tasted them myself) wines. Altogether, I estimated fifty to sixty wine tasters to be in the room.

With assistance from his crew, Mr. Cline, the owner himself, conducted the wine tasting. I was amazed at how he described each bottle of wine from memory: its content ratios, what type of customers it has appeal to, what kind of grapes it comes from, and which grapes grow best on certain soils.

Mr. Cline exports wines to different countries in the world. Our guide related that while Mr. Cline tends his home and company in California, he and his family also maintain a residence in Italy, enabling him to keep a modern feel of the wine industry in Europe and North America.
He did not appear to be a man of stature; he was humble, unassuming, and very courteous, yet I understood, his products appeal to the taste buds of wine lovers of the world.

The next stop on our excursion was at the Sebastiani winery which looked to be an even bigger winery, and where activities appeared to be more businesslike and formal. Like the Cline Winery, this winery exports wines to different countries in the world.

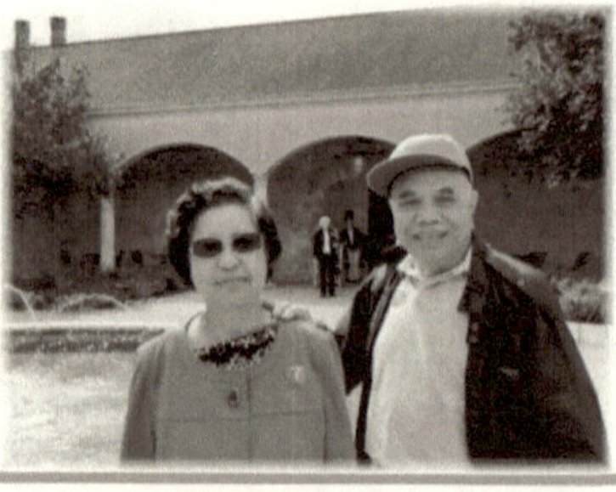

At Napa Valley Wineries, California

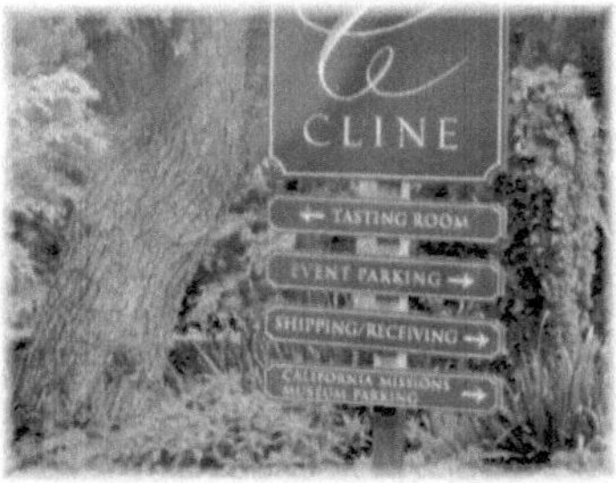

Wine tasting at the Sebastiani winery was conducted by members of the staff in the company, with wine tasters initially gathering around and standing, taking their cups of wine thereafter. Unlike in the previous winery, the tasters walked around as they pleased with cups of wine in their hands, and even while tasting was going on.

The store has a huge showroom in addition to the general store which is fully stocked with anything relating to wines. But to me, the stealer of the show was the 59,000-gallon wine barrel, largest in the winery. I was not sure if it is the biggest in the industry, this tour being only second of my rare wine tasting experience.

We headed back to the ship after having a successful wine tasting experience. The ship was already preparing to sail for the next stop on our itinerary.

As an afterthought, every cruise ship also has its wine tasting schedules confined to a limited space, and not as elaborate as the ones we just had. What we just witnessed in addition to wine tasting, were sights of real barrels of wines stocked to the ceilings, fields of grapes as vast as the eyes can see, and field and brewing equipments to produce the wine from planting to brewing.

Having been residents of Southern California during our entire life in the United States, we cherish the experience of visiting one of the popular destinations in Northern California, the Wine Country.

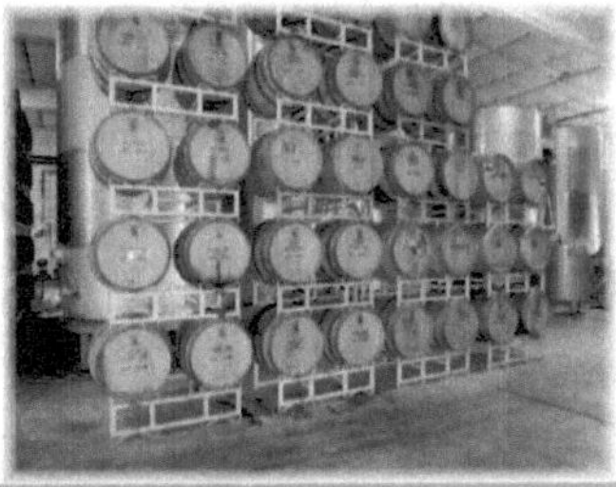

At City of Monterey, California

At City of Monterey, California

Coming down the California coast from San Francisco, the City of Monterey was our next stop. We did not plan on joining an excursion in the city because Amelia was not feeling well due to stiffness from the previous excursions. However, she was open to the idea of walking on the wharf. After all, we have never been to Monterey and never would be unless we purposely endure the long drive to the city from Southern California.

As soon as the ship got the clearance from customs to allow tourists to disembark, passengers immediately formed a line stretching from the hallway down two flights of stairs through another corridor onto the deck overlooking the gangway. Unable to keep pace with the rushing passengers because of Amelia's disability, we waited until she could grab the handrail and had space on the stairs to come down.

The ship's crew helped Amelia down another flight of stairs to the deck where the gangway was located. The 30- to 45-degree angled stair leading to the tender was steep for a healthy person, extremely more so for Amelia. Had we known earlier how difficult it was to disembark from the ship to the tenders we would have given up the idea of walking on the wharf.

It was low tide when we approached the dock. The increasingly rising steps leading to the landing on the dock went up in one direction and turned around in another before finally ending. After we had surveyed the long inclining climb towards the dock, Amelia decided she would not be able to make it even if assistance was offered. We waited for the next tender to take us back to the ship, Amelia unable to even step on land in the city.

At City of Monterey, California

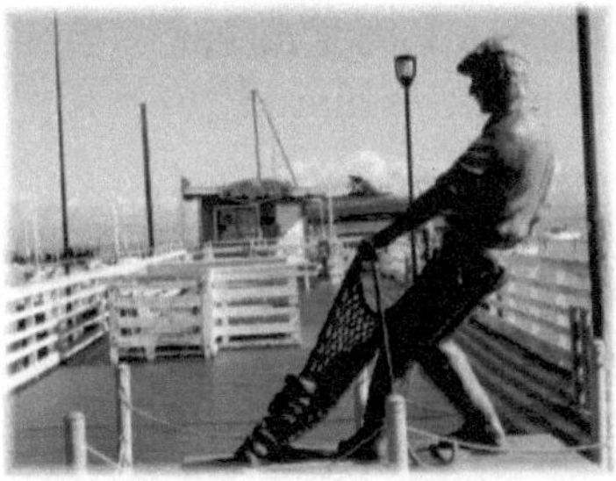

The transfer to the ship was not difficult for Amelia this time because the passengers were lead on board the ship from the tender which was leveled with the lower deck. She needed very alert assistance though for safety reason because the tender was swaying quite wildly from the ocean waves. Instead of retracing our way back when we disembarked, we took the elevator to the promenade deck where Amelia recovered from the earlier disembarking struggle.

Amelia always felt safe and comfortable at the promenade deck because it was where most activities were taking place and where she met new friends. After seeing that she was comfortably seated at the customer service area on the ship, I took the next tender back to the city, promising her that I would be gone for only two hours.

At the Fisherman's Wharf, some children were dropping food crumbs to the sea lions triggering the creatures to howl nonstop. I have never been to a place noisier from the barks of sea lions than at the City of Monterey. While children were having fun with the animals, other people including me were offended by the deafening noise.

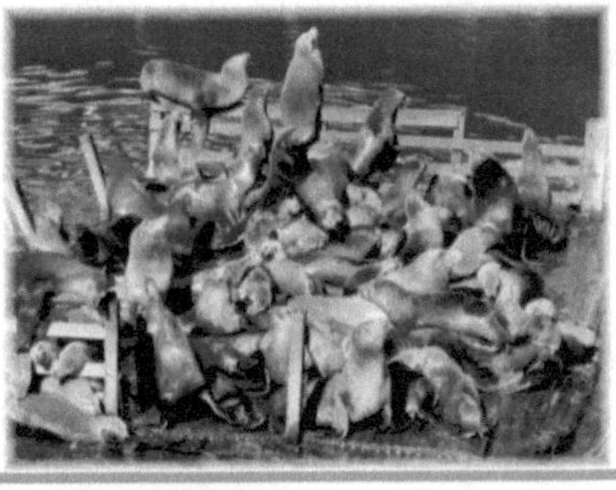

From the few sculptures on the wharf, one can tell that the city has a history as a fishing port. With tourists from our cruise ship and others reaching the city by other modes of transportation, the wharf appeared to be more crowded and oriented to tourism. In fact, it is in another newer dock, which I did not have time to visit, that real commercial fishing activities are conducted.

The harbor of the city is dotted with yachts of different sizes, an unmistakable sign of the city's share of economic wealth. Not too many huge cruise ships are stopping at the city, so when they do, the tourists are keen to see how the city of Monterey looks, its history being well-known.

One only needs to walk around the Custom House Plaza to gain knowledge about the city's history. At the Monterey State Historic Park, stands the old Customhouse, designated as the first California Historical Landmark. The Stanton Center, a maritime museum, also occupies a major area of the plaza. Other buildings of obvious historical importance at the Monterey State Historic Park are too numerous to notice carefully in the two hours that I allowed myself.

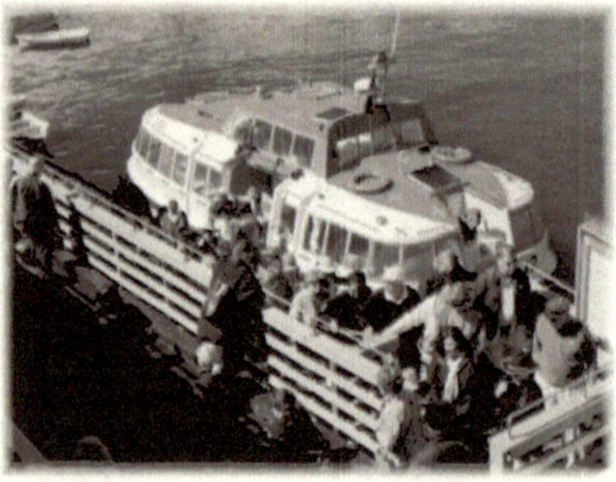

A metal plate on a wall in the plaza briefly summarizes the important dates and changes that the city had undergone to make it what it is today. The Monterey Jazz Festival, one of the most consecutively run jazz festivals, was prominently advertised by postings in the plaza. Postings of the Japanese American Heritage Days to be held at the Old Fisherman's Wharf were evident as well.

To cover as much area in two hours without being far from the wharf, I walked along the beautiful Fisherman's Shoreline Park which offers an excellent view of the marina. More relics and historical points of interest are identified in plaques and plates for

At City of Monterey, California

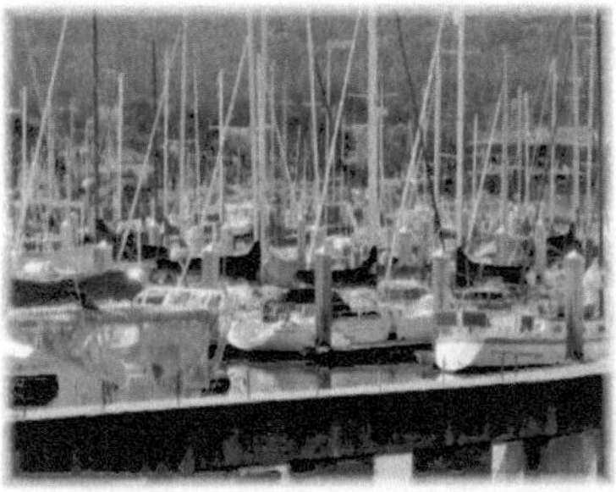

tourists to see. It would take many days to appreciate even a short period of the City of Monterey's history.

Not evident from the pier area but on many publications, the city also has a history of added affluence, being the preferred residence of some famous celebrities from different events and endeavors. It is also the home of the world-famous Monterey Bay Aquarium and one of the most popular golf courses in the world.

My impression of the city as a tourist destination is limited to the pier area. By all accounts from the media and many events, the city is one of the priciest and most prestigious in the United States.

At City of Monterey, California

Chapter 9 – Destination New York

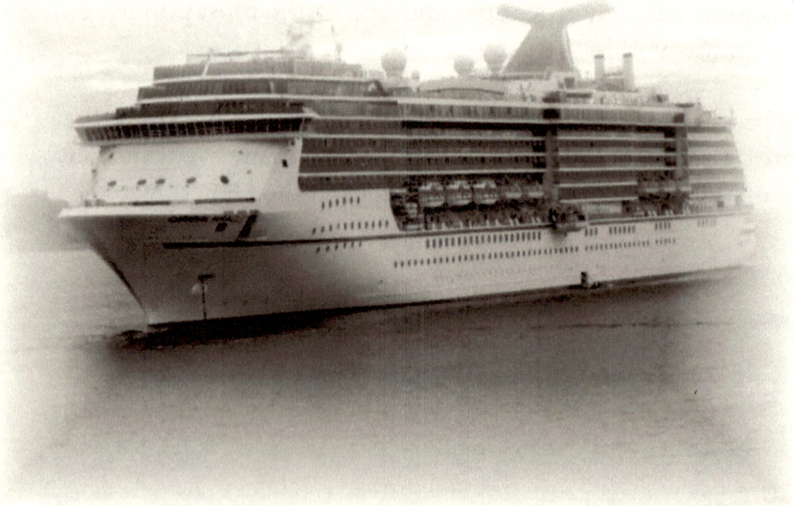

At New York, New York

At New York, New York

As far as Amelia and I are concerned, cruising is a remedial and therapeutic kind of vacation especially that she has a physical disability arising from strokes. I do not want to rush and spoil it, for it is short and soon it is over before too long, defeating the purpose for which it is intended. Allowing two to three pre-sailing days would give me time to react and adjust should changes in schedules occur beyond our control. Our cruise to the Caribbean was not an exception; we flew into New York City by way of Newark Airport in New Jersey three days ahead of the scheduled embarkation.

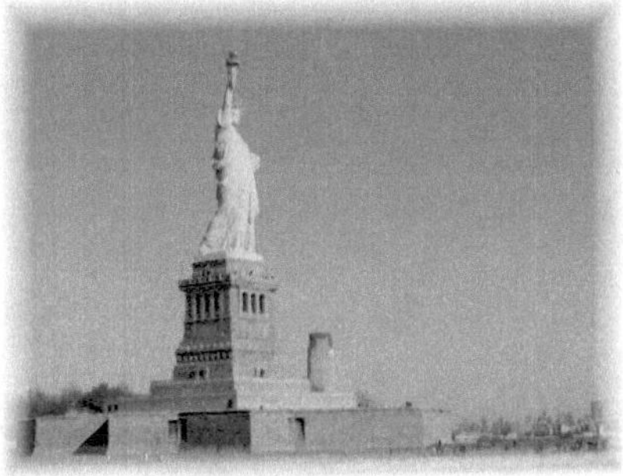

Even before depositing our luggage at the hotel on the first night of our stay in New York City, Dolly's niece treated us to a dinner at a Japanese restaurant, which we graciously enjoyed despite being weary from the five-hour flight. Although already late at night immediately after dinner, we shopped for clothes suitable for New York's weather, we having arrived wearing clothes appropriate for California's climate.

Free only this night to show us around New York City, Dolly's nephews took us to ground zero, the grand central train station, the New York Waldorf Astoria hotel, and the family-owned flower shop. We were also shown apartment living condition as a way of life in New York City, one of Dolly's nephews having been living in one shared with another tenant.

At New York, New York

The following day, we had a guided tour of New York City. Though it was impossible to remember what the tour guide narrated, the tour was a memorable experience for us who are unfamiliar with the city. Then for our unguided experience, we took the public transportation buses to different places of interest like the Rockefeller Center, the Empire State Building, Central Park, United Nations Building, Columbia University, St. Patrick's Cathedral, and other places too numerous to remember and mention.

Interestingly and to our surprise, the parish we go to in California is Saint Elizabeth Ann Seton Church. At Manhattan, the actual residence of the saint is one of the places that the buses were passing by; every time we drove by it, we experienced reverend feelings towards the residence which appeared to be under renovation and reconstruction.

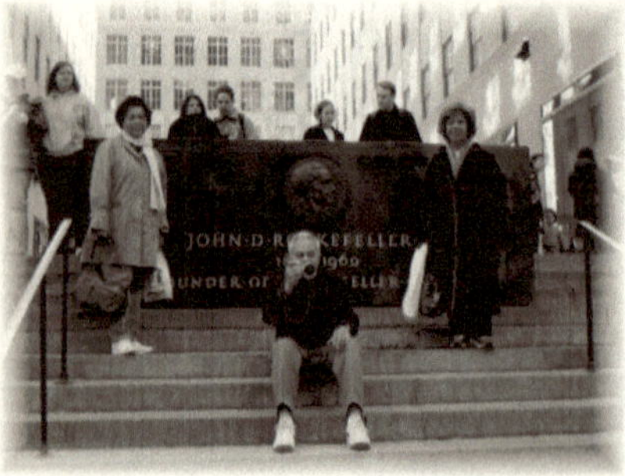

Tired and devoid of more energy, we retired to our hotel located at the foot of the Brooklyn Bridge. As advertised, the hotel location itself has enough history to it; I booked it based on its glowing historical details.

Up to this time, our knowledge about Manhattan was limited to news about Wall Street, but when we looked around, we gained ever so minuscule perspective of the city. We watched the ferries loading and unloading passengers to and from the city. Having recovered our stamina slightly, we dined at a restaurant at the dock area close to the hotel, planning for the next day's activities.

At New York, New York

The following morning we took the tender to the Statue of Liberty. Honestly, I did not like the climb for fear that if there was an emergency and because of the tight space, the only way for the climbers to be out of the statue was last in first out, the first one on the top being the last one to get out. We had fun nevertheless, and we boasted to friends back home that we did climb the statue.

Coming back from the Statue of Liberty, we took the ferry to Ellis Island, the island where the first immigrants to the United States flocked through. Being displayed in rich historical and educational relics, are the primary roles the Island played in making the United States what it is today. I imagined the romance, challenge, and relief of those who had gone through the immigration process in the island, being triumphantly happy and feeling unshackled in the new motherland.

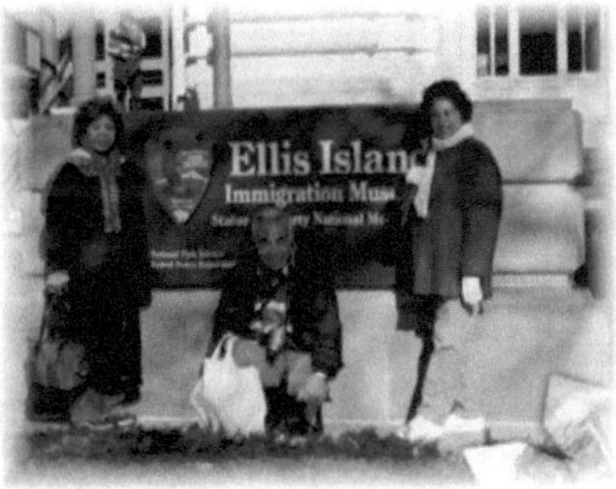

To my joy, all the time that we were exploring the Statue of Liberty and the Ellis Island's relics, Amelia was quiet and unconcerned. She liked the tours as well, only needing to be watched for the appearance of the hunger syndrome which causes her glucose level to drop and make her shake and uncomfortable. We dined at a restaurant in the same dock area near the hotel to avert Amelia's ailment, finally ending the last pre-sailing hectic but worthwhile day.

Back at the hotel, we prepared for the embarkation onto the cruise ship the following day. As a pass-through city, we made the most out of our three-day stay in New York. It would take a concerted effort and a considerable time to get familiar with New York City.

At New York, New York

Having been residing in the Los Angeles area of Southern California for most of my entire life as an immigrant, the comparison between the two cities could never be more different. Various factors determine one's preference between the two cities. My family's preference is principally determined by the weather condition.

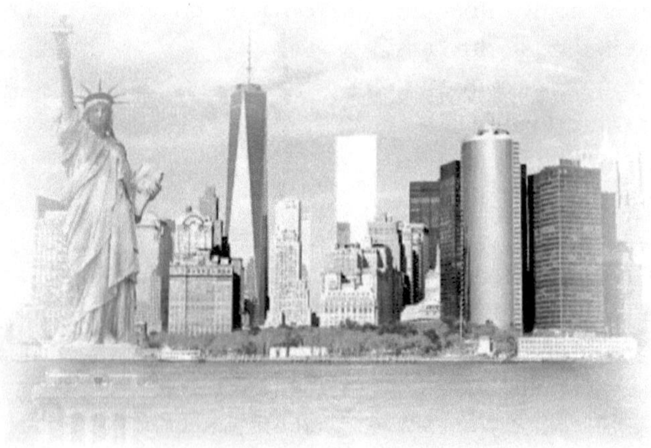

At New York, New York

Chapter 10 – Destination The Caribbean

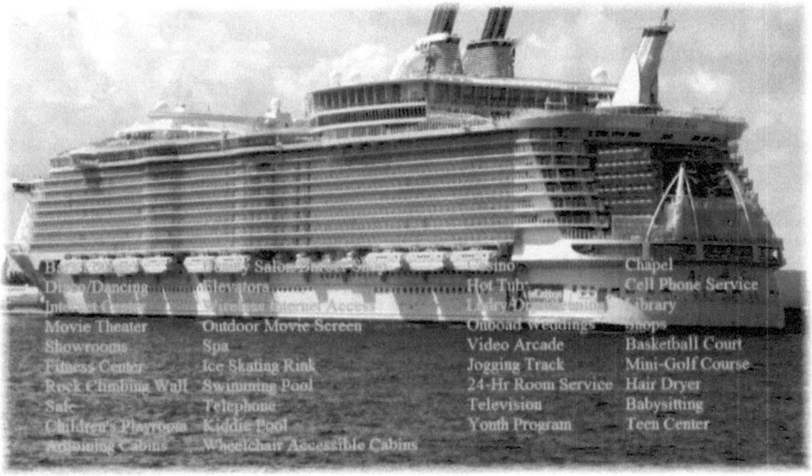

At U.S. Virgin Island, United States

Amalie, in the United States Virgin Islands, was one of the scheduled stops on our itinerary. Its popular Skyride was the talk of the tourists on board the ship and during the tender ride. Having heard about it from friends who were at Amalie before, it was one in this cruise that I did not want to miss. The starting platform for the ride was not too far from the harbor; it did not take the tour bus long to get there.

Having started late and still being kept on the bus, our group did not get to the base of the platform until almost noon. When we were finally let off the bus, it was lunch time, but we figured that

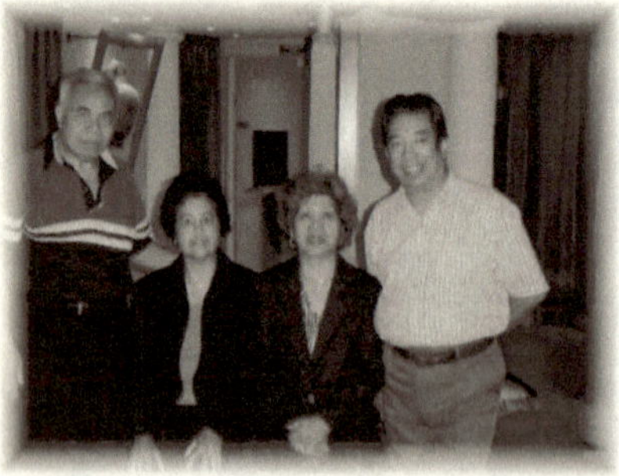

we would eat lunch at the endpoint of the Skyride. Owing to a large number of tourists taking the ride, we had to wait a few more minutes for our turn during which an unfortunate incident found us missing the ride after so much anticipation.

Due to the heat and the long wait while standing, Amelia felt dizzy. She needed to sit down, eat some snacks, and drink some liquid which was available on vending machines nearby. We had to give up our precious positions in the queue of tourists waiting to take the ride while I had to take care of her. Despite eating some snacks and drinking soda, Amelia felt she could not get into the queue again and wait for the Skyride, passing it entirely in favor of a bus ride. Accordingly, we turned back and found the tour bus that brought us to the base earlier and took it to Paradise Point, the end of the Skyride.

At U.S. Virgin Island, United States

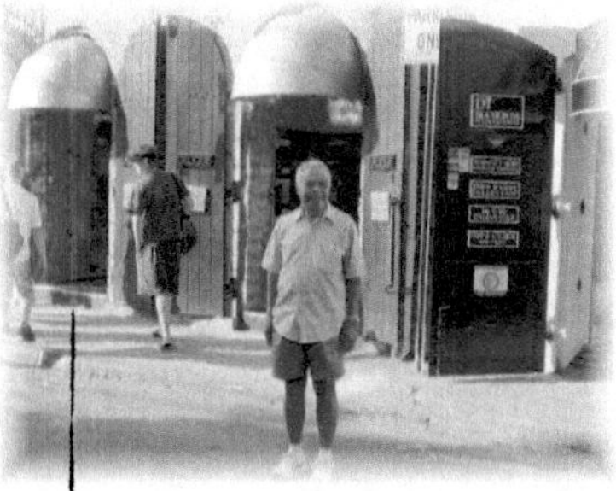

The route to Paradise Point by bus was probably not as scenic as that on the Skyride, but exhilarating just as well. We had a panoramic view of the harbor dotted with hundreds of yachts and sailboats, and the blue horizon yonder partly shrouded with fine mists. Our huge cruise ship, anchored beyond the harbor area, was very distinguishable from among the few that were closer and docked along the piers. As the bus inched farther and farther up, we felt like we were traveling on top of trees because of the scenic route carved from the mountainside, finally ending at Paradise Point.

An otherwise frustrating excursion turned out to be as exciting as any we had in previous cruises. Paradise Point lives up to its name but because of my fear of height, I could not turn my back towards the steep mountainside for picture taking. Neither did I encourage Amelia to do so because of her physical condition; a slight misstep could mean real emergency. Fixed sturdy platforms with handrails around the structures at Paradise Point failed to boost my confidence and appease my fear, either.

We took the bus back to downtown Amalie where tenders were unloading late sightseers and picking up returning ones. It did not matter how many times one could go on and off the ship because it was anchored at Amalie one full day. An abundance of tourists from few cruise ships made downtown Amalie crowded and in a festive mood. While enjoying the

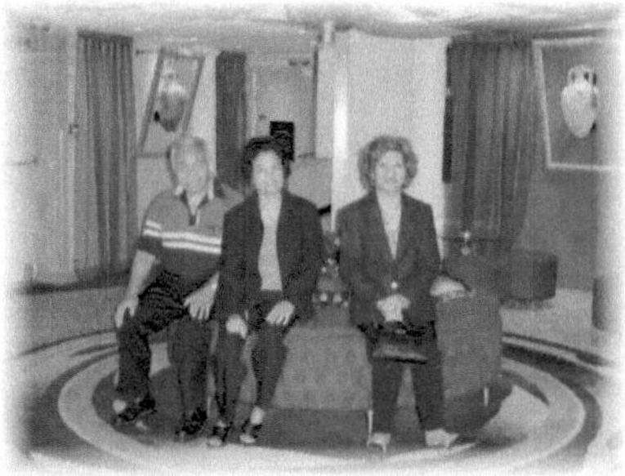

At U.S. Virgin Island, United States

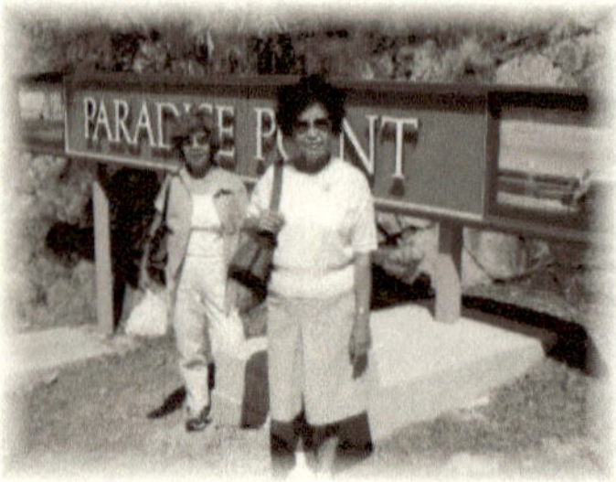

spontaneous festivities caused by arriving visitors we shopped around for souvenirs before taking a tender back to the ship.

After seeing to it that Amelia was comfortable on the ship I took a tender back to the shore to shop for some compact discs that we heard being played when we arrived. I did find the store that was selling the discs and purchased four of them; half of the contents stopped playing when I tried them at home.

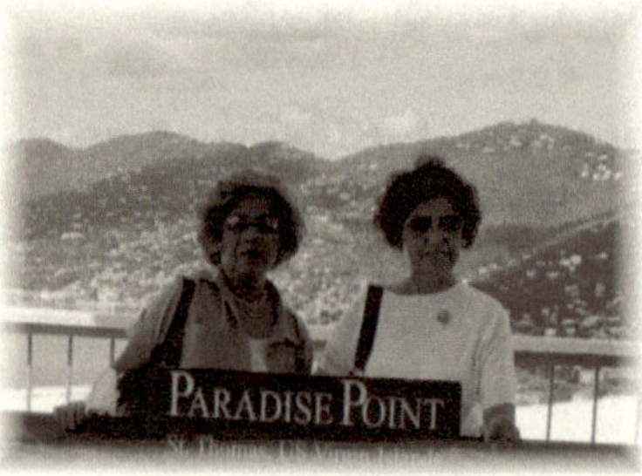

Having the United States Virgin Islands tucked into our record of visited places, we spent the rest of the day resting and relaxing, deciding which of the ongoing entertainments to watch before retiring early to our cabin. We needed enough rest because we would be waking up at a different port the following day, and possibly joining another excursion.

The United States Virgin Island is one of the Caribbean islands that I would not hesitate to recommend to anyone to visit. It is different in many ways than the places in the United States mainland like the Los Angeles metropolis.

At Martinique, Martinique

The cruise ship dropped anchor way outside the harbor at Fort de France, Martinique, for whatever reason we did not know. It did not matter though because the ocean was very calm while the tourists were being tendered to shore.

In the tender they were identified and grouped together to be sure each group belonged to a target excursion on shore. Ours was one that first went by boat to a marina opposite Fort de France for transfer to a tour bus. On the vessel, passengers were treated to cold refreshments and a variety of goodies while some were dancing to lively music in unison with the boat's swaying motion along the ocean waves. Our excursion appeared to be in a good start, I could tell.

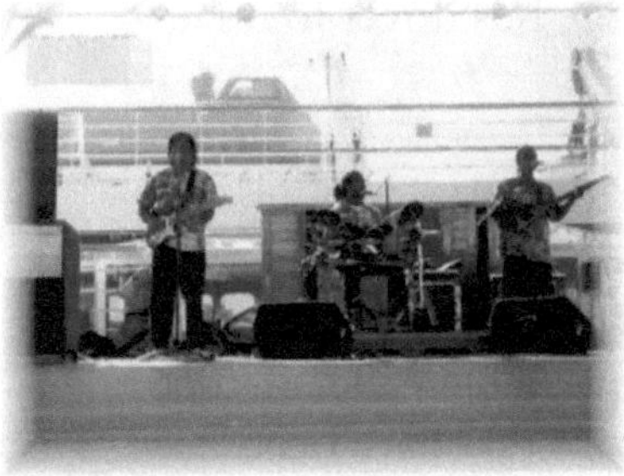

The tour bus drove up to the backwoods of Martinique. Though French, our tour guide spoke fluent English and was able to describe most of the vegetations along the route. It being in the tropical zone, Martinique has an abundant population of tropical animals and creatures; we observed lizards and other creatures climbing trees while some were unhurriedly crossing the roads unmindful of our presence.

Towering trees of tropical classifications flank the roads on both sides making the roadway somewhat dark and misty.
After two to three hours of bus ride, we gladly stopped to eat and rest at a general store which sits on a wide and well-manicured lawn. From the location, we had a full view of Mt. Pele, the volcano that killed 30,000 people on its last destructive eruption in

At Martinique, Martinique

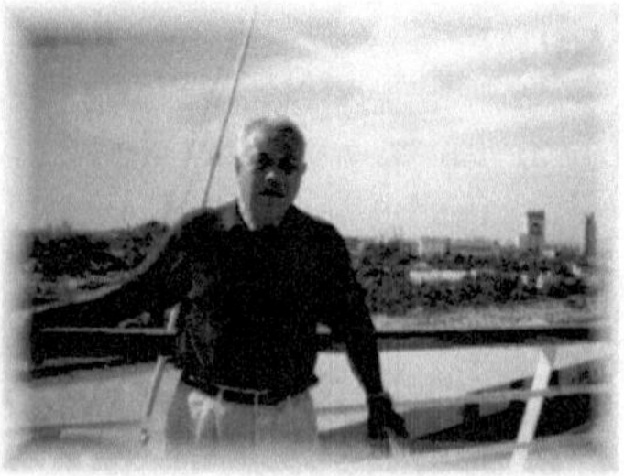

1902. Actually, the general store is located in the hinterlands, a location that showcases the lush and tropical jungles of Martinique. Inside the general store is a winery which offered free wines and ice creams, courtesy of the tour company.

Well fed and rested after an hour, we climbed back to the bus for the return trip to port by way of the coast. This time additional attribute of the island was showcased in the form of beautiful coastlines. White beautiful beaches stretch for miles and miles along the coast. The sight of many parasailers, surfers, and kayakers, delighted us that we prompted the bus driver to drive slower to allow us to take some pictures.

Opposite the ocean side of the road and towards the mountains, we could see more tropical plants with cattle and horses grazing at the corralled green grassy areas at the fore lowlands. Finally, we were about to finish our tour of Martinique, a once in a lifetime experience for us, considering the handicaps that have been bothering Amelia for some time now.

The tour bus stopped at the small marina where our excursion started from or close thereby. The marina was where Amelia's hunger syndrome began to make its presence felt; she started to stutter and could hardly walk straight without assistance. Her hands were cold, her complexion pale, and she was sweating liberally. It was past her lunch time, and she needed to eat food and drink liquid, I knew. Dolly, Dennis, and I were

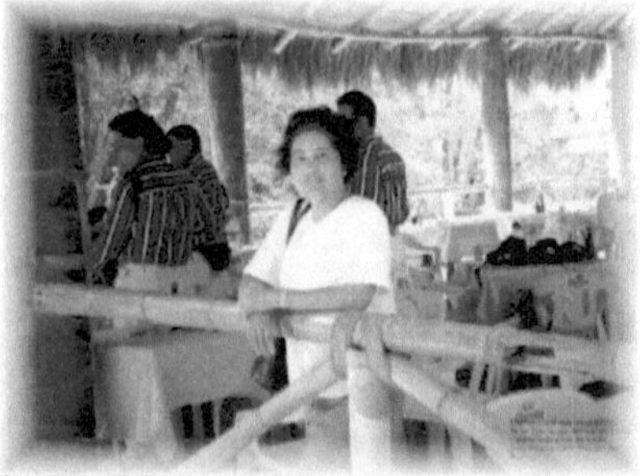

At Martinique, Martinique

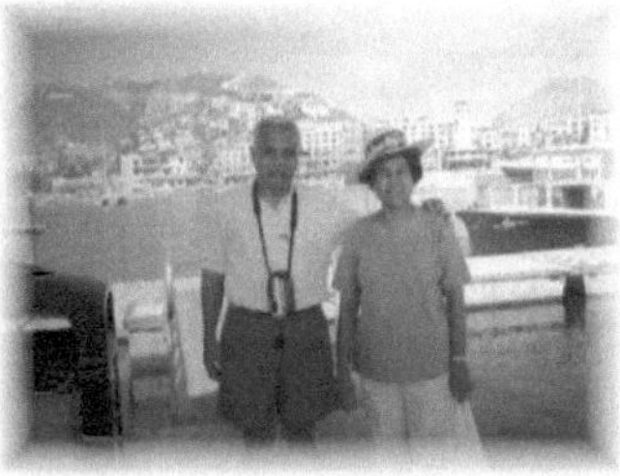

hungry too, but hunger affected Amelia more so than others because of diabetes.

It took us about fifteen minutes to find an eating place which turned out to be serving American food also. Hurriedly, I ordered food just for Amelia bypassing the customers ahead of us, who understood the circumstance for my rudeness. When Amelia finally got her food and drinks and started eating, her complexion returned to normal. She stopped perspiring and could stand and walk steadily without assistance again. Meantime Dolly, Dennis, and I waited for our turn in the queue to get food.

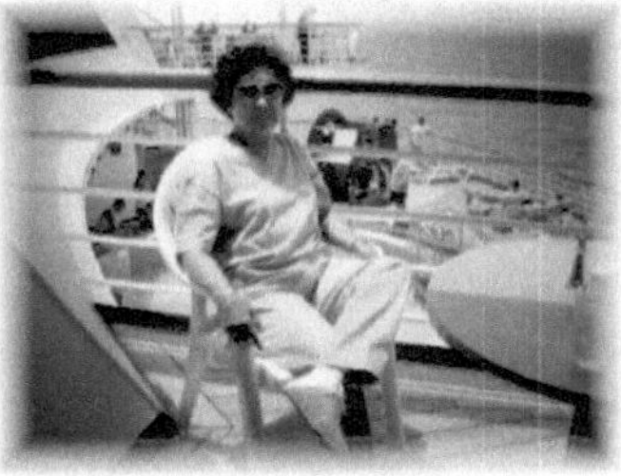

The day's excursion already fulfilled, we were anxious to get back to the cruise ship. We boarded the boat that took us to Fort de France whence the tender took us back to the cruise ship. We finished the day resting and relaxing on the ship, deciding what type of entertainments to watch before retiring to the cabin.

Overall, the tour of Martinique was an absolute success. Without reservation, I recommend the tour to anybody because it is fun and different, Martinique being geographically located in the tropical zone. Martinique and the Caribbean have elements of romance in their names and sounds.

At Barbados, Barbados

As usual, a cruise ship sails during the night and docks at a particular port early in the morning to allow tourists to enjoy enough daylight for sightseeing. This morning we found our ship docked at the pier at Bridgetown, the capital of Barbados.

The capacity of the dock to take on our cruise ship which was the largest at the time, with enough space to spare for other ships was an indication of how big the city of Bridgetown is. The ship alone was more than twice the length of a football field. Docking the ship at the pier favored the tourists because they did not have to be tendered.

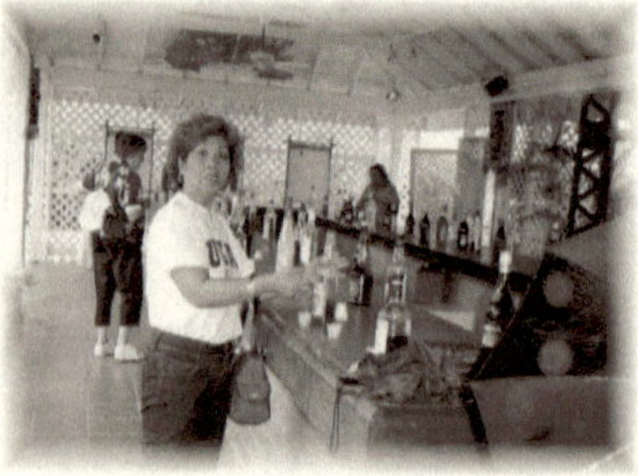

At Barbados our excursion was to a winery for what else - rum tasting - located about three hours away from the wharf. But first, we had to walk the length of the pier to the customs area to join the group. The long walk was all right with me; my concern was Amelia's inability to walk long distances. Slowly and carefully and with a little assistance from me, we reached the customs area and got clearance to board the tour bus for the trip to the winery.

Along the route, the bus made frequent stops for the tour guide to describe scenic areas and historical sites which depict some of the struggles that Barbados had to fight to gain its independence. The tourists who were keen on buying souvenirs for their loved ones back home were able to do so at souvenir shops. Not knowing whether eating facilities were available at the winery, we ate lunch

At Barbados, Barbados

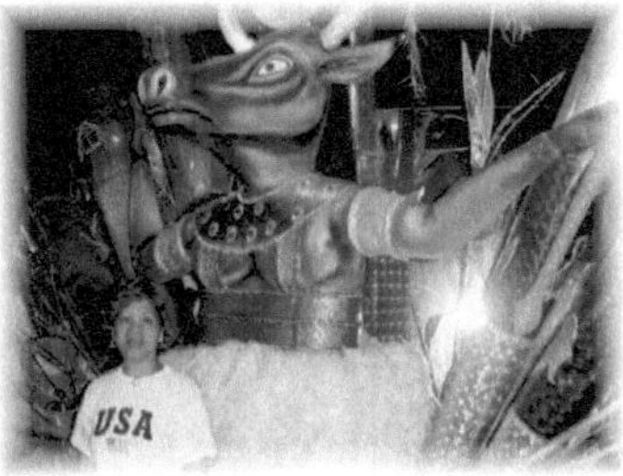

instead of shopping to avert the fluctuation in Amelia's glucose level.

The demonstration of the brewing process was just starting when we reached the winery few minutes past noontime. Not wanting to understand the process thoroughly and trying not to appear rude, we had to listen and watch the demonstration of how rum has to undergo, before it becomes a beverage. After all, we just had a moderately heavy lunch before we arrived and were ready to taste the rum for which we came.

After the demonstration which lasted about twenty minutes, we were taken to a huge area where bottles and barrels of rum were stored. We were told that the place exports rum to countries all over the world and that what we saw was just a small part of the extensive rum inventory. Adjacent to the area was small rum tasting building which was just filling with tourists not only from our ship but also from other places arriving in different modes of transportation.

It was unbelievable how many tourists were in the brewery for rum tasting. For the first time, I tasted fresh rum from sugar cane, and I honestly liked it. Judging from the expressions on their faces, I could tell similar approbations from other tourists. It was not unusual to see some visitors going for more than one round of tasting, each round tasting one kind of rum; there were several kinds, and tourists were not limited in the number of times they went around.

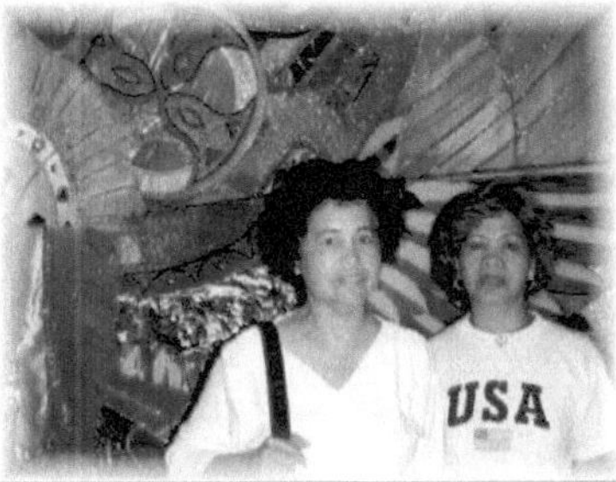

At Barbados, Barbados

After the rum tasting which lasted about two hours, we were ready to get back to the ship on a different route from the one we came through. Along the way, we passed by St. John's church where we stopped for fifteen to thirty minutes allowing us to say some prayers. The route took us through the vast expanse of sugar cane plantations, the source of rum. We also drove by old and abandoned cannons, testaments to Barbados' historical and turbulent past.

Back at the ship, we rested and relaxed waiting for nightfall to find out what entertainments to watch or hear. We considered the excursion entertaining, educational, and historical. It demonstrated how an industry of the rum type, could help a country's economy and independence. With the diminished demand for sugar, product like rum from sugar cane is an absolute substitute industry.

At Targoles River, Costa Rica

The day before we boarded the cruise ship we joined an excursion promoted by the hotel to the Florida Everglades, to watch and hear accounts of how alligators survive and react when humans get close to them. And here again on the cruise ship, I was reading a brochure of the excursion to watch the same, but different size species of animals in their habitat at Targoles River, Costa Rica.

Whereas the smaller alligators at the Everglades tend to hide below the surface of the water these giants of creatures, the crocodiles of enormous size, are seen in the open along the banks of the river unperturbed by the presence of humans. Out of curiosity, I signed up for the excursion.

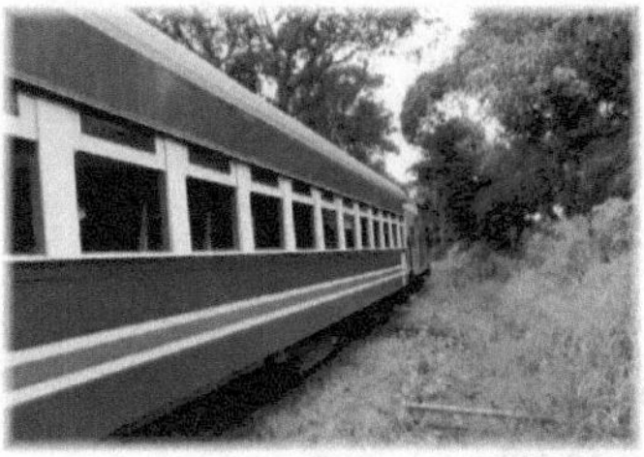

Getting to Targoles River was a short story by itself. From Puntarenas pier, we boarded a comfortable air conditioned bus to hook up with a train that took us deep into the jungles of Costa Rica.

The train was of the old types depicting Costa Rica's colonial history and its progress into the current century. The train ride was very uncomfortable - it was meant to be such to recreate history - because of heat, noise, humidity, and rocking motion. Nevertheless, we made the ride to Targoles River in about two hours.

In a market where fresh fruits and drinks were served, the tour guides - some of them from different groups - were giving last minute instructions to the tourists, in effect saying, 'keep your hands to yourself inside the boats.' The warning, though simple, was very sinister and easily understood by the tourists; they already had mental pictures of the huge crocodiles.

At Targoles River, Costa Rica

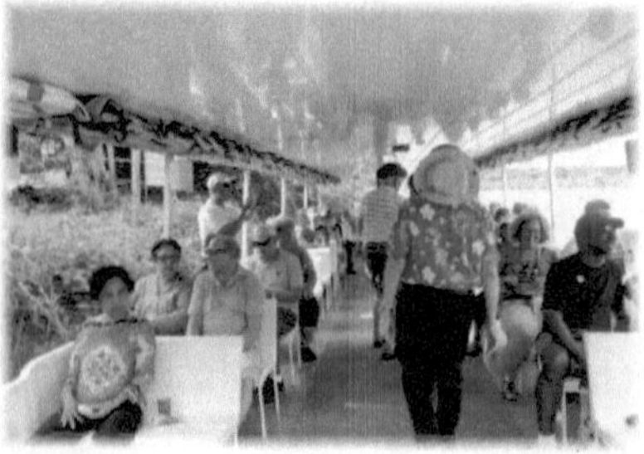

If there was an indication of the popularity of the excursion, it was the significant number of river boats all ready to pick up the tourists coming from all directions by different modes of transportation. The market place was very crowded; there was hardly a vacant space for parking. Long lines formed at the hospitality areas and snacks and sodas were selling as fast as they were restocked.

Our boat was about a dozen steps down from the river bank at about 40-degree incline. Amelia was helped down by two assistants, one each on her sides. We left her walker securely kept at the platform.

Before sailing, nicely printed brochures describing the different kinds of birds and mammals that inhabit the river, the river banks, and the trees farther inland, were handed to us. Our tour guide who majored biology in college, appropriately made use of her degree as a narrator during the trip, effortlessly describing and comparing each creature in the area against the pictures in the brochures.

We were not even fifteen minutes into our river excursion when ahead at the river bank, basking in the late afternoon sun, oblivious of the few birds near it, an enormous crocodile was observed. The tourists in our group - some fifty of them or so - eager to take pictures of the reptile, tended to crowd the boat on one side. Though I was sure that the flat bottom boat would not tilt over and sink, the tour guide jokingly reminded the tourists that swimming

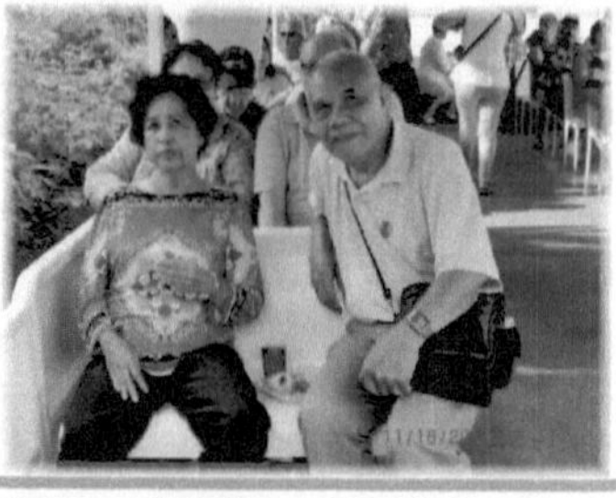

At Targoles River, Costa Rica

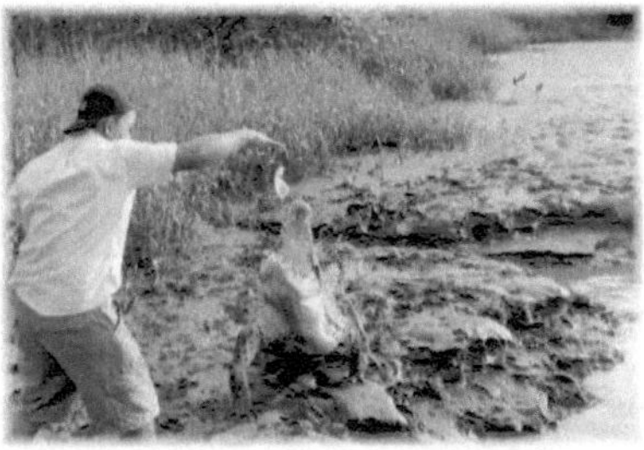

in the river was not an excellent idea, in case it did capsize.

Farther ahead, the pilot edged the boat to a clearing on the river bank, got out and fed some crocodiles with dead chicken. The crocodiles were unafraid of humans, snatching the chicken from the pilot's hand. I assumed that the pilot made a living out of his courage to feed the crocodiles, and therefore he was well trained in the dangerous art. The same death-defying feat was being performed for other groups a few hundred feet ahead and yet another one farther away - all three performances happening at the same time.

After the crocodile demonstration, the boat turned around to take us towards the wooded area of the river where flocks of birds of different kinds, perched. Taking control of the microphone, the tour guide in a classroom-like scene, led the tourists in matching them against the brochures.

The tour turned into a matching puzzle, adding more fun and excitement to the passage through the dangerous Targoles River. It was getting late in the afternoon and was time to head back to the tourists' assembly area where the tour bus picked us up.

The tour bus dropped us almost at the gangway of the ship, a favor we highly appreciated because of Amelia's physical disability. Except for the train ride, Amelia did not experience any discomfort during the excursion which I felt vindicated for its selection. We spent the rest of

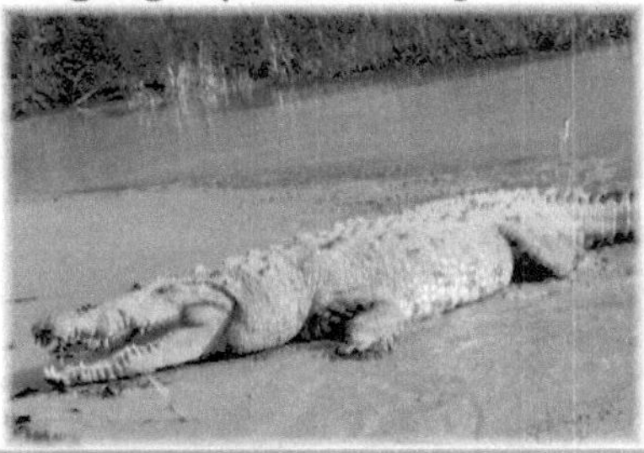

At Targoles River, Costa Rica

the day resting and relaxing, waiting for the night entertainments.

To the wildlife lovers, the Targoles River tour is one that should not be missed. For a small country, Costa Rica is rich in history and adventure.

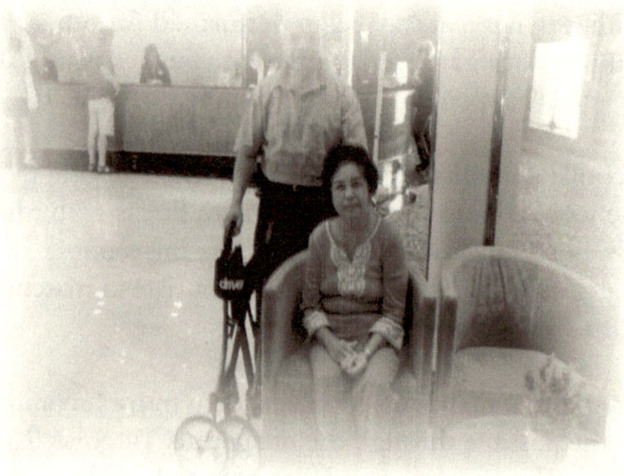

At Haiti Coast, Haiti

We opted for this shore excursion over few others because of its moderate physical demand; it only required being settled on the motorized boat during the entire time of the outing.

Due to the distance from the ship to the assembly area of the excursion, we did not make it to the 9:15 AM sailing despite the help of a paid wheelchair pusher. Had we made it, the 2-hour duration of the excursion would have allowed us to return to the ship in time for lunch.

In the meantime on the shore, heat and humidity were sapping our stamina especially Amelia's, she having diabetes, had multiple strokes, has Alzheimer's, and diagnosed with congestive heart failure. The cruise ship even arranged for bottled water distribution right on the shore to alleviate the passengers' misery from the weather.

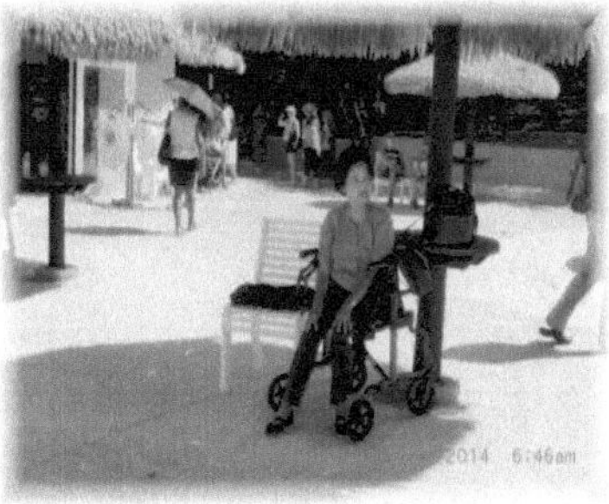

When the announcement came that we would be boarding the next boat at 11:15 AM, we were relieved. The boat was large enough for a group of about 15 passengers, so we did not have to bump into each other even when we moved around to take pictures. In constant motion, the boat helped in the passengers' catching the colder ocean breeze.

The boat first maneuvered to offer the passengers a different view from the ocean side, of our imposing cruise ship. It then veered towards the coastline and traveled for a short distance so that certain points of interest were visible while being described by the

At Haiti Coast, Haiti

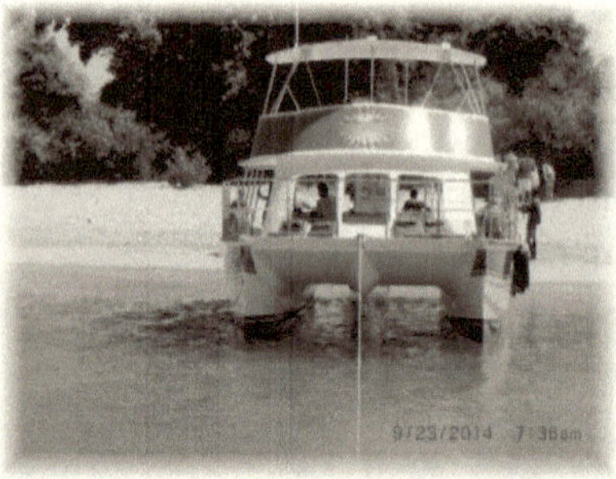

tour guide. Slightly veering out towards the open ocean again, the tour guide pointed out the reefs where shipwrecks lie beneath the surface.

The shipwrecks were part of the excursion for a unique reason. They have been creating a lucrative business, their metals being pilfered, salvaged, and hoarded for export by local nationals. The business has become very popular that well-financed enterprises have gotten involved in it, creating the impression that shipwrecks are wished to occur and welcomed in Haiti. On a clear day the skeletons of the ships can be seen by the naked eyes without being in the water, the tour guide narrated.

The boat then proceeded to a small wooded islet, less than five acres in size. The islet is surrounded by a wide span of white sand visible from a distance. During the day, sightseers and picnickers visit the islet, leaving it uninhabited during the night. Maintenance of the islet is provided by local nationals who depend on donations from visitors and sightseers. Keeping the islet clean is an incentive for more tourists to come and donate more, which in turn provides the incentives for the local nationals to keep it clean constantly.

The tour boat traveled a short distance from the islet to the bay where Columbus sought refuge from a storm. The bay protected Columbus' ships but had no source of fresh water. It had to be fetched from another area of Haiti towards

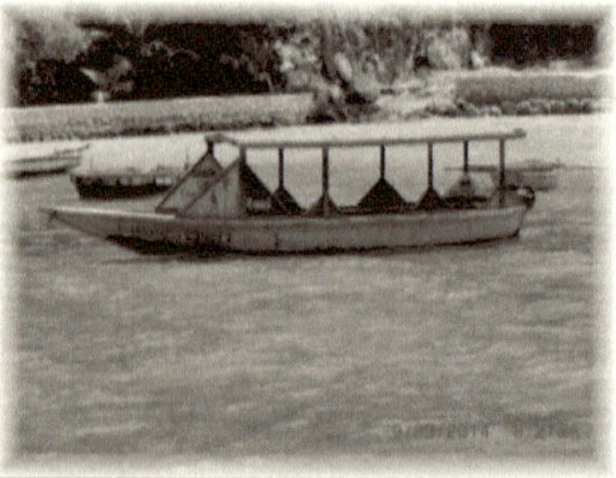

At Haiti Coast, Haiti

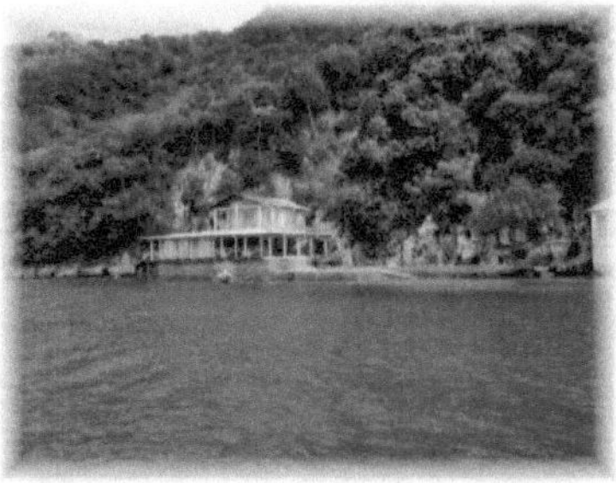

the pier where currently our cruise ship was docked.

The tour guide narrated that on a clear day - not during this particular excursion - the Citadel of Haiti could be seen from where our boat was temporarily stopped. Built to protect Haiti from French invasion after its newly gained independence from France itself, the Citadel was the largest fortress in the Americas at the time of its active commissioning.

With nothing else in the itinerary and with the wind starting to blow stronger, we turned around and headed for the cruise ship. The boat, working against the wind, was kept close to the coastline for the return trip.

Fishing boats were meandering their ways along the coast as well. Fishing being the primary source of income along this area of Haiti, fishermen equipped their boats with oars and sails. When the wind blows against their direction, they row, when it blows in the same direction as theirs, they raise the sails. Evidently, they work very hard either way.

More points of interest were pointed out to us, providing more photo opportunities. With high rugged mountainsides immediately rising from the ocean's edge, motorized land transportation like cars is non-existent. As close as we were to the coast, not one car was observed; boats are the traditional mode of transportation for residents including some from other countries who established residences of their own along the coast.

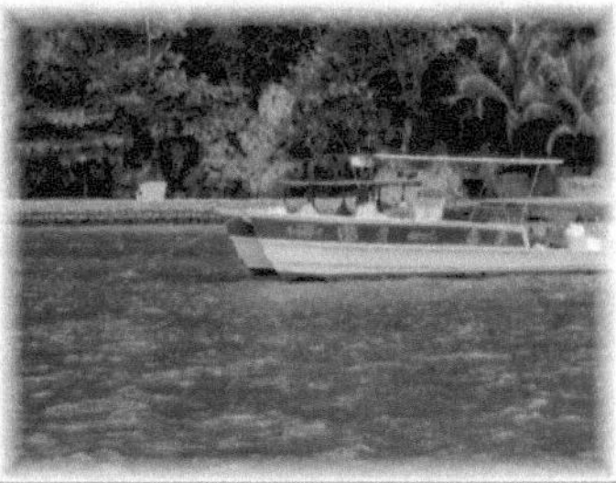

At Haiti Coast, Haiti

We got back to the cruise ship mid-afternoon, ready for late lunch or early snacks. The heat and humidity were still so intense to make one feel exhausted, tired, and drained of energy. We rested the rest of the day and waited for the night time shows.

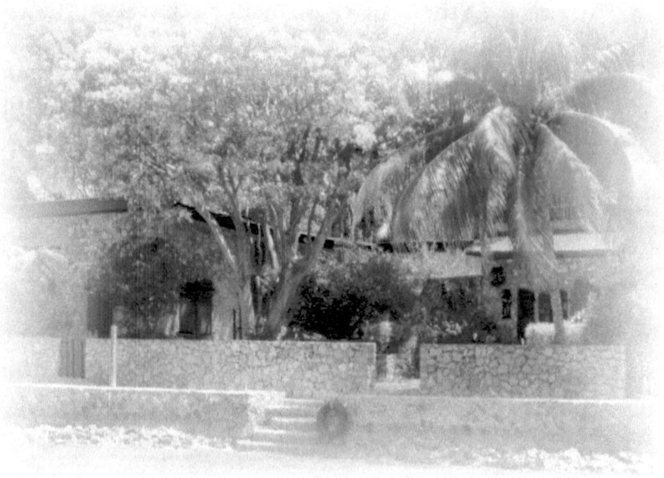

At Falmouth and Montego Bay, Jamaica

In all excursions, timing is always an issue for us because Amelia uses a walker which significantly hinders our ability to move. So it was a unique advantage when the gangway on the cruise ship opened on time to let the passengers off for various reasons. Ours was to be at the peach-colored building at noon, at the port area to join the group excursion to Montego Bay. To reach the building, I had to push Amelia on her walker for less than a mile from the ship. Past the customs area, the streets are cobbled or paved with tiles of slightly uneven heights causing me some maneuverability problems with the walker.

We made it to the peach-colored building fifteen minutes before departure time, where a sports utility vehicle which held fifteen passengers was waiting. Not needing the walker because wheelchairs were provided at Montego Bay, we left it at the building under the care of tour personnel.

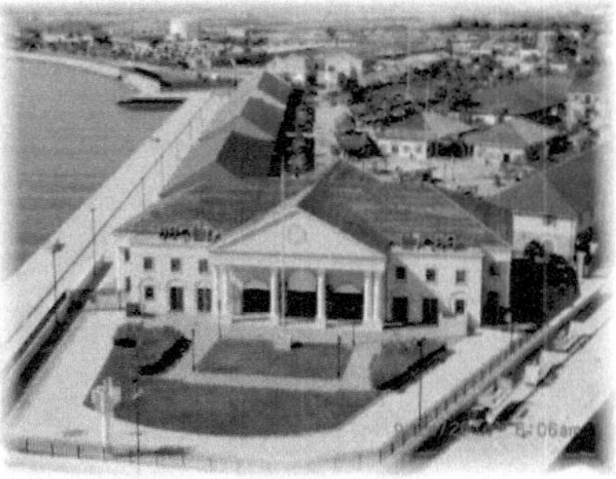

The first thing I noticed as the vehicle started to move was the side of the road the vehicle was being driven. On both two-lane and multi-lane highways, the opposing traffic was coming on the right lanes. Jamaica, having been a British colony, still manifests British colonial vestiges including vehicular travels. It was not surprising then that the steering wheels of the vehicles are on the right side. It took me a while to get rid of my cringy feeling of seeing from my perspective, cars driving on the wrong side of the road.

At Falmouth and Montego Bay, Jamaica

Along the Caribbean Ocean on one side and the hillsides dotted with beautiful mansions built during the plantation era on the other, we drove through a smooth, excellent, and well-paved highway. In one section of the motorway, cement trucks were lined up to deliver their cargoes, an evidence of many new constructions - some by foreign investors - being built along the highway.

The area where the song "Day-O", made famous and popular by the widely-acclaimed artist Harry Belafonte, was pointed out to us by our tour guide, and so was the rose-painted high school buildings where Usain Bolt, one of the fastest runners of all time, practiced barefoot on the school's track and field.

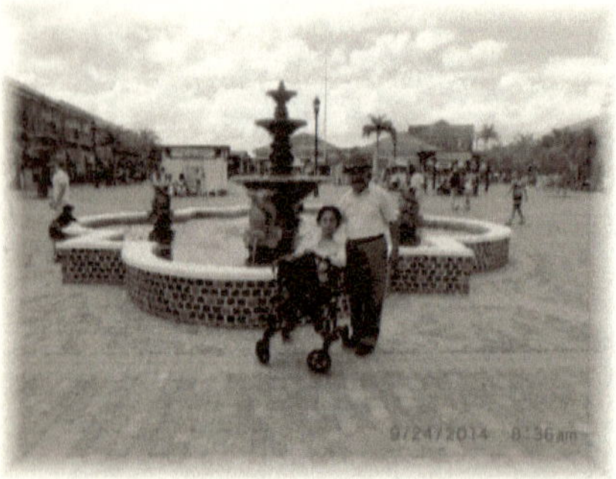

On the Caribbean Ocean side, large hotels and commercial buildings were visible, an indication of Jamaica's transition from the plantation era to a contemporary bastion of commerce. We drove by an airport where huge FEDEX planes were parked, yet another evidence of Jamaica's share of the global economy.

At a location where we made the turn from the highway towards Montego Bay, a row of old high school structures was being demolished and in its place a huge call center building was being constructed. We drove by Rose Hall, one of the most famous historical attractions in Jamaica where many sets of the James Bond movies were taken.

At Falmouth and Montego Bay, Jamaica

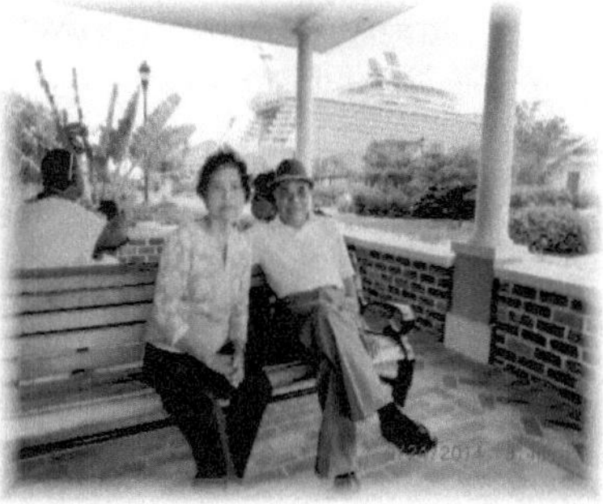

We arrived at Montego Bay Marine Park, our primary destination, at the designated time. But with visitors trying to avoid the rain, every possible space inside the building was taken, making it look extremely crowded.

Due to Amelia's physical disability, we decided to stay in the vehicle to avoid accidental slippage on the wet pavement. The rain was on and off, and the incline from the pavement to the park was treacherous even with the help of some park personnel. Our tour guide kindly brought us some very strong Jamaican Blue Mountain Coffee and delicious banana bread, the same treat that the tourists inside the park were enjoying. When the rain let up for a short time, I stepped out of the vehicle and took some pictures.

Across the bay are Jamaica's largest airport and most major shopping centers. When completed, Jamaica will also have the biggest cruise line terminal in the same general area. Unfortunately due to the haze caused by the heavy rain, vision across the bay was obscured at best.

I considered the excursion to Montego Bay very successful despite the disappointments caused by the rain. The tour personnel were very knowledgeable, courteous, and friendly. Our trip back on the same route offered more photo opportunities on the other side of the highway.

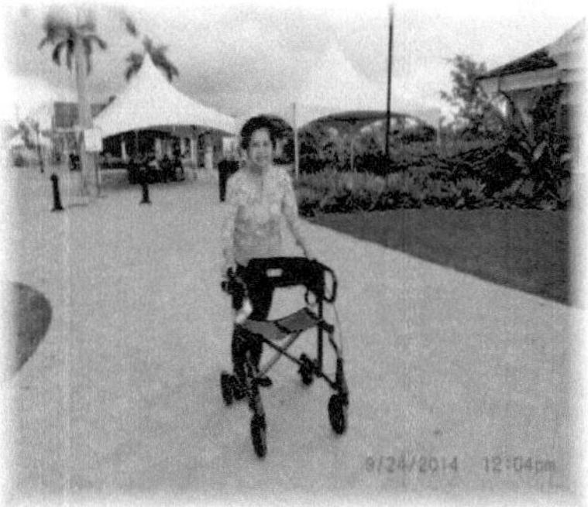

At Falmouth and Montego Bay, Jamaica

Jamaica has more to offer than what can be observed from a moving tour vehicle. We boarded the cruise ship at Falmouth in time for dinner. We rested the rest of the day in the comfort of our temporary home, The Allure of the Seas.

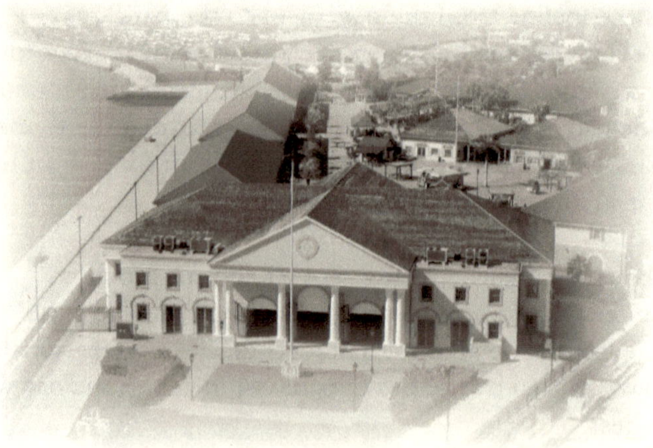

At Mexico Park, Mexico

If what the newsletters on the cruise ship said about Mexico Park were true then it was one which I had not seen any likeness before. The newsletters sharpened my desire to explore Mexico from the comfort of a single trip, by way of Cozumel's miniaturized representations of the country. The miniaturized reproductions are called maquettes. It is impossible to appreciate Mexico's diverse culture and vast territory by attempting to visit its places of interest. A miniaturized Mexico therefore, would suffice my curiosity about the country.

The departure time for the excursion was at 10:30 AM, but we started early as soon as the gangway on the cruise ship opened, to allow for our slow pace on account of me having to push Amelia on a walker. The walk covered slightly less than a mile from the ship, farther beyond the pier area, with the trip being slightly uphill between 5 and 10 degrees.

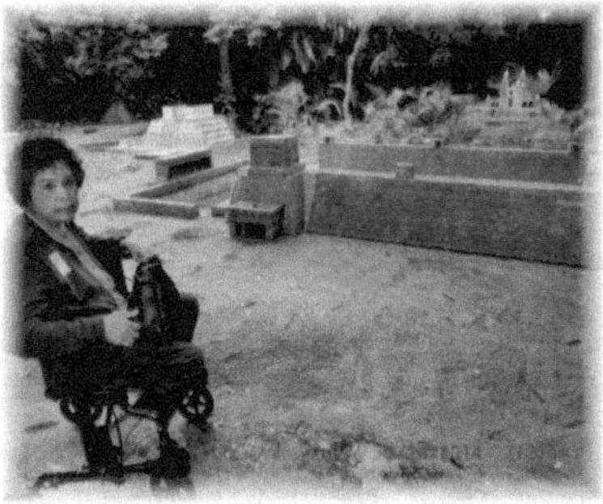

We arrived early at the assembly point in the shopping area of the port. The crews from the ship were on hand to help the tourists assemble their groups. Due to a light drizzle, we had to endure a slight discomfort even though enough tents were set up for the tourists who sought refuge from the rain.

It only took about 20 minutes to drive from the port area to Mexico Park. The tour guide first took us to a huge darkened museum where videos of the points of interest in the Cozumel part of Mexico, were playing. Thence, we were led to the displays

At Mexico Park, Mexico

of different artifacts, each group of artifacts representing a particular culture. There were the Inca's, the Mayan's, the Azteca's, to name a few that I could remember. Due to the darkened hall, we only took random pictures which did not turn out clear, to my disappointment.

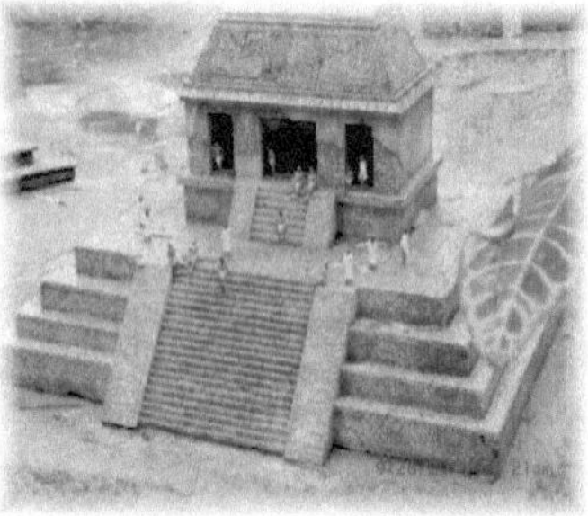

We exited the museum on to the park. The pathways on the park are graveled, so I had a minor problem negotiating them with Amelia's walker. The park consists of miniaturized replicas of all that is Mexico with respect to culture and era. The scale of miniaturization is 1 to 25, each inch in a maquette representing 25 feet in actual edifice or ruin which measured probably in millions of feet.

Because we were always left behind the crowd, I had more time to take pictures of the maquettes. The maquettes representing the ruins of a particular culture alone took an hour or so to admire, study, and peruse. I imagined that the engineering employed in the construction of the actual edifices without the benefit of heavy equipment was astonishing if not daunting.

We rested for about half an hour to eat lunch and hydrate ourselves. While doing so, we watched locals hand painting tiny multi-colored artifacts with uncanny precision. At first, I thought that the art of painting was just to make the locals' time worthwhile. To my admiration, just a short distance away, there was a store of thousands of these

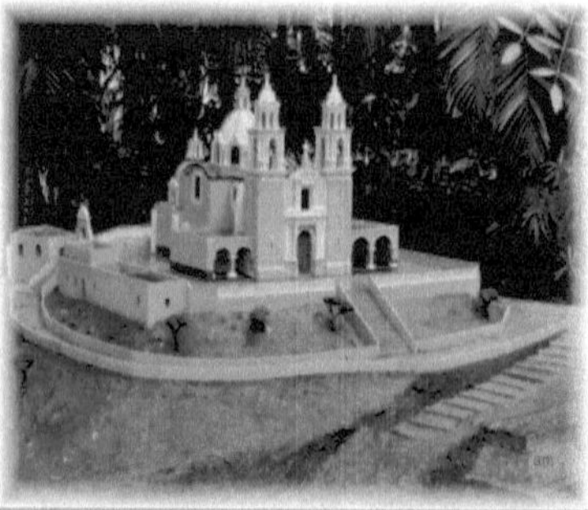

At Mexico Park, Mexico

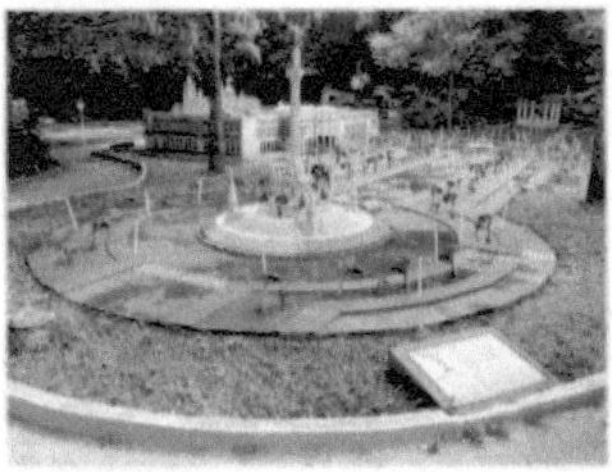

artifacts in various shapes and colors produced in the same meticulous and tedious way - hand painting.

After lunch, we moved on to the part where modern Mexico is again represented in exact miniaturized replicas. Famous buildings, mostly sets of government at different points in time, are precisely replicated. Some buildings housed famed Mexicans who had influence in making Mexico what it is now.

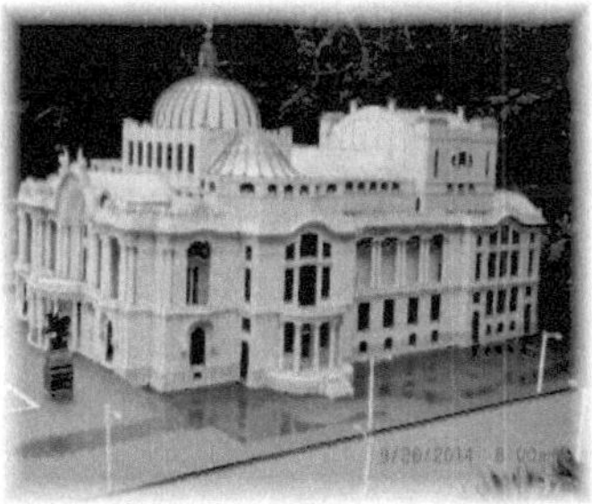

I considered the excursion historical, educational, and successful. Cozumel truly presents Mexico in a nutshell. The fact that the different cultures and cities of Mexico complete with edifices are represented in a single park made me wonder whether this was not the best way to represent a country. How the maquettes were precisely built to scale is mind boggling especially to one without engineering training.

The tour guide had us taken back to the port area. We boarded the cruise ship in time for late lunch. Then we rested the rest of the day and waited for the night to fall which ushered new types of entertainments. It was seldom that a type of entertainment is repeated unless it was very popular often indicated by public demand.

At Mexico Park, Mexico

Chapter 11 – Destination Florida

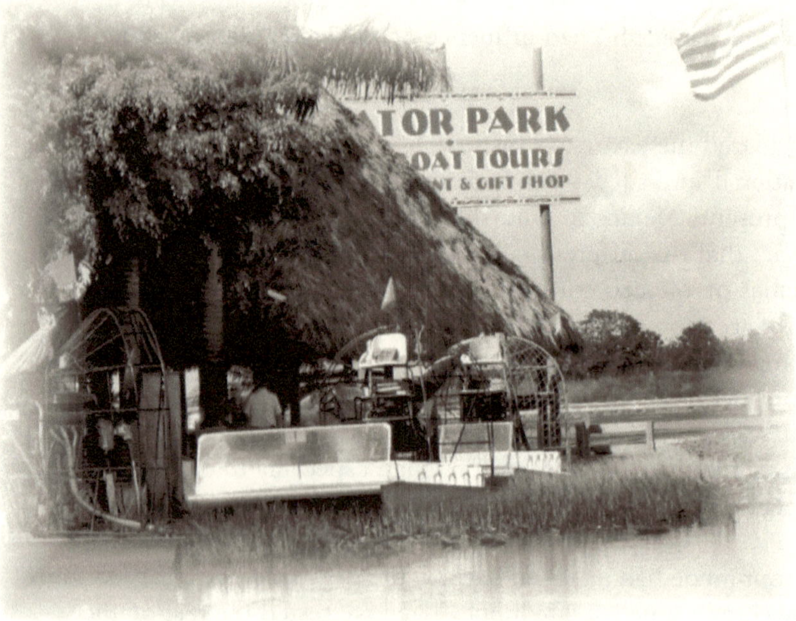

At Miami International Airport, Florida

Substitute photographs (picture-taking not allowed at the airport)

The president of the United States was coming to Florida a few hours behind our arrival at Miami International Airport. Traffic was just beginning to be rerouted as usual for his arrival, and supposedly our checkout from the airport was expected to be slightly stressful.

After six hours of flight time, I could see that Amelia was uneasy and tired. Just on the third month of recovery from her most recent stroke, she could hardly walk even with a walker, but with encouragement, she made the distance to a small airport store where I had her sit down and drink a fresh bottle of water. Humidity was exceptionally bad that she felt slightly dehydrated. While taking care of her, I asked around and found out that the baggage claims area was one level down, accessible by elevators from our current location.

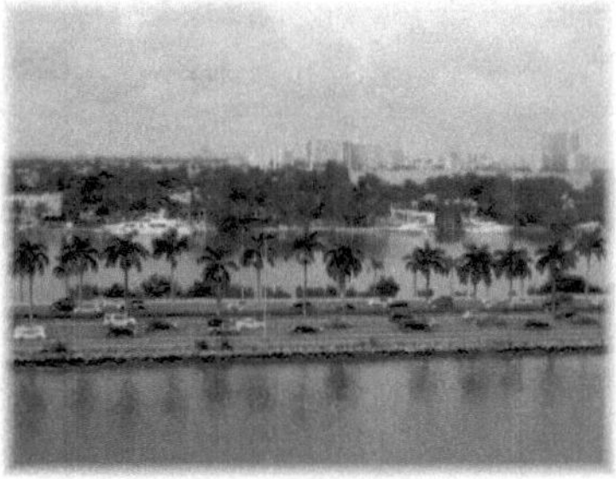

With enough coaxing again, Amelia made the distance to the elevator, and we descended to the baggage claims area. I had her sit down on her walker at a corner about thirty feet from the carousel where the pieces of luggage were rolling out. I covered the distance back and forth several times to check if Amelia was all right and if our luggage had already rolled out.

At Miami International Airport, Florida

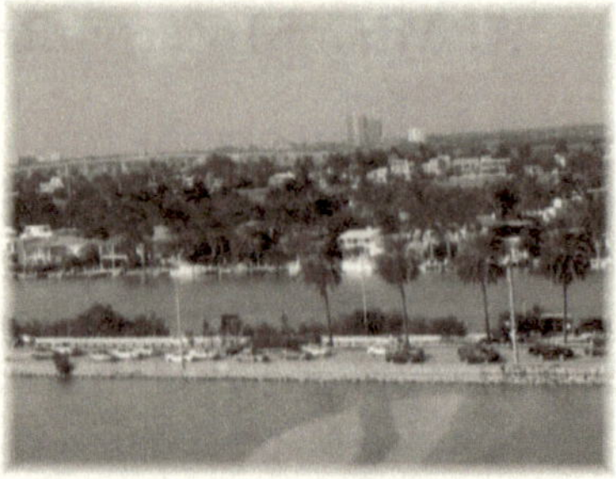

Finally, I gathered our luggage and deposited them close to Amelia while I contemplated our next move. How to pull two pieces of 50-pound luggage and carry a backpack while tending to Amelia on a walker, was a developing problem at hand. The elevators to the second level were very crowded; it was not a good idea in our case to rush along with other passengers who were in a hurry to avoid the expected traffic jam.

I saw an opening, and while encouraging Amelia to follow, I let go one piece of luggage, pushed the elevator button, and picked up the luggage again, just to get in. It did not work; Amelia was being squeezed out and left behind. We had to wait till we could have the elevator almost by ourselves.

After most of the passengers had been gone, we made it to the second level where the courtesy bus stop was just across the doorway. However, we had to cross a wide and busy traffic lane to get across. First, I crossed the lane with the two pieces of luggage and the backpack and left them at the curb by the bus stop, walking back thereafter, to get and push Amelia on her walker across the lane.

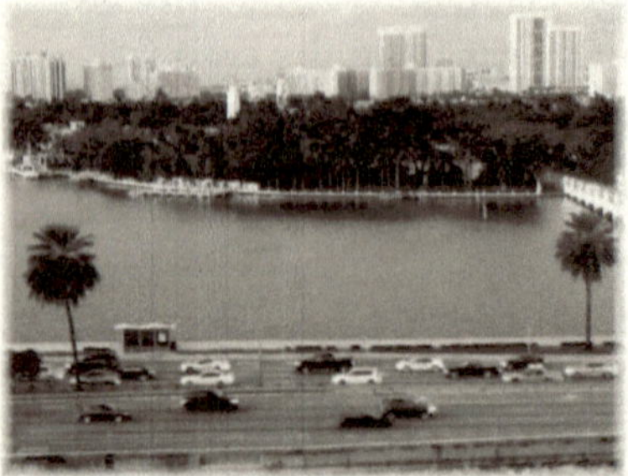

We waited close to forty-five minutes for the hotel's courtesy bus to arrive. While waiting, I had to take care that Amelia was comfortably seated on her walker under the humid air. Fearing that she might get dehydrated, I kept a bottle of cold water always

At Miami International Airport, Florida

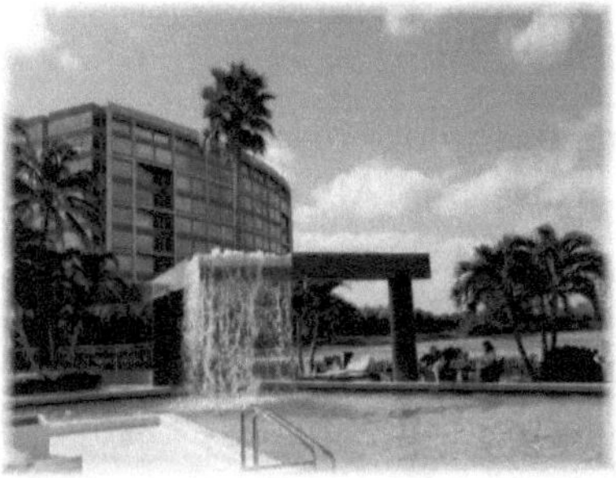

accessible to her. The courtesy bus finally arrived, taking us to the hotel.

We settled at the hotel exhausted because of the experience at the airport, but were thankful that nothing serious happened to Amelia. She rested until dinner time while I walked around to take a few pictures of the landscape around the hotel.

The airport experience was daunting, but if it was to fulfill Amelia's desire while she could still travel, I would not hesitate to do it again, for I feel that any of her wishes and requests could be her last before she finally succumbs to her ailments.

At the Everglades, Florida

Pre-embarkation excursions allow tourists to explore places in the vicinity of the port before boarding the cruise ship. My practice is to join with one if it is available, be it as an offer by the hotel or as part of the cruise vacation package.

Before we flew to Miami from Los Angeles for our Panama Canal cruise, I booked to join the excursion to the Florida Keys with a company apart from the cruise lines. However, from the information I gathered at the hotel, the long round trip to the Florida Keys would be afflictive to Amelia, considering that she was just three months into recovery from a stroke, her third. So we abandoned the trip to the Florida Keys, forfeiting the fees; instead, we joined the excursion to the Everglades.

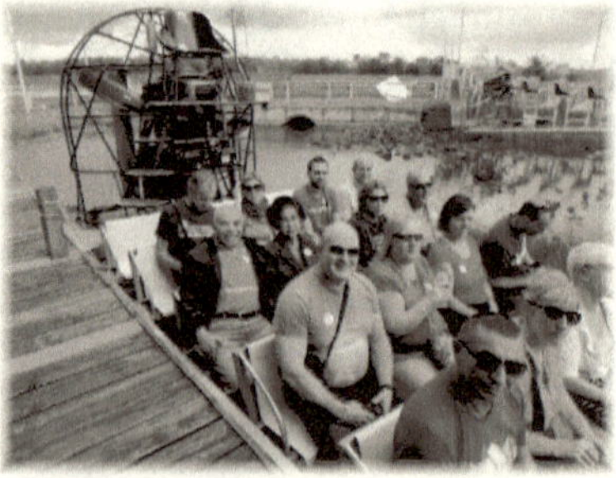

The trip to the Everglades took less than two hours. Though the sports utility vehicle did not have designated seats for passengers with disability, the Australians who made most of the tourists in the vehicle moved over and made room for Amelia. We were in a group of fifteen with Amelia, me, and a Spaniard being the only non-Australians. It was about 9:30 AM when we arrived at the Everglades and food was announced to be available at the stores before boarding the boat that would take us through the Everglades.

We passed up eating at the store so we could take the early boat ride and head back to the hotel as soon as the Everglades adventure terminated. Getting onto the boat from the platform was a struggle

At the Everglades, Florida

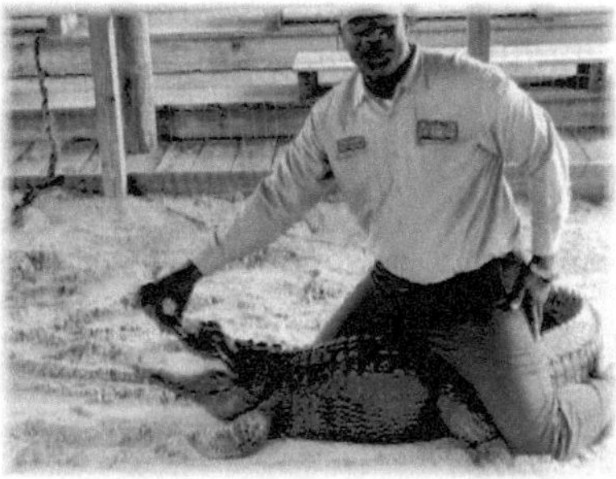

for Amelia even with my assistance. Thanks again to the Australians they helped her get into it.

I could observe Amelia's dread of riding on an unfamiliar boat. We were handed ear plugs to protect our ears from the loud and deafening noise generated by the engine. Amelia did not want to use them and threatened to throw them away into the water, an apparent violation of park regulations, not to mention the potential damage to her ears; I had to force her to use them. After listening to some precautions to be observed during the ride, the boat proceeded very slowly at first then it accelerated.

The boat glided through the Everglades forward, sideward, then forward again, at a very rapid rate of speed, then suddenly stopping, making the passengers lurch forward. The motion was repeated a few times that the passengers close to the side of the boat had to cling on to the rails and grab bars to keep them from being dislodged and thrown overboard. I had to hold Amelia because from her looks, she was even more concerned and afraid, wondering when the ride would end.

Asking her later at the termination of the ride if she enjoyed it, she nodded in approval. However, she could not move her right leg, the one weakened by the stroke, and she was on the way for the other passengers to disembark. For the third time, the good

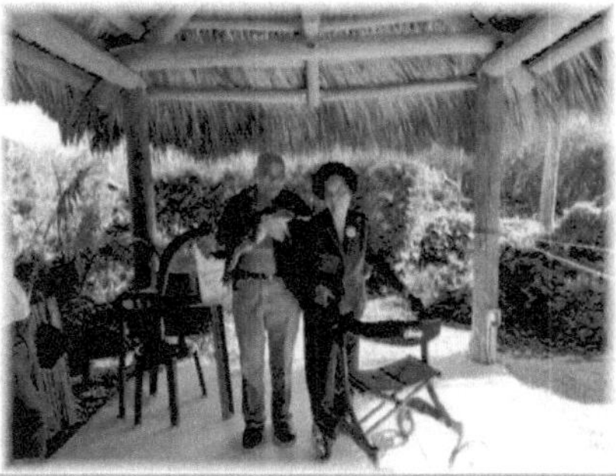

At the Everglades, Florida

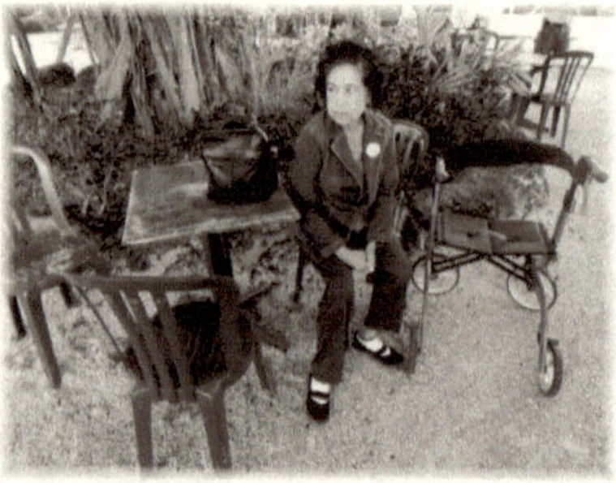

Australians came to the rescue; they helped her out of the boat again. By then we were ready for lunch.

I was not sure if it was serious or just a joke that we heard from other tourists in the stores that the sandwiches and hamburgers were of alligator meat. Upon hearing this, no amount of encouragement could convince us to eat the food at the stores. We ended up eating some crackers that I always carry along for Amelia on long trips.

The excursion was over, and we could then go back to the hotel. But, since the excursion was on contract, we could only head back to the hotel if all the passengers were ready. Some were not, so we spent the rest of the time watching alligator shows and displays of animals that inhabit the Everglades, until everybody was ready.

During the trip back to the hotel Amelia, exhausted and tired, slept soundly until we arrived at the hotel where we were dropped off together with the Australians; they were staying at the same hotel, and they turned out to be taking the same cruise vacation we were taking, the Panama Canal Cruise.

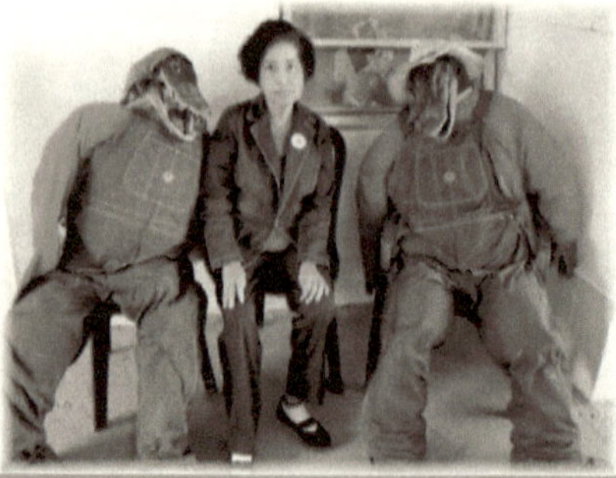

At the hotel, I asked around about transportation to the port for the following morning's embarkation. We had to take a taxicab to the port of embarkation, I was told, because I booked our cruise package with a travel company

At the Everglades, Florida

apart from the cruise lines, making us ineligible for free pickup by the courtesy bus. But, through the intercession by a friend who booked theirs direct with the cruise lines, we were accommodated in the courtesy bus the following morning, saving us the trouble of taking a taxicab.

All went well, and we appeared to be on our way to a very memorable 15-day Panama Canal cruise vacation, traversing the Caribbean Ocean on one side of the Americas and the Pacific Ocean on the other.

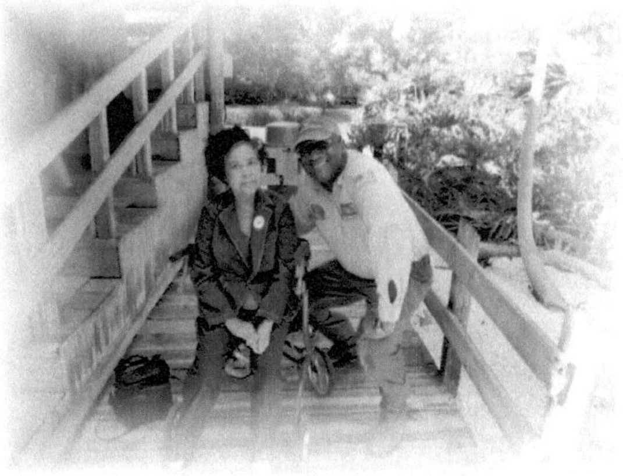

At Ft. Lauderdale Land and Sea, Florida

At Ft. Lauderdale Land and Sea, Florida

The $80.00 price for this excursion was smartly recouped in value of experience returned. First, we had the privilege of disembarking ahead of most passengers, second, we had the four-hour land and sea tour of Fort Lauderdale, and third, we were dropped off at the airport at the end of the excursion, together with our luggage. The drop-off saved us the trouble of temporarily staying in a motel or hotel to wait for our flight on the same day, and of hailing a taxicab.

Lauderdale Land and Sea was a four-hour post cruise excursion consisting of land and coastal tours of Fort Lauderdale. After a week of regular and fun activities on board the cruise ship except on days spent on excursions, we needed a break from the monotony of ocean sights and the lulling effects of the waves.

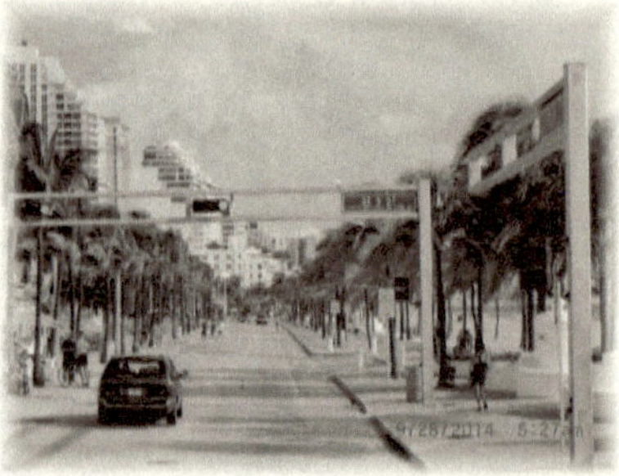

The land phase of the tour took us along S Fort Lauderdale Beach Blvd for a few miles with long stretches of white sand on one side and high rise buildings on the other. The day was moderately warm. Few canopies started being set up on the beach while beachgoers began to flock in bicycles, skateboards, and other modes of transportation. I did not know whether it was low or high tide; all I could see was hundreds of feet of white sand from the edge of the ocean to the wall separating the boulevard and the beach.

Many buildings, the tour guide pointed out have historical significance relating to the development of Fort Lauderdale. In fact in my personal observation, if the tour guide was right, all the buildings except for very few, would qualify as historical landmarks.,

At Ft. Lauderdale Land and Sea, Florida

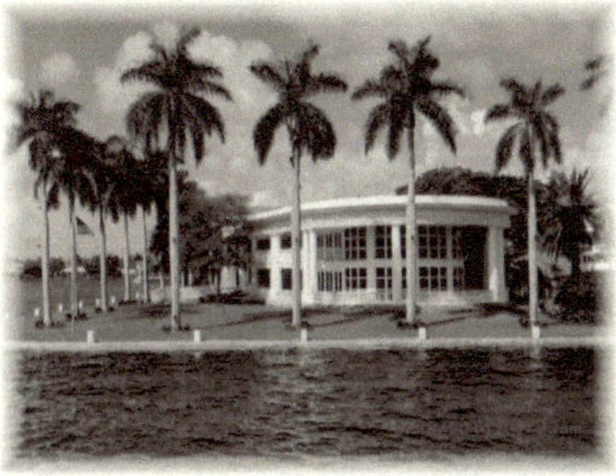

requiring a concerted effort to catalog and record to be remembered by generations to come.

While the land tour was going on, the tour guide related more stories about Fort Lauderdale, from its very beginning to what it is now. The one I vividly remembered that she narrated was how the city got its name; the name was after Major Lauderdale who was sent by General Jackson to fight and subdue the Seminole Indians, unsuccessfully. We visited a few more landmarks before we proceeded to the dock where a Mississippi paddle-wheeler style boat was waiting for us.

The boat has a kitchen from which we ordered sandwiches, hot dogs, sodas, and beers to be sure we were amply fed and hydrated during the excursion. When it appeared that no more passengers were coming on board, we proceeded with our sea tour of Fort Lauderdale, the Venice of America, on the Intra Coastal Waterway. First, we had to go through a series of narrow canals lined by moderately impressive homes and other structures on both sides, before we exited to the main Waterway.

On the way out towards the open ocean, we had a view of the Millionaires' Row, with unbelievably beautiful homes lining up both sides of the Waterway. The right-of-way rule required that our tour boat stay closer to land on the right side, allowing tourists to

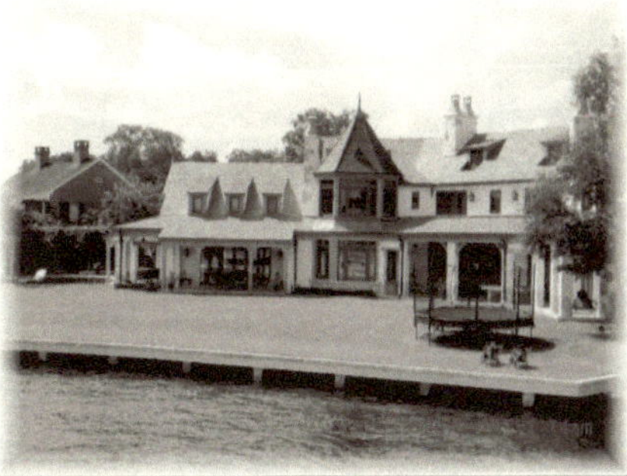

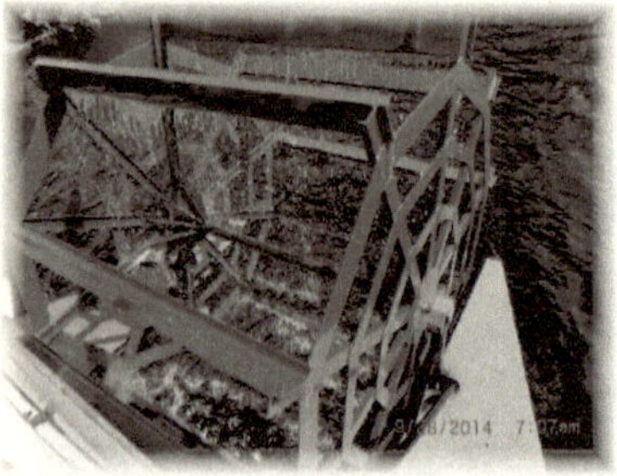

get closer to homes for photo opportunities. Each home has its dock naturally, enabling the owner to dock a yacht which, in some cases, amounts to few million dollars. At one point of the tour, the fastest yacht in the world was pointed out to us by our tour guide. Fort Lauderdale is the yachting capital of the world, we learned from him.

To put this display of wealth in perspective - we were sailing for about an hour one way in one direction at ten to fifteen miles per hour with occasional stops, and all we could see on just one side of the Waterway are mansions of enormous value and surreal beauty. We sailed under a draw bridge and as far out to the tour limit before the boat turned back. The same display of wealth is repeated on the other side of the Waterway.

"Lavish" was an understatement to brand this type of living as far as I could imagine. Contrasting our first and last excursions was heartbreaking. Back in Haiti, our first excursion in this particular cruise vacation, people were rowing strenuously and vigorously against the wind just to catch a fish for a chance to survive another day. In this part of Florida probably people are working just as hard, but more so to create wealth and bolster their holdings to create even more wealth.

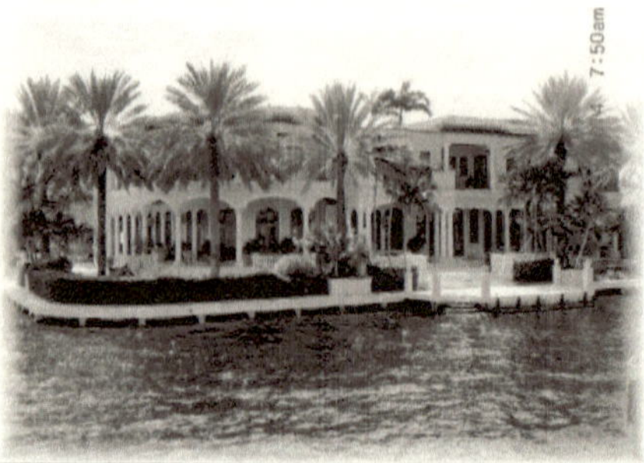

Unfair, yet it is true! The uneven distribution of wealth inflicts miseries to some people while it implodes

At Ft. Lauderdale Land and Sea, Florida

extreme happiness to some. It is easy to get carried away in comparing the disparity between the people of extreme wealth and the people of abject poverty, yet the reality is that some people are luckier than others. The more successful ones tend to be endowed with more luck while the unlucky ones tend to be more hapless and destined to be eternally that way.

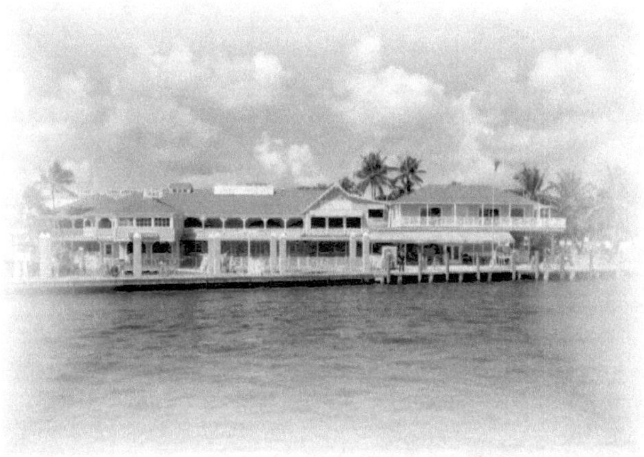

At Ft. Lauderdale Land and Sea, Florida

Chapter 12 – Destination France

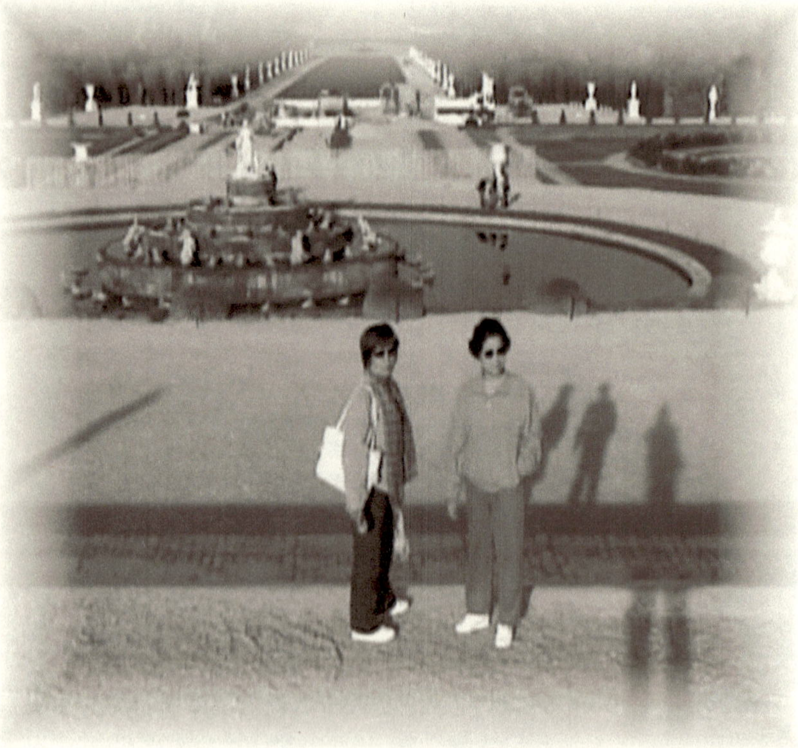

At Palais Longchamp, Marseilles

Where we were headed in this particular excursion was confusing at first. Palais Longchamp was not mentioned in the brochure; if it was, perhaps we missed it because we rushed signing up for the excursion to Notre Dame De La Garde before tickets would sell out. It came to pass that Palais Longchamp was included in the excursion package; we learned later when we boarded the tour bus.

Palais Longchamp was the stop that our excursion had to make before proceeding to Notre Dame De La Garde. It was a very nice stop it turned out, for the trip was reasonably comfortable except that the bus had to negotiate very narrow uphill streets among apartment buildings. Sometimes it needed to back off then push forward to make very sharp turns on street corners. Evidently, the tour bus driver has been making several of these trips for he maneuvered the bus unconcernedly even with some sense of hurriedness to reach the destinations on time.

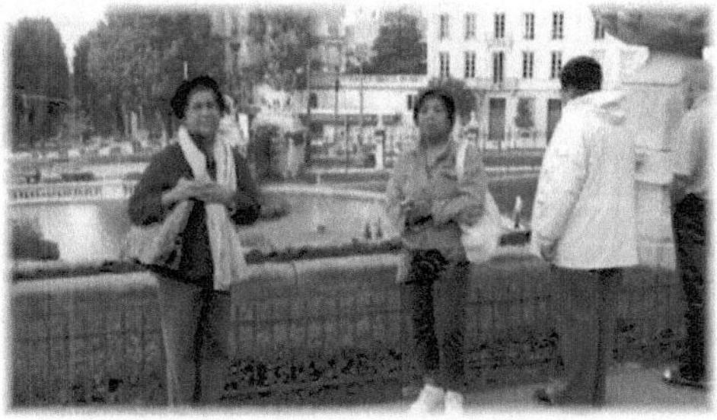

We arrived at Longchamp already crowded with tourists. With numbered placards raised overhead, tour guides from various excursions assembled their groups to orient them about the palace before proceeding on a short tour. Unfortunately, our tour guide was way ahead of us on a rise of the landscape which Amelia could not make quickly in time for the assembly. They proceeded with the tour of the palace without us because of Amelia's physical condition.

At Palais Longchamp, Marseilles

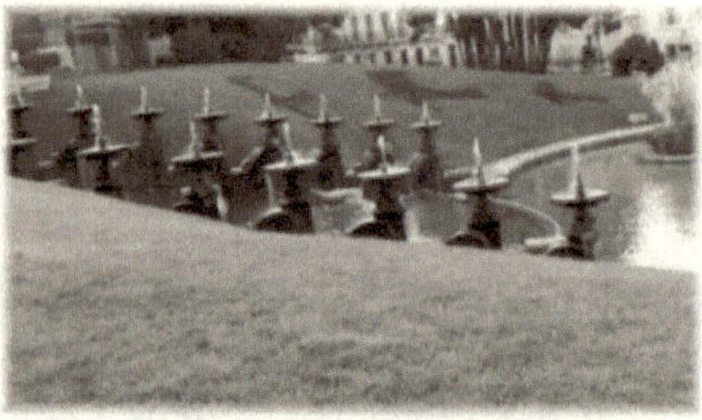

We hoped to rejoin the group when it came back from the short trip. Making sure that Amelia was comfortable with the slight rise and fall of the landscape, we opted to stay at the base of Longchamp. It has enough attractions to satisfy a tourist's curiosity and admiration from all angles after all. We were just as happy resting at the base as we would have been enjoying the uneven path taken by the tour.

Water is abundantly flowing from a huge lofty waterfall in front of the palace. A lake nearby with symmetrically arranged water-suspended balls is itself a tourist attraction; water fountains are spouting and seemingly sucking the water back in unison. I could not help wondering how so much water was able to be directed to the palace a hundred years or so ago with probably using the bare minimum of equipment.

Leaving Amelia at the base, I climbed the stairs of the palace where I was even more surprised and impressed at how sturdy and wide the walls are. From my vantage point, I had a panoramic view of the water being dispensed from the palace. The sound of the waterfall was even more distinct and naturally semi-thunderous as it cascades to the fountain at the base. The tourists at the base all appeared to be looking up making them including Amelia, a real target of excellent photography.

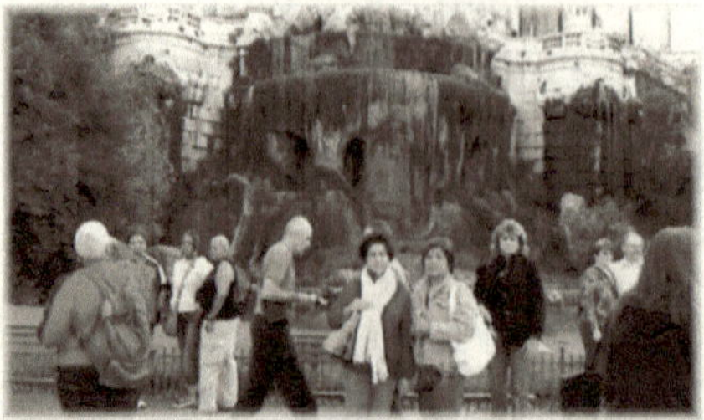

The area around the palace had sheltered some rowdy characters for a while, our guide told us. But the government has started taking back control of the city. The

At Palais Longchamp, Marseilles

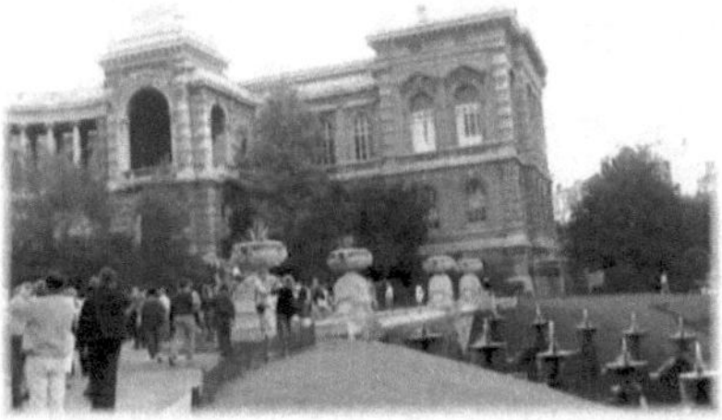

streets are starting to be widened and cleaned; trash has begun to be picked up regularly.

Businesses have begun to come back, and the government started earning taxes from the tourists, for the improvement of the area around the palace. Evidently, with the number of tourists visiting it, the palace ought to support a growing economy in the area. We rejoined our group and boarded the bus for the next stop, the Notre Dame De La Garde.

At the Louvres Museum, Paris

Our target for sightseeing this particular day was the Louvres Museum located at the banks of the Seine River in Paris. The hop-on-hop-off bus that would take us to the museum was at the Triumphal Arch at the center of Paris, which was about thirty minutes away from our hotel. Dolly, Dennis, and I did not have any problem covering the distance whatsoever, but to Amelia, this short trip on foot was tiring because of her physical disability.

The museum was very crowded. The ticket counters and entrances are located below the street level, accessible only by using the escalators. Always looking for a chair or bench where Amelia could sit, I found none, to my disappointment. I was concerned about Amelia's ability to remain standing for an extended period, without having some type of discomfort arising from her ailments. The lines and wait times at the ticket counters were long, only breaking when some tourists gave up waiting, or when they opted for different but shorter tours. Dolly and Dennis decided to take the longer tour while I chose the cheaper and shorter one.

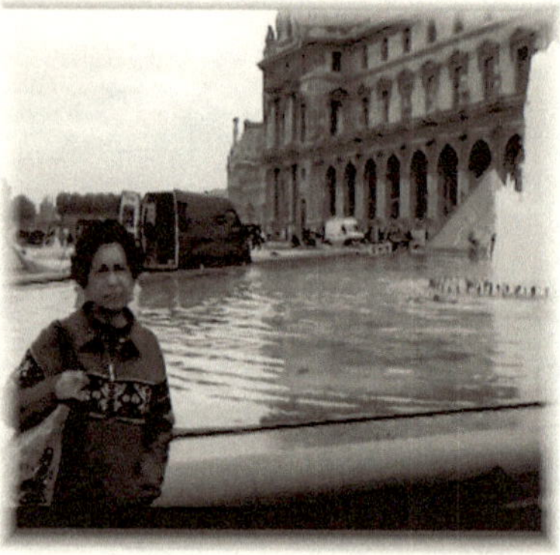

Amelia argued with me that we should have joined Dolly and Dennis in order to have company during the tour of the huge museum. I explained to her that her inability to walk long distances was the reason we took the shorter tour. Apparently she was not convinced, fearing that we could easily get separated and lost in the crowded and busy museum.

At the Louvres Museum, Paris

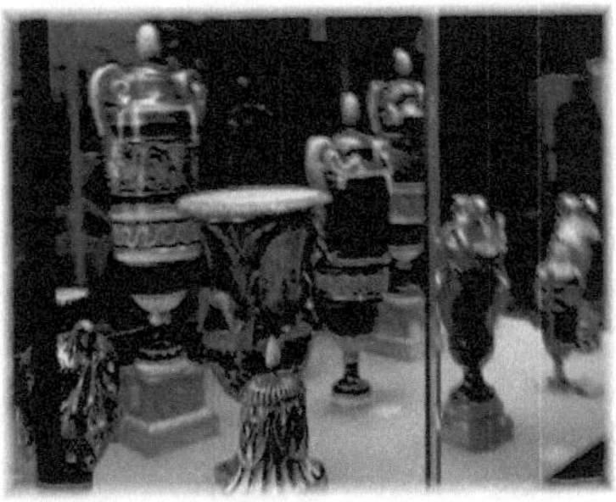

We finished the tour, disappointed that picture taking was not allowed inside the museum. Even with the shorter tour, we ended up exiting at the far end of the building which, to my estimation, must be more than one hundred fifty yards from the museum yard where tourists were congregating.

By then the museum yard was so crowded that the only place to sit down was on the fountain rim. I could tell that Amelia was exhausted, tired, and hungry; her hands were noticeably shaking. Fearing that her glucose level might have gone down, I fed her with fruits which I carried around to combat her hunger. But she needed water or juice which we did not have anymore, having consumed all of them earlier.

Buying water from the vending machines located at the museum entrances would take me longer than twenty minutes. I did not want to leave Amelia alone in her slightly unstable condition, lest she might have an emergency without me around. Noticing my predicament, some kind tourists offered Amelia some orange juice, which we thankfully took and acknowledged. Amelia gradually recovered; her energy was evident again.

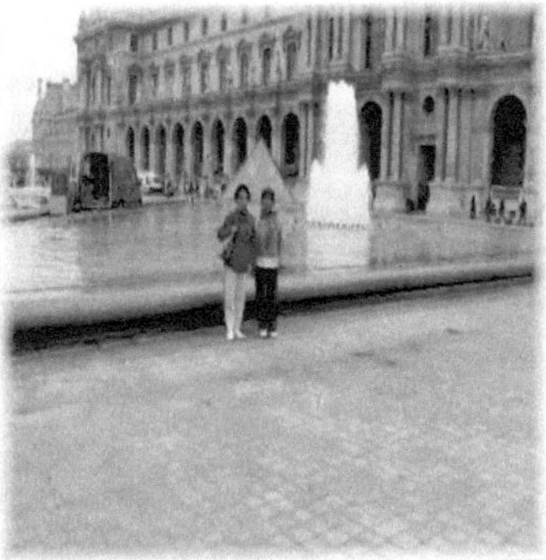

While mulling about whether we had enough energy to fill the rest of the day with activities, we were joined by Dolly and Dennis at the fountain. They considered their longer tour a success. Ours was equally pleasant

At the Louvres Museum, Paris

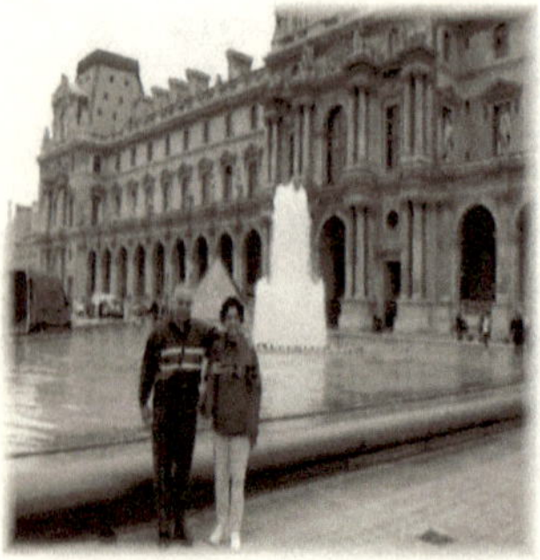

and successful, except for Amelia's slight emergency.

During lunch at a restaurant near the museum, we concluded, after confirmation with Amelia, that we had enough strength to go on another tour. Amelia was always the determining factor on whether to take on an excursion because she was the weakest in the group owing to her ailments. Since there was sufficient daylight to spare, we proceeded to our next target tour, Notre Dame, which is only a short distance away from the Louvres Museum.

At Versailles, Paris

With a full day under our disposal, we walked to the Triumphal Arch area of Paris where the underground train station is located. Without uttering a word, we pointed out on a map, to the ticket counter staff where we wanted to go - the Versailles. Not knowing how much the tickets cost, we placed enough Euros on the ticket dispenser to be sure the cost was covered. I did not know if we overpaid for them or not because we did not know where the change if any, was coming out and the gate restrainer was already opened for us to get in.

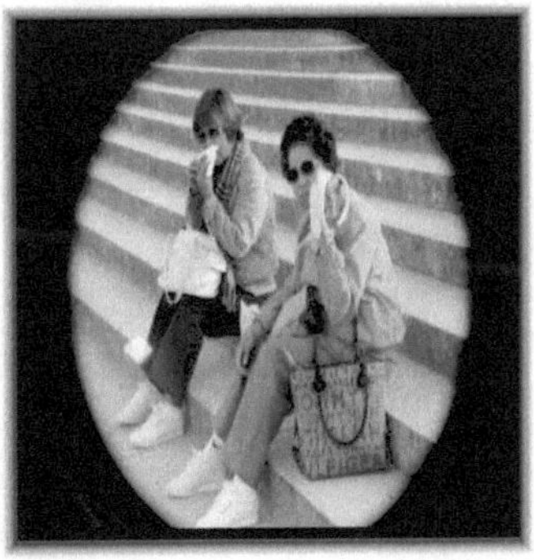

We thought that by asking fellow passengers, we would know which station to get off the train to go to The Versailles. Evidently English was not the language for asking direction; we traveled past The Versailles by three stops. We kept looking at the overhead map and finally a passenger who spoke English asked where we wanted to go. When he learned we were heading for The Versailles, he said we passed by it three stops ago. He advised us to take the opposing train and get off at the third stop. That was what we did, thanks to the kind passenger.

We had to walk a few blocks from the train station to the Palace of Versailles, stopping and going to adjust to Amelia's pace. The palace location was unmistakable because the large crowd of tourists was moving in the same direction. Instantly at the entrance to the palace ground, one could see the cameras popping out; tourists were snapping pictures of the expansive building. I have taken a limited number of pictures myself, limited because I was

At Versailles, Paris

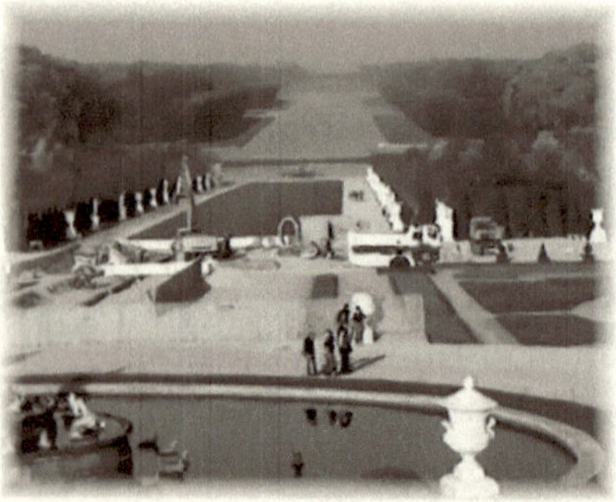

carefully helping Amelia negotiate the cobbled yard which is hard for people unused to cobblestones.

At the end of the yard close to the ticket window, a long line of tourists was already forming even though the palace was not opened yet. We thought we would make it to the head of the line by starting early, but other tourists had better ideas and started earlier than we did. Touring the palace interior was no longer an attractive choice because of the long wait; instead, we decided to explore the palace gardens which are free of admission fees and are prettier beyond compare with any garden we had ever seen before.

The garden area starts on the same level as the palace, descending several feet down by way of negotiable slopes and concrete steps. On the palace level are water fountains, gargoyles, and numerous sculptures. Below are more sculptures, well-trimmed bushes, shrubs, and trees. Because our visit was on a hazy day, the vast lake appeared to extend to the horizon. Tall trees bound the lake on all sides. From what I learned, the lake and the ground provided hunting places for the royalties.

Dolly and Dennis decided to explore the gardens below, including what appeared to be a smaller garden within the palace gardens itself. Amelia and I stayed and sat on the steps overlooking the lake. Even though I was

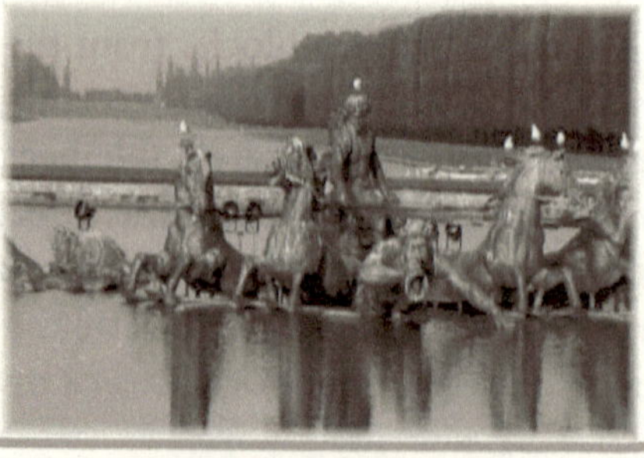

At Versailles, Paris

disappointed for failing to join Dolly and Dennis in their exploration, I felt grateful that at the time that Amelia was feeling tired and hungry, I was able to readily assist her. I had her eat fruits, and drink water which I carried around on this particular trip, anticipating that her hunger syndrome might make its presence known. When Dolly and Dennis rejoined us, they too were tired, so we decided to take off for our hotel.

Before we could make it to the train station, we all felt starved on account of the constant walking at the palace gardens. The effect on Amelia was more evident than on the three of us. We looked around for a place to eat, and though very crowded, we found ourselves waiting to be seated at a Vietnamese restaurant. The wait was not particularly long because diners were leaving in groups.

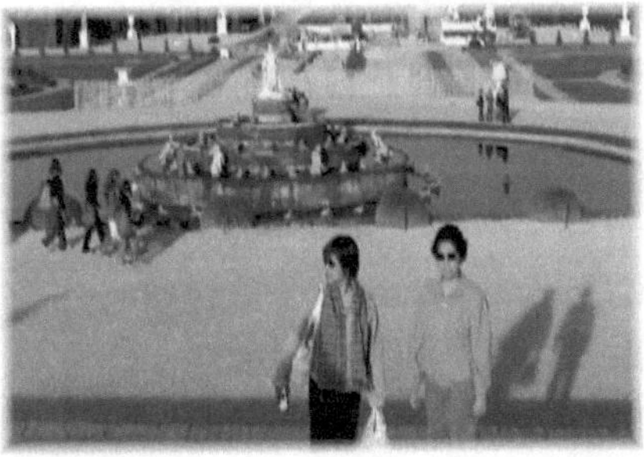

While dining, we reflected on the value of having gone through the trouble of visiting a historical and out-of-the way place like The Versailles. Even though we were tired, we were in good spirit and feeling lucky to be healthy enough to visit famous places away from home. We had enough fun for the day; we were happy traveling back to the Triumphal Arch area of Paris and ultimately to the hotel.

As usual, for dinner our favorite place this segment of our European tour was at MacDonald's at the Triumphal Arch area of Paris. It was the only place we could readily order food to our liking without the fuss of reading menus in French. We never did learn how to order food in French. We walked back to our hotel and rested the few hours left of the day before retiring and admiring from our hotel window the lighted Eiffel Tower.

At the Triumphal Arch, Paris

For the four of us - Dolly, Dennis, Amelia, and me - this was our first morning and day in Paris. After confirming our reservations at the hotel, we relaxed and contemplated what to do with the rest of the day. According to the members of the hotel staff, with just regular pace, we were about thirty minutes away from the Triumphal Arch. That being the case, we made our first venture out in the streets of Paris, towards the arch.

We decided to have breakfast close to the arch; our breakfast turned out to be at MacDonald's which is just a few hundred feet from the landmark. After breakfast, we took pictures of the arch at different angles and of ourselves with it as background, all the while delighting in the fact that we were at the center of the city of lights, Paris, in this very early morning; twenty-four hours ago we were in California.

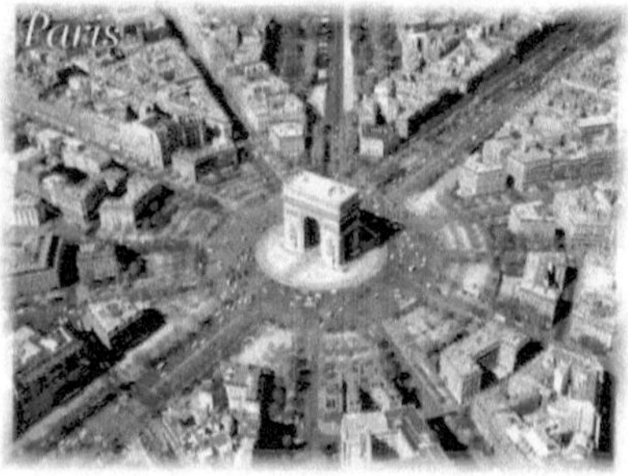

More than a dozen major streets radiate from the arch. From what I could tell, traffic was confusing and dangerous, with vehicles circling the arch and fighting for their rights of way. Watching out for errant vehicles, we crossed to the base of the arch nevertheless, with no traffic lights, police officer, or crossing guard to help pedestrians.

There was plenty of room for visitors to gather at the base of the arch. However, crowds of tourists started forming causing accidental collisions among them including us. It was easy to get bumped while focusing a camera. Nevertheless, we were able to

At the Triumphal Arch, Paris

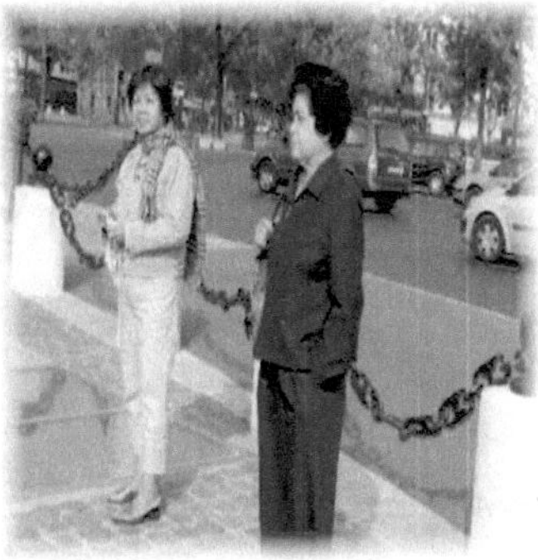

take pictures of the sculptures on the arch without backing into the traffic lanes.

A war history lover, I felt excited about the arch because of its role in welcoming the liberators of France during World War II. It was hard for me to believe that right now, this very moment, I was in the place where history was made more than sixty-five years ago.

The base of the arch is not a small area for one with a physical disability like Amelia, to walk around. By now she was getting tired, I noticed. I had her sit on a bench while I was going around for more pictures. Finally, I decided to go down to explore the chamber of the arch telling Amelia that I would be back in a few minutes. She did not like the idea of being left alone in an unfamiliar place; she wanted to come along, and I was glad she did. We climbed a few steps down with Amelia holding on to the rails with both hands and having no issue whatsoever.

I did not realize how big the underground chamber of the arch is until I was there. Murals on the walls are wide and long. As circular as the outside base of the arch is, so is the chamber. I felt the reverberations and heard echoes as people spoke. We took some more pictures of the murals and other sculptures in the chamber, losing my sense of direction while doing so.

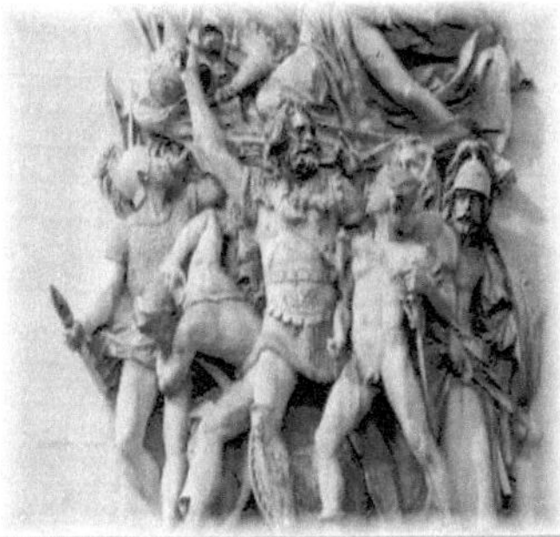

Because Amelia was already fatigued and apparently having some phobia being underneath the arch, she asked

At the Triumphal Arch, Paris

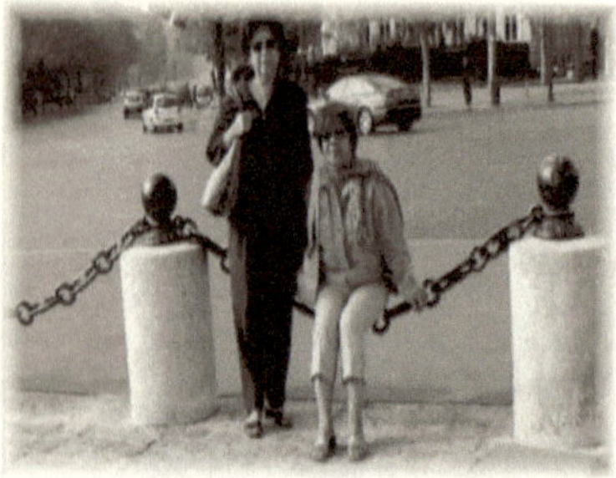

that we go back up, and that was when a slight problem occurred. Instead of heading to the entrance where we came through, we were headed towards the other side of the chamber. We were already so many feet into the wrong direction before I realized the mistake; I had to slowly lead Amelia back in the right direction. We finally got out of the chamber with Amelia exhausted, and made the daunting traffic crossing from the arch towards the stores and sidewalk areas.

We went to MacDonald's again to have snacks of coffee and pastries. We spent the rest of the day gawking at various places around the arch. Then we headed back to the hotel and waited for our luggage to arrive; they did not come on the same flight that we took to Paris; they came in the evening from London on a different flight. We retired to our hotel rooms and planned for the next day's activities.

At Notre Dame, Paris

Notre Dame is a short distance away from the Louvres Museum which we just finished touring. After eating at a restaurant close to the museum and with still enough daylight to spare, we took the first hop-on-hop-off bus that arrived, to Notre Dame. We wanted to be there, finish the tour, and catch the last train that would take us to the Triumphal Arch area whence we would walk to the hotel.

The bus dislodged its passengers at the bus stop along the side of Notre Dame, from where we could see a crowd forming in front but far from the door of the building. Through hedges, we followed the slightly winding path to the crowd. Joining the tourists, some pushing their babies on baby walkers, some in wheelchairs, and some just leisurely walking along, we became part of the crowd. We did not know what to expect at the end of the procession.

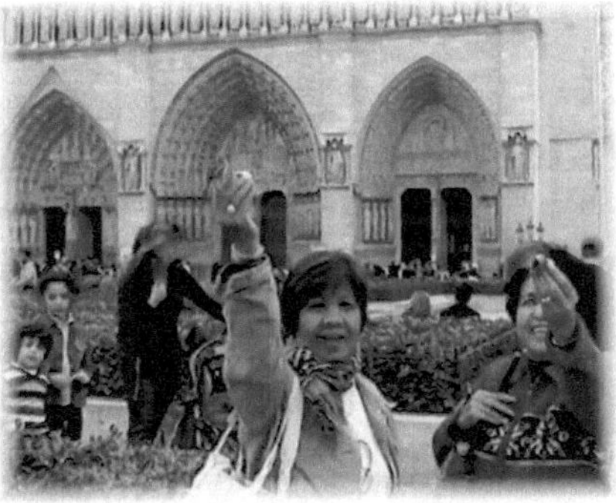

By now the crowd had grown to a few tens clustered around a man with a small bucket in his hand, and with birds all over him, on his hands, on his shoulders, on his head, and on wherever the birds could roost. In unison, the birds in hundreds would fly away from and back to him. The flybys were repeated for as many times as the man held rice in his hand. He would cast the rice into the air and hedges, and the birds would swoop down to catch the food. I was thinking to emulate the man. If he could do it like magic with a short stroke of his hands and had fun at the same time, anybody could do it as well.

At Notre Dame, Paris

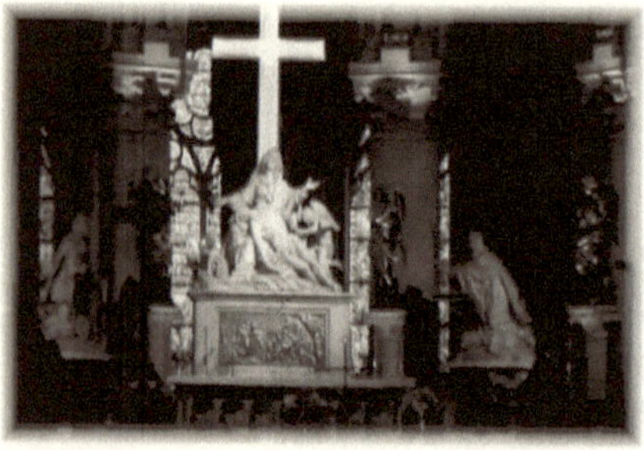

Upon inquiry, we found an enterprising man on a corner of the yard farther from the crowd, selling rice for feeding the birds. We did not know whether the man feeding the birds and the man selling the rice, were in some form of advertising arrangement. For five Euros we got some rice ready to feed the birds. We picked a spot on the yard farther from the crowd, where Amelia and Dolly started feeding the birds. The birds did not care on which part of the yard the rice was available - they too appeared anxious to entertain the tourists.

Although we were tired from the previous tour of the Louvres, I've never seen Amelia and Dolly so tickled and laughing until their rice was all consumed by the birds. Like on the man who attracted the crowd in the first place, the birds were all over them, on their heads, hands, shoulders, and arms. They hovered over them waiting for their turns to pick the food from their hands. Amelia even raised her right arm and hand - her weaker side - higher than what I would usually observe. She could have closed her hand and caught one of the birds, and what an excitement that would have been if she did.

To my delight, the birds appeared to have a therapeutic effect on Amelia. I did not realize how happy she and Dolly would be, feeding the birds. I would have been tickled and exhilarated myself were I to hold the rice with hundreds of birds coming so close to me. Having to photograph the spectacle, I did not have the chance to do it. For Amelia and

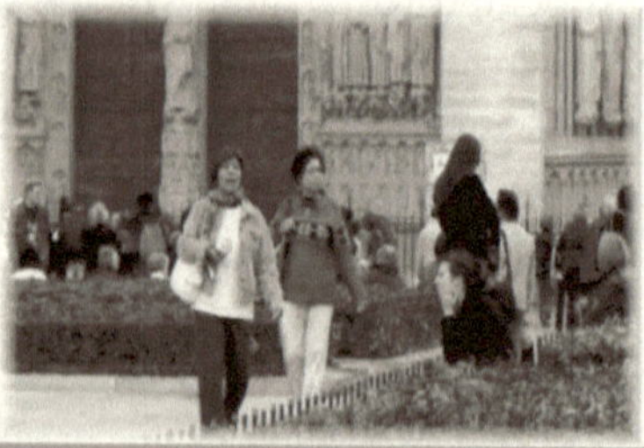

At Notre Dame, Paris

Dolly, experiencing it in Paris with Notre Dame in the background, away from home, was certainly an unforgettable moment, though it is possibly happening in the United States too with a different background.

After the birds and rice excitement, we went inside the building and joined the tourists touring Notre Dame. Immediately what came to my mind was the movie 'Hunchback of Notre Dame', after witnessing the enormous construction of the building. Just looking at the displays, one would be able to recreate part of the history of France. Joan of Arc, one of my favorite heroines in movies, was prominently sculpted. Small replicas of Notre Dame are also in display. There are hundreds of displays depicting notable moments in history that helped in shaping modern France.

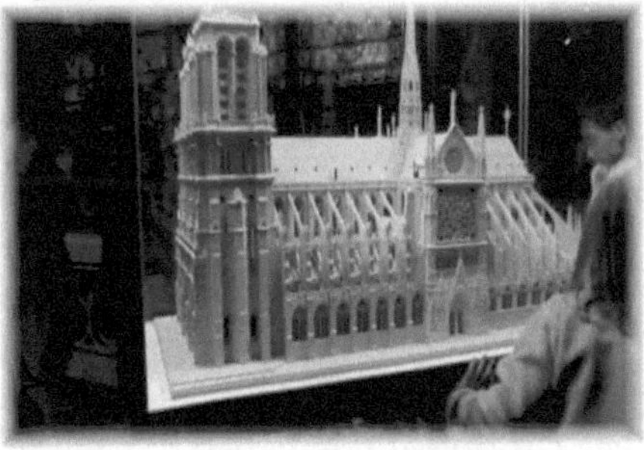

After the tour, we took the train that stopped close to our hotel. We relaxed and planned for the next day's activities. Notre Dame, known throughout the world, was now an important item in our list of places visited as part of our quest for travel. Under duress from Amelia's physical and mental condition, the trip would seem impossible, but we made it as I vowed to do, while she can still appreciate her surroundings.

At Notre Dame De La Garde, Marseilles

At Notre Dame De La Garde, Marseilles

Notre Dame De La Garde is probably one of the most popular tourist attractions in France as evidenced by the huge crowd of tourists speaking different languages and wearing distinct costumes. Its strategic location in the Mediterranean makes it an attractive destination for tourists visiting by land, sea, and air. We were coming by one of the many buses that picked up tourists from two or three cruise ships docked at Marseilles harbor. Along the way, we toured Palais Longchamp.

The Basilica is located at the end of a winding road overlooking the Mediterranean Sea. The road was so crowded that some tourists including us ignored the signs to proceed orderly, and took the steep shortcut to the yard ahead, bypassing the regular roadway. With my help, Amelia was able to negotiate up the slippery slope but by the time we reached the yard she was panting and exhausted. I felt, it was payment in kind for our lack of politeness in bypassing the crowd ahead of us.

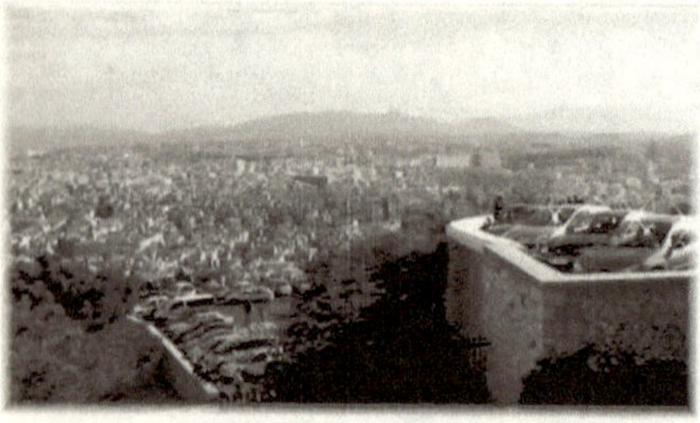

We rested at the yard enjoying the partial view of the Mediterranean Sea. From our location which was still distant from the Basilica, we could see the tourists climbing up and down the tower like ants. While Dolly and Dennis were already on their way to the tower, Amelia and I were still in the yard.

At Notre Dame De La Garde, Marseilles

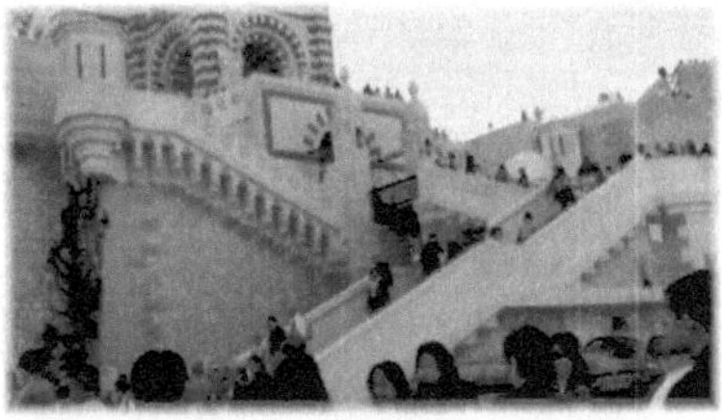

I was watching Amelia for any sign of discomfort, and it did not take me very long to notice that she was very sick and needed some food and drinks which I learned, were available at a restaurant in the Basilica. Very slowly this time, we made it to the Basilica, politely excusing ourselves when we passed some tourists ahead of us, indicating to them that Amelia was not feeling good, and that we needed to reach the restaurant as quickly as possible.

At the Basilica we were told that the restaurant is on the upper level which could be reached by elevator just a few feet away. We made it to the restaurant all right, but not having a menu to point out what we needed, and unable to speak French, I could not readily order food. Some customers ahead of us obviously had a similar problem. Compounding the problem was the fact that only one person was manning the eating place. Looking around for someone to help us, I caught the attention of our tour guide sitting at a corner of the restaurant.

She interrupted her lunch and kindly helped us get food, indicating to the customers ahead of us that Amelia was sick and needed food and drink immediately. She was the only one among few people at the restaurant who spoke English. By then other customers not particularly from our tour, also started asking her for help, evidently trying to get out as fast as possible to enjoy the view outside.

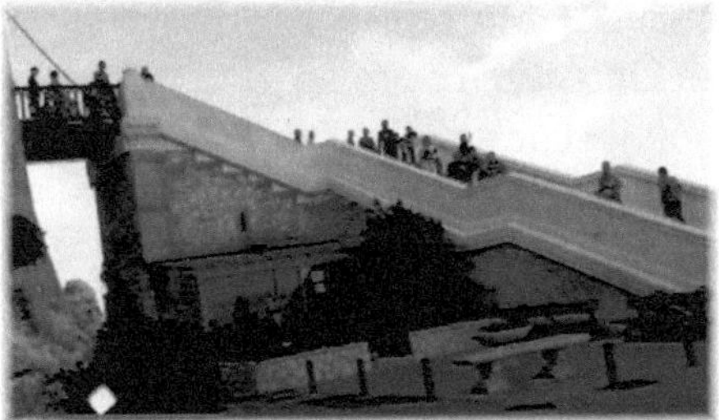

After eating the French food which Amelia did not like, but which relieved her hunger nonetheless, we were told by the tour guide that we could rest at the restaurant; she would come by to let us know when we were ready to leave. That was very kind of her, and when she mentioned that she planned to come to Los Angeles for a vacation and to visit a friend, I offered her some hints of places to visit in the area. As tour guides changed buses, that was the last time we saw her.

The most precious moment of the tour was having a complete view of the Mediterranean Sea from atop the tower, but to my disappointment, I was not able to do so because of Amelia's condition. On the other hand, Amelia was able to say her prayers at the Basilica, a very precious moment as well.

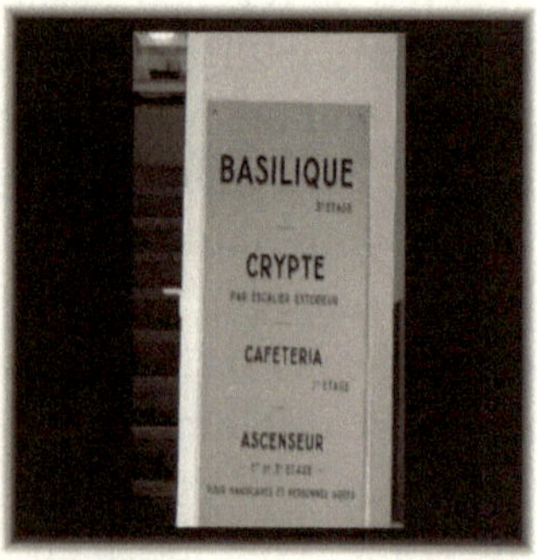

Dolly and Dennis described how spectacular the sight was from the tower, and I believed them. The Basilica reaches only one-third the height of the tower and already offered some nice perceptions of the region; its full height then must offer a 360-degree bird's-eye view of the tower's surrounding, the ocean, and beyond. With telescopes and viewing platforms, the Basilica's yard was the favorite location for those who did not want to climb the tower for fear of height.

We regarded our tour to be very satisfactory and informative, considering the historical significance of Notre Dame De La Garde as a lookout point for protecting the city of Marseilles. I recommend the tour of Notre Dame De La Garde to anyone, without reservation. The tour bus took us back to the ship at Marseilles, where we rested and relaxed for the remainder of the day.

At the Eiffel Tower, Paris

The Eiffel Tower was not far from our hotel. From the balcony window of our hotel room, we had a perfect view of the tower, especially at night when the tower's lights were on. Its rotating brilliant and radiating lights would keep me awake for a few hours before going to sleep. The Eiffel Tower appropriately represents to the world the city of lights, Paris. Missing the Tower while in Paris even for a short stay is an unforgivable misgiving.

The Eiffel Tower looks the same from many angles of photography. But the well-lighted public area which has a plaza, stands, benches, vending machines, and ticket windows for the ride up the tower is where tourists mostly congregate. Incessantly taking on visitors during the day and well into the night, the area looks alive and bustling. Picture taking is a major past time especially at night when the images are prettier than those taken during the day.

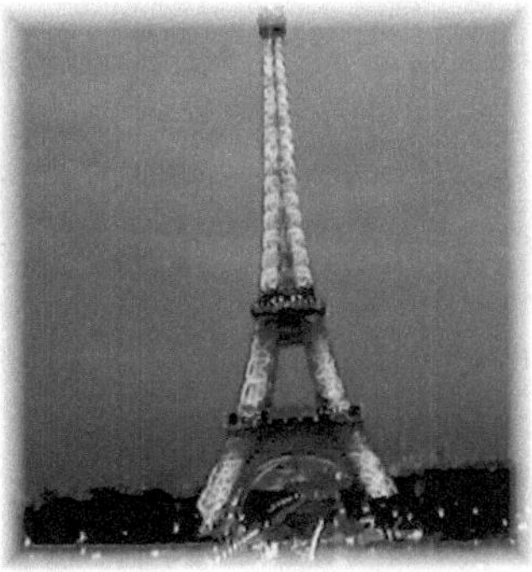

Contrary to some rumors and cautionary advices, the area around the tower appeared to be safe. However, like many travelers around the world, we had to carefully hang on to our identity papers in case we needed them for any reason. It is very easy to be carried away and become careless and vulnerable to bad elements outside the public mainstream especially when excitement tends to loosen personal safeguard. Visitors can quickly lose attention and be easily distracted while looking up at the tower most of the time.

The Eiffel Tower served us in a special way in this segment of our European tour. During the first two or three days of our stay in

At the Eiffel Tower, Paris

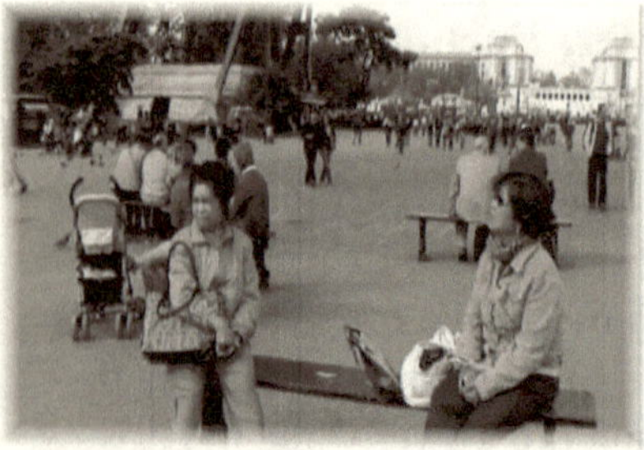

Paris we often got lost, and asking directions from strangers was difficult because of language difficulty. What we would normally do was to look yonder for the tower as our beacon. At night when the lights were turned on, the tower served us immensely, but during the day we had a slight difficulty unless we could see the tower top. All we had to do was proceed in the direction of the tower, knowing that it is only a short train ride from it to the Triumphal Arch whence we would walk to our hotel.

The underground train station near the tower was our transfer point going to and from the Triumphal Arch area of Paris, which was close to our hotel. When taking the hop-on-hop-off bus, we would also stop by the tower. Not constrained by time, we would usually spend hours at the Eiffel Tower before heading to our hotel. Only when we got tired and when the night turned to be unbearably cold for Amelia would we longingly leave the tower.

Each time that we stopped by it, the tower appeared to have a new appeal. Such is its beauty and attraction that we never stopped appreciating it. When illuminated, the surrounding areas of the tower are by themselves tourist attractions. The buildings and their architectures tend to be emphasized and inspiring when viewed during the night. The city of light, Paris, is portrayed and exemplified by the Eiffel Tower and its surroundings.

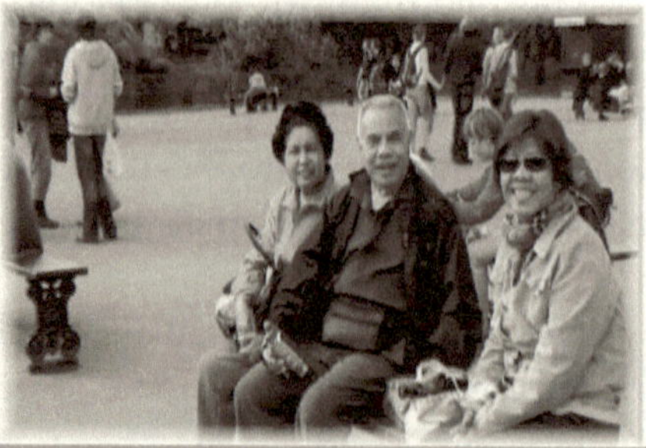

Only needing warm clothing at nights, Amelia had no problem at all stopping by and

At the Eiffel Tower, Paris

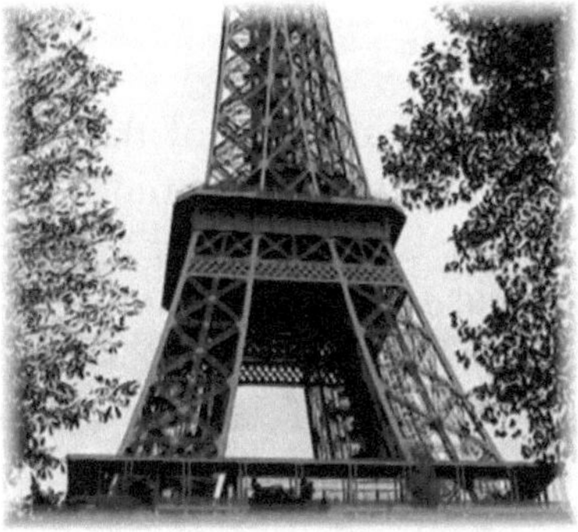

going to the tower. Her dislike for French food though, necessitated that she ate American food, MacDonald's to be specific, before venturing to the tower. Our excitement about the place was limited only by Amelia's cheerful attitude owing to her mental and physical condition; this time she did not fail us.

We had a good time in Paris. The Eiffel Tower is as iconic as it is beautiful; it is a tourist attraction one should not miss while in Paris. There are plenty of attractions in Paris, but the Eiffel Tower is a national symbol recognizable all over the world. That is why I unequivocally recommend the trip to the Eiffel Tower to anyone who happens to be in France.

At Monte Carlo, Monaco

At Monte Carlo, Monaco

Monte Carlo, Monaco, was one of the stops in our itinerary of the Mediterranean cruise. The name 'Monte Carlo' is amusing to some, it being associated with romance and adventure. Depicted in different kinds of merchandise and products like cars, games, and hotels, it is almost a household name. Not only is it a place of implied romance and adventure, but it is also the seat of administration of the sovereign principality of Monaco.

In the morning of our scheduled stop, we found our cruise ship docked at Nice, the seaport where passengers and cargo bound for Monte Carlo, are discharged. As Nice has its own tenders with conspicuous colors and markings different from those of the cruise ship, passengers were transported to and from the shore with them; no tenders from the cruise ship were put into service in this regard.

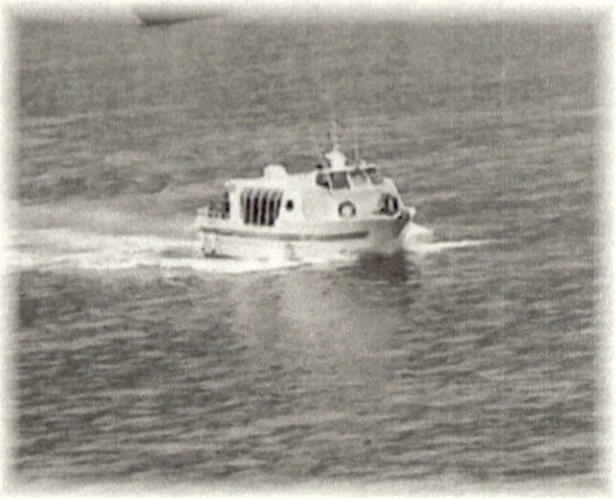

We were then transported by bus from Nice to Monte Carlo. Along the way, we stopped at a lookout point where tourists alighted from the bus to take pictures of the panoramic view of Nice and its harbor. Initially arriving on a very bright day at Nice, there was no need to use the stationery telescopes available at the point. It was easy to make out even the small yachts out of hundreds dotting the harbor.

Further along the highway and getting closer to Mont Carlo, the driver pointed out ahead the site on the roadway where Princess Grace met her tragic death in a traffic accident. With requests from the passengers to slow down at the location, the driver obliged and allowed the passengers to gawk at the roadside. Grace Kelly, later

At Monte Carlo, Monaco

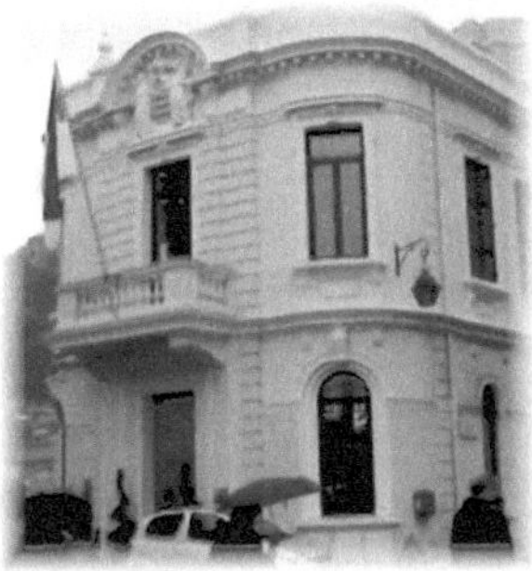

known as Princess Grace, was one of Amelia's favorite movie stars; she was mine too, and from the reaction of the passengers, she might be theirs likewise. In fact, some passengers were visibly unable to hide their commiserations for the noble family.

It was lightly raining when we arrived at Monte Carlo. Part of the tour I believed, was for the tour bus to take us along the shoreline where the Monte Carlo Grand Prix is held every year. Not fond of the sports of racing, this part of the tour did not interest us much, nor it did other passengers. Monte Carlo, the city, was the ultimate destination for most of us especially when the rain started to get heavier and the sky was getting darker.

Finally, we stopped at a huge parking structure where other tour buses were discharging their passengers. Taking the escalator to the street level, we finally and officially arrived in the city of Monte Carlo.

On the open yard were two colorful guards pacing towards then away from each other, who did not mind having their pictures taken with Amelia and Dolly in the foreground. Like the good soldiers they were, they minded their soldiering business and did not care to talk to strangers.

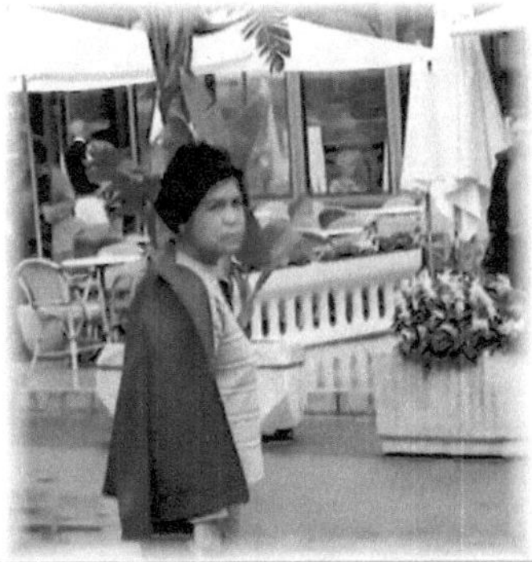

The weather was not cooperating; the rain was turning to a light downpour and the wind was blowing harder. Whereas Dolly and Dennis trotted

At Monte Carlo, Monaco

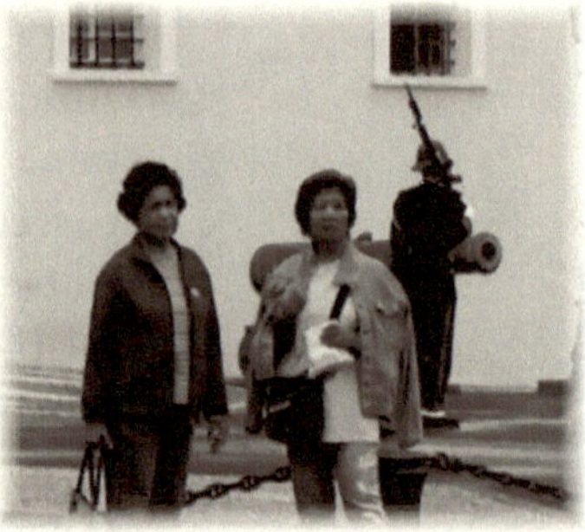

from one place to another to skip the rain, Amelia and I could not do it due to Amelia's physical condition. But as usual and though struggling, Amelia always made it albeit slightly wet, to whichever side of the streets we wanted to go.

When the rain let up and while we were crossing one of the streets, our tour guide pointed out to us the temporary residence of the princesses marked by the official flag of Monaco. For a residence of nobilities, the place is relatively small tucked in a business district. I presumed that is one of the reasons for the closeness and popularity of the royalty among its constituency.

We visited St. Nicholas Cathedral, which is not colossal as some cathedrals are. Therein, a crowd formed around an inscription which I believed, is that of Prince Rainer and Princess Grace. With the reflective mood of the attendees and the conversations almost down to a whisper, we found it rude to pass by the seated congregants to get behind the crowd surrounding the inscriptions. We did not try; instead, we left the cathedral and continued on our tour of the city.

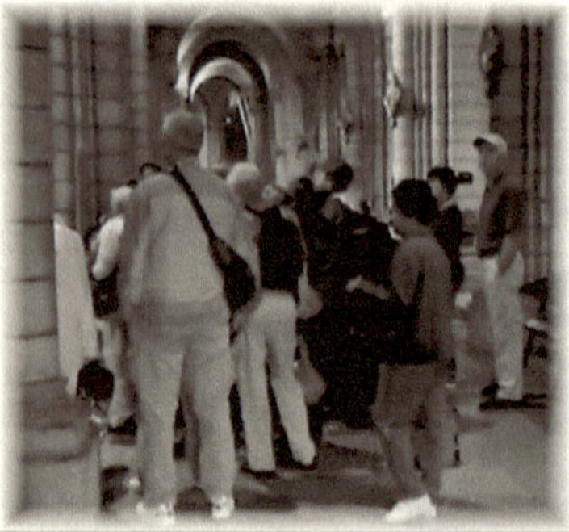

Despite the rain and with brisk walking we made it to the biggest casino in the city. Gambling was not in our agenda, so we stopped short of the entrance to the casino. Keeping an opinion to myself, I concluded that the casinos in Monte Carlo are significantly smaller than those in Las Vegas.

At Monte Carlo, Monaco

Starting with the beautiful city of Nice through the picturesque roadsides where special events are celebrated, and the tour of the city of Monte Carlo with its important landmarks, we ended the tour happy and exalted despite the rainy day. The tour bus took us back to Nice where tenders were waiting to take us back to the cruise ship. We spent the remainder of the day relaxing and waiting for the nightly shows and other entertainments.

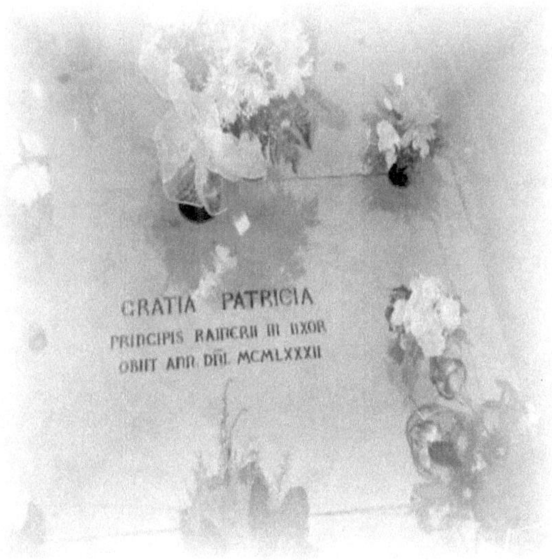
GRATIA PATRICIA
PRINCIPIS RAINERII III UXOR
OBIIT ANN. DÑI. MCMLXXXII

At Monte Carlo, Monaco

Chapter 13 - Destination Hawaii

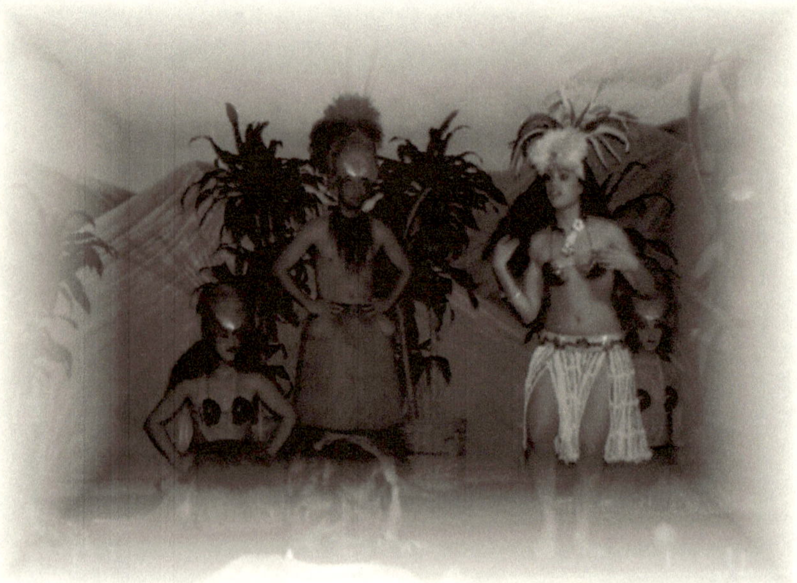

At Iao Valley, Maui

At Iao Valley, Maui

Not having been to a rainforest for a long time, the entrance to Iao Valley immediately aroused our interest and feel of the environment. The temperature noticeably changed to a comfortable level from Lahaina's warm and summery weather. The valley being the habitat for various species of tropical animals, glimpses of wild animals such as land lizards crossing the road were frequent. Incessantly crowing wild roosters seemed to announce our arrival, while monkey-like and cuckoo cries could be heard from a distance.

Fresh drinkable water is continuously flowing from small tributaries feeding the main brook. Sustained by cloud covers on top of the mountains which provide enough moisture and rain to keep the water flowing into the stream, Iao claims to have the second highest rainfall among the Hawaiian Islands.

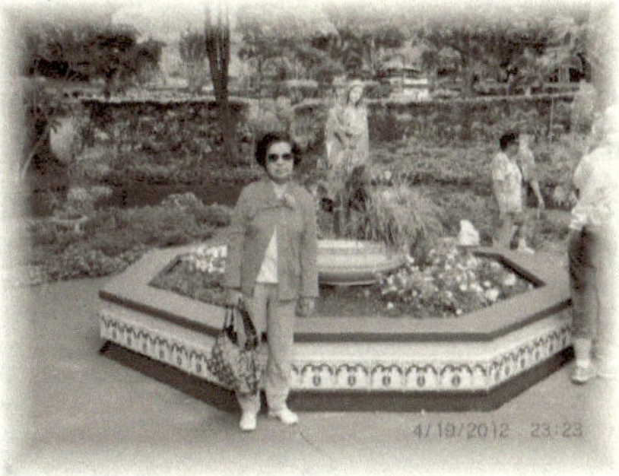

Deeper down the valley from where we stopped - no further encroachment into nature's beautiful landscape - was where a bloody battle between Kamehameha's army and Maui's army under Kalanikupule occurred, the tour guide narrated. No trace of the encounter is evident from the viewing site ending at a bridge.

A rickety rope ladder which is climbable only by a trained person and not by casual tourists like us, was observed immediately following the bridge. Other than the site of the beautiful valley including the fresh flowing water and the lush rainforest covering the slopes of the mountains, there is not much in the way of

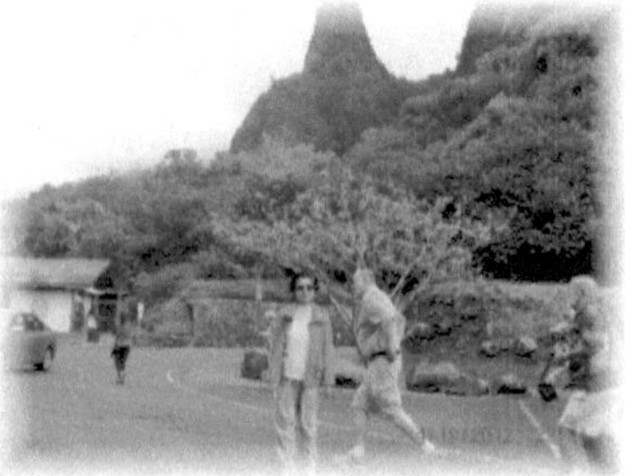

entertainment. The valley is a showcase though, of what an unimpeded nature looks like – green, lush, fresh, and primitive.

Going back towards Lahaina from where the tour started, we retraced our route coming into the valley for a short distance then branched into a highway leading to the Heritage Gardens. The Gardens made up for the lack of entertainment in our previous stop.

There are beautiful cottages, villas, and pagodas, so on so forth, of different ethnic groups that settled in the valley, clustered but distant from each other, in a well-arranged pattern. History was made in the Heritage Gardens late in the eighteenth or early nineteenth centuries. The ethnic groups each with its cottage or pagoda, represented in the Gardens were Filipinos, Japanese, Portuguese, Chinese, Koreans, Americans, and Hawaiians. It took us an hour or so to explore and admire the Gardens.

While others were exploring the Gardens, Amelia's hunger was acutely overwhelming her. Her last memorable stop in the Gardens was at the location where there is a statue of the Virgin Mary. From there we selected an isolated spot at the picnic area where she ate her supply of fruits I brought along from the ship. I could see that she was not satisfied with fruits for lunch, so I promised her that at the first opportunity where food was available, I would buy lunch.

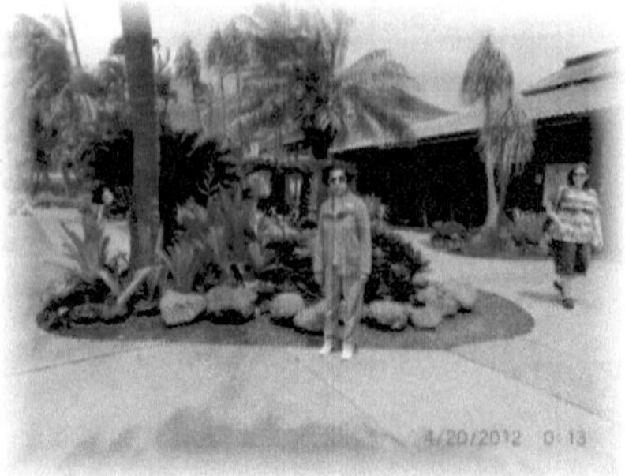

At Iao Valley, Maui

The first opportunity to buy lunch came at the Tropical Plantation almost an hour drive from the Heritage Gardens. I hurriedly bought lunch almost bypassing people ahead of me on the queue because Amelia had her hunger episode and her glucose level was down, I believed. After she ate lunch and recovered, I asked her if she wanted to take the tram on a tour of the plantation. Not wanting to be left alone, she forced herself to agree.

At the plantation tour, I could see Amelia's lack of interest. She stayed on the tram while tourists roamed around, taking pictures, and admiring the different plants including pineapples, taro, squash, sago so on so forth. She was eager to go back to the ship, an option hardly feasible considering the distance from the Plantation to Lahaina where the cruise ship was docked; it was probably a two-hour long drive. We let the tour take its course and only left when everybody was ready to leave.

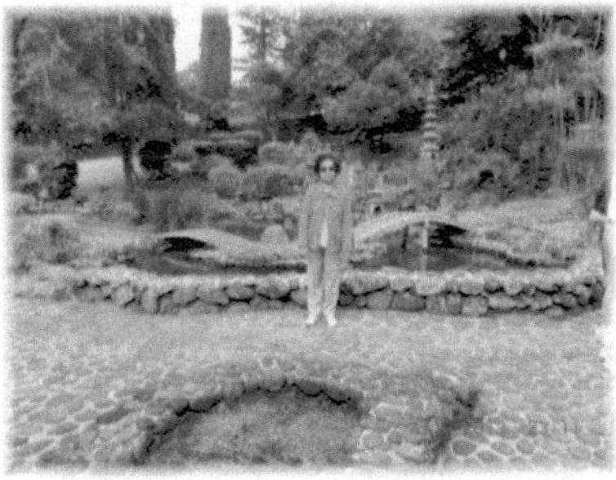

Notwithstanding Amelia's slight discomfort, the excursion ended on a very positive note. It was quite an experience unmatched by other tours we had on the mainland because of the difference in climate zones. The history of Iao Valley is clearly etched in the form of magnificent cottages that transcended ethnic divisions.

At Waimea Canyon, Kauai

Waimea Canyon, known as the Grand Canyon of the Pacific, was our destination on this particular excursion. From the number of tourists booking the excursion on the ship, I could tell that it must be as grand as its namesake in Arizona. I barely got our tickets before the excursion was closed for overbooking. It is a must-see tourist destination while on Kauai, according to the staffs on the ship.

The tour bus took us through some beautiful rainforests. Being the wettest spot in the world, Kauai boasts of lush green hillsides and abundant plant life on the roadside. So-called wild roosters did not appear too wild at all; they came very close to the tourists not hesitating being fed. Other wild animals were darting across the road avoiding being run over.

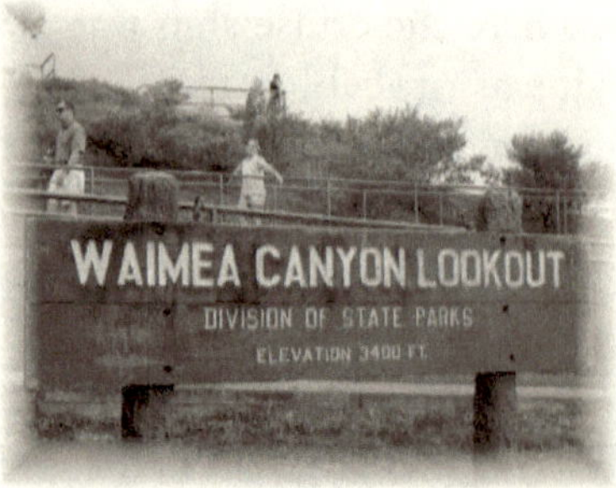

The bus ride which took us through a Filipino community did not appear to affect Amelia. In all of our trips, her condition is always my concern, she having diabetes, having multiple strokes, has Alzheimer's, and with a failing heart. Nonetheless, Amelia was delighted to hear the bus driver talking to the residents about the church nearby and the activities going on. The parishioners were dressed up for a wedding, and the bus driver evidently knew many of them by the way they exchanged congratulatory remarks.

At lunch time we found ourselves at the Waimea Canyon, the Grand Canyon of the Pacific. Fearing that her hunger syndrome might make its presence known, I bought some drinks and food for Amelia from a vending machine at the visitors' bureau since the

At Waimea Canyon, Kauai

store was not open yet, giving me a chance to look around and stretch after the moderately long ride. At lunch time the visitors' bureau which is situated very close to the edge of the canyon, still appeared to be empty making me think that it is true, Hawaiians coolly take their times.

Though dubbed as the Grand Canyon of the Pacific, Waimea Canyon is not as grand as its namesake in Arizona. It is significantly smaller in comparison, yet it is equally dangerous and deadly relating to injuries caused by falling.

To my surprise in spite of her disability, Amelia walked to the very edge of the canyon and had me take a picture of her. Though she did not know how to handle a camera, she unsuccessfully asked me to turn around against the rail so she could take a picture of me in turn. With the rail just about waist high, I did not dare get close to it with my back turned against the canyon; I refused her offer to take a picture of me.

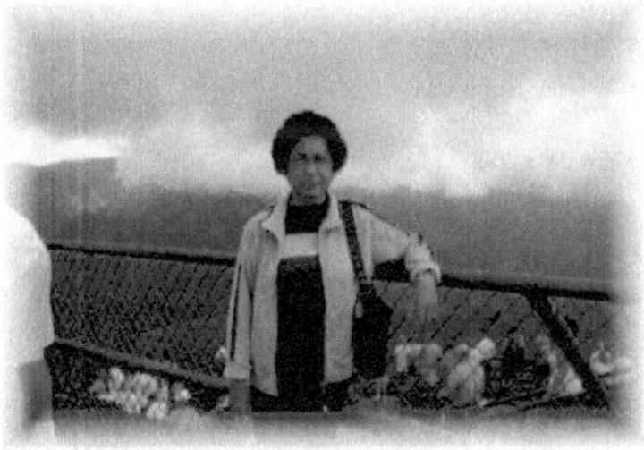

I felt that the canyon has more vegetation than the Grand Canyon in Arizona, obviously because of the abundant rainfall in the island. For trail seekers, there are plenty of hiking trails with plenty of precautions as well. One particular warning is that because of the drop in the canyon if one ended up at the bottom, the only way for him to be extricated is to walk back up if he is fortunately not disabled. Otherwise, it would be a case of search and recovery. Some hikers did not mind the warning; they came in groups ready to test the canyon's challenge. As the day went by, more and more tourists came by cars and buses.

At Waimea Canyon, Kauai

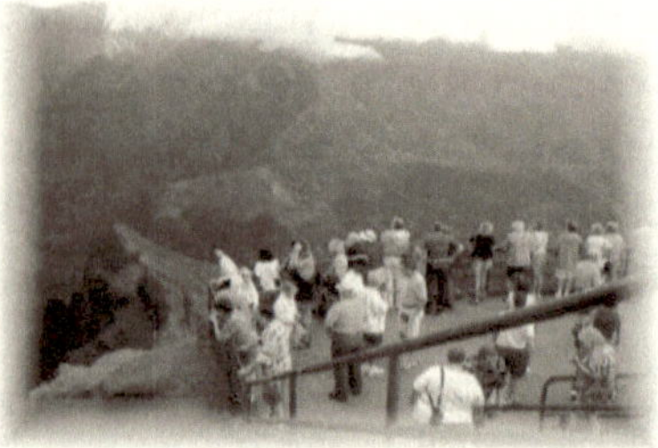

Another display of Hawaii's allurement, Waimea Canyon does not disappoint visitors especially ones who have not been through rainforests. Having two grand canyons, one in the mainland and one in the Pacific, the United States covers a very broad area of free natural pastime. No other country has the bragging right to have two such similar coverage on a very grand scale.

I considered our excursion very successful, which ended when later in the day, the tour bus took us back to the ship where we rested, relaxed, and waited for the nightly entertainments

At the USS Arizona Memorial, Pearl Harbor

We had to leave early for the USS Arizona Memorial to avoid the crowd which I understood, to be always present at the site. Since Amelia was moving ever so slowly, we were the last ones to get on the bus, leaving us no choice of seats except the very last ones. The arrangement was all right so we would not be on the way when the passengers got off the bus.

Despite our early start though, the parking lot at the tourists' processing area was already very crowded when we arrived. The bus did not have the chance to drop the passengers with disabilities at the designated place and was required to park some distance away from the entrance to the processing center. Being the last ones to get off the bus, I somewhat served as the end marker of our group of some fifty passengers. Ahead of us were two or three groups making the line even longer and requiring Amelia to stay standing for an extended period.

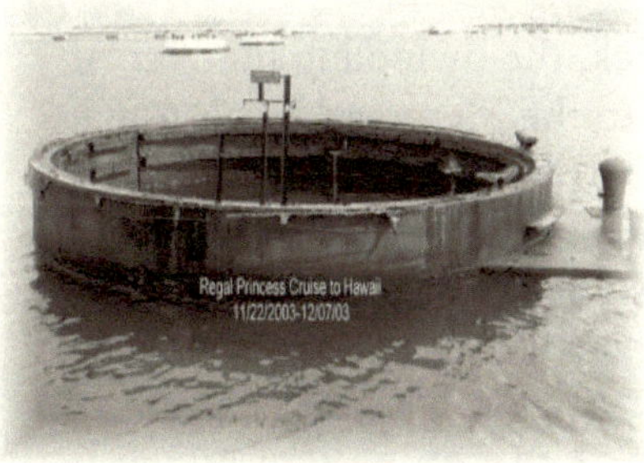

Thirty minutes went by before we finally reached the processing desk. It was a requirement that we attend a presentation of what to do during the tour of the Memorial. The presentation included the events that started the war with Japan.

Briefly, the surprise attack on Pearl Harbor on December 7, 1941 plunged the United States into war with Japan. The surprise and devastating attack prevented the United States from retaliating immediately. Most ships of the United States Navy were anchored,

At the USS Arizona Memorial, Pearl Harbor

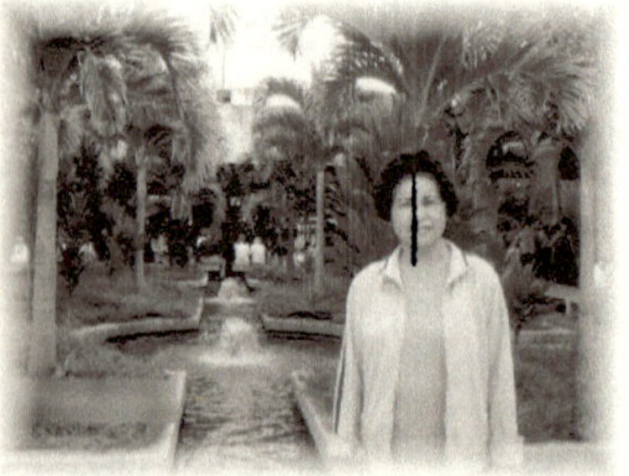

concentrated, and caught off guard at Pearl Harbor making them easy targets from the air.

One of the Navy ships caught like a lame duck, the USS Arizona, thought to be the best equipped and most invincible, was attacked without let up until it sunk. Only a handful of its crew and sailors survived the attack. One only has to look down the sunken ship's turret to imagine the sufferings of the sailors in their watery death. The USS Arizona Memorial lists the names of the sailors who died in the attack and entombed with the ship.

Commemorating the events of the attack, the dwindling number of survivors of the attack annually comes to the Memorial to bestow honors to the sailors who perished in the tragedy. Even the few surviving Japanese attackers come to join in the commemoration of the event that plunged the world into one of its darkest moments, the attack on Pearl Harbor.

There are other sunken navy ships in the harbor being memorialized as well, but the USS Arizona is the main one. On the days that the Memorial is open, there is no shortage of crowd; it is exceptionally and naturally more crowded on Memorial Day.

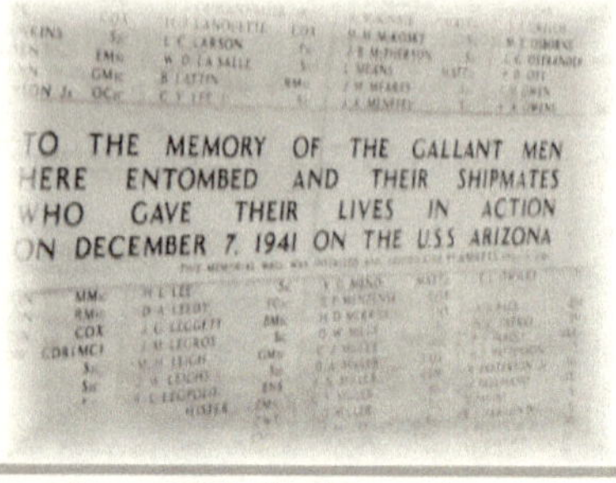
TO THE MEMORY OF THE GALLANT MEN
ERE ENTOMBED AND THEIR SHIPMATES
HO GAVE THEIR LIVES IN ACTION
N DECEMBER 7, 1941 ON THE USS ARIZONA

The Memorial is visited through tenders that require visitors to go through checkpoints before boarding. Furthermore, visitors are compelled to behave in certain ways consistent with applicable military regulations. As the Memorial filled with more visitors,

At the USS Arizona Memorial, Pearl Harbor

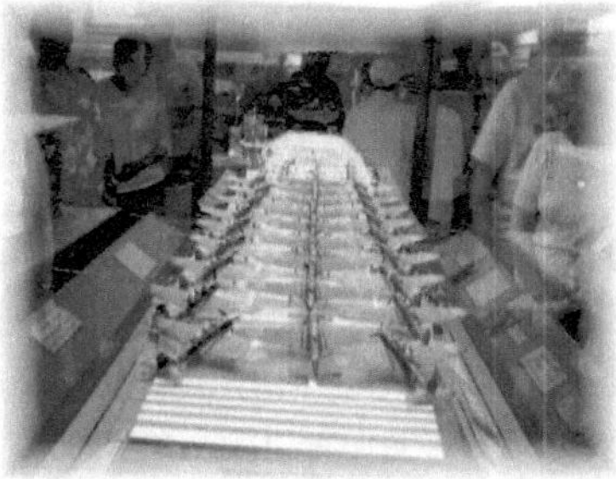

trips by tenders tended to be more frequent. After forty-five minutes in the Memorial, we took the tender back to shore.

After the tour of the Memorial, at our request we returned to the cruise ship because Amelia was not feeling good; other tourists continued to other attractions on the island. We rested and relaxed at the cruise ship, waiting for the nightly entertainments.

The USS Arizona Memorial is a reminder to all people of the futility of war because even the best laid out plan can turn into a tragedy. The USS Arizona Memorial showcases the ship's failed invincibility and the fate of its sailors. Avoiding war must be the prime goal of all nations, for even the slightest semblance of hostilities can provoke retaliation of unimaginable result.

At a Luau Party, Lahaina

The excursion was on our first trip to Maui, Hawaii; we had made three trips to the island so far. The sea was very calm in the morning when we found ourselves waking up with the cruise ship anchored outside the harbor at Lahaina, Maui. There was no indication that our appointment with an outdoor luau party scheduled for late in the afternoon was going to be interrupted at all, giving us some time on shore to shop for souvenirs.

The luau party was not in Lahaina itself. We were taken by bus to a specially configured hall to handle big parties, about an hour drive from Lahaina. Eager to see more of Hawaii's famed surroundings, we favored the long drive as the driver who turned out to be one of the performers, described the landscapes along the way. There was only a light drizzle when we left Lahaina, not enough to disrupt the luau party.

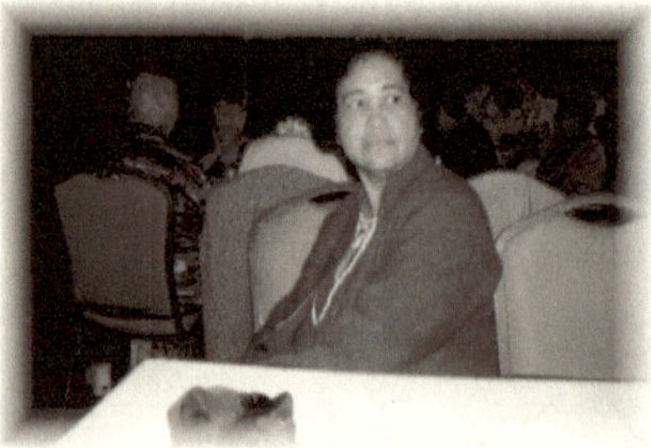

Three busloads of partygoers to the occasion appeared to be a large crowd by most standards but average for a luau party, the driver told us. As if by prearrangement, the rain started to come down very hard as we reached the place for the party. The tarp covering the party supplies, chairs and benches, and the pit was no match against the rain. The party organizers waited for the rain to stop, but it kept coming down even harder.

The party organizers concluded that the party would have to be held indoor. They brought the food back in and rearranged the place so that people could eat their food on the tables. Earlier, the food was expected to be eaten outside so that party goers would be

At a Luau Party, Lahaina

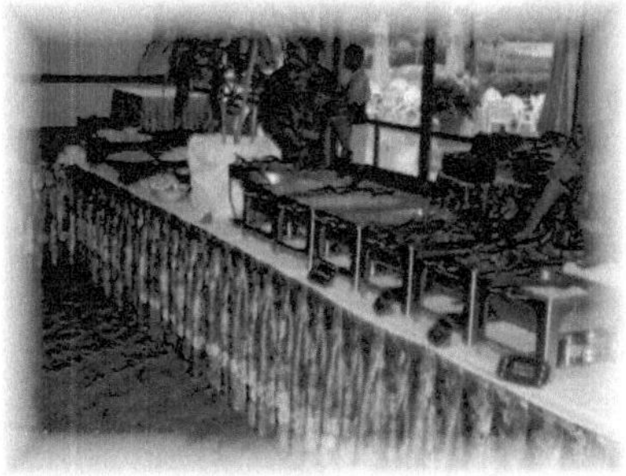

able to roam around and mingle with everyone else having fun. With the uncooperative rain, that was no longer possible.

As the stage was being prepared for the show, the main attraction of the party, tourists started to get their food and settled on the tables to eat. Food of course, is what luau party is mostly known for, and plenty of it was available for the taking. Starved tourists including me ate their food with gusto. On the other hand, Amelia only tasted some cookies and refused to eat, coming up with the excuse that she would have plenty of food choices on the ship. Her attitude towards food had noticeably changed since she had massive strokes.

As if to defy the merriment inside the building, the rain came down even harder as the show started. Having come with the first bus, Amelia and I were able to avoid the drenching rain while some latecomers arrived thoroughly wet and dripping.

Once the stage show, mostly with Polynesian dancers, got started, it went on uninterrupted completely ignoring the torrential rain outside that was coming down with a vengeance. The crowd was continuously applauding, only stopping when there was a lull in the performances.

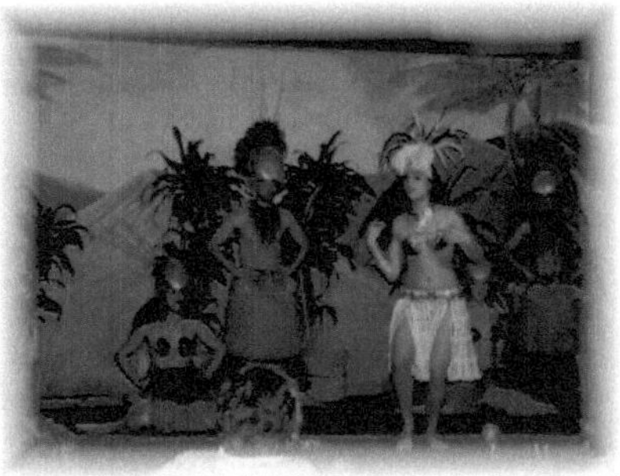

The party lasted about two hours with the intermittent rain keeping the party goers within the building until departure time. Because of Amelia's

At a Luau Party, Lahaina

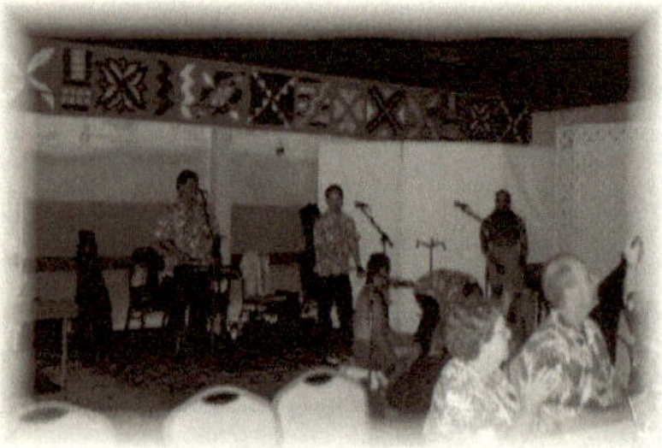

disability, we had to walk slowly to the bus, and that was when we got drenched. The rain continued until we reached Lahaina. At Lahaina we had to skip from store to store just to get closer to the pier area from where the tender took us back to the ship.

At the ship, we immediately changed to dry clothes followed by a trip to the food deck for steamy hot coffee and dinner. Notwithstanding the rain, the luau party was very successful. I recommend it unequivocally to anyone while in Hawaii.

For what Hawaii is known for, luau unites people through their taste buds and interests in the Hawaiian form of entertainment. Luau has now been migrated to different activities like luau retirement party, luau homecoming, and luau anniversary. What comes to mind first at the mention of 'Hawaii' is 'luau' for some people. That is how the term has transcended the Hawaiian form of entertainment.

At Kona Submarine Ride, Kona

After the previous day's tortuous excursion we were somewhat indisposed to go on another one, preferring to stay on the ship, relax and hydrate ourselves. Our muscles, needing much rest, were hurting at the slightest movement. Amelia refused to commit to another excursion because her legs were devoid of power, so she said.

But, as they happened in many previous occasions, while cruising things could suddenly change. With most of the passengers gone ashore, the ship looked utterly lonely; not too many new activities were going on for lack of audience. We changed our minds and decided to go ashore as well.

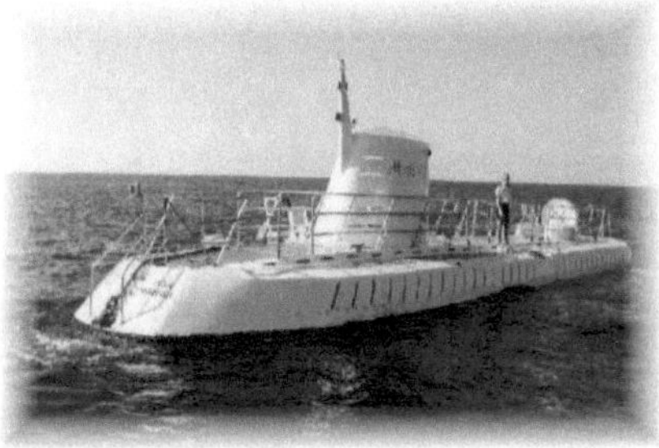

We went to a small shopping center by taxicab and spent an hour there before going back to the dock to look over the place after all. We still had about five hours to spare before the last tender would depart for the cruise ship, a pretext on my part to convince Amelia to go for whatever event was happening near the dock.

The Atlantis was docked at the end of the pier, maybe fifteen minutes of walking from where we were at the last store. From the picture of a submarine on a huge billboard, I right away knew it to be the one utilized to entertain tourists with what is happening below the surface of the ocean. Somewhat excited, I bought tickets for the ride.

To our surprise there were already few tourists who were waiting to get in the ride, hoping that the submarine gets filled right away,

At Kona Submarine Ride, Kona

since it would not leave until every seat was allocated to a passenger.

The members of the submarine crew were real submarine officers before retirement - that was how they were introduced. Military courtesy was observed, naval jargons could be heard, and salutes were executed where appropriate. I was sure that part of the courtesy was for showmanship. Safety was strictly enforced as the passengers were led into the submarine down a very steep and narrow stairs.

Each passenger was assigned a seat with a glass porthole for viewing the creatures below the surface of the ocean. The seats were so close together that the passengers were almost touching each other. Amelia and I did not mind the condition knowing that we would only be there for less than two hours.

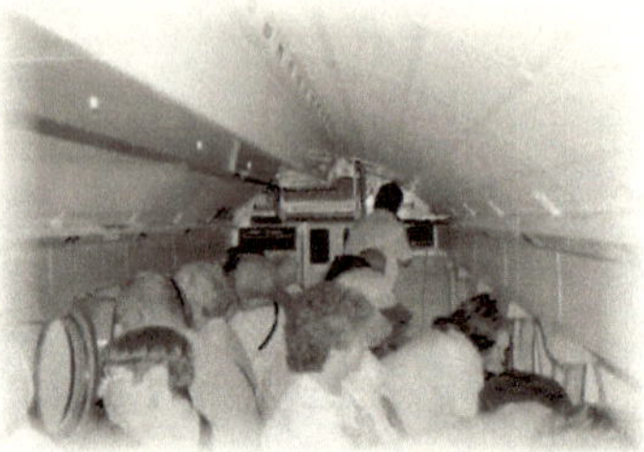

As the submarine started to move forward a few hundred feet out to sea, it began to descend. As it did, some fishes appeared to fly by, the appearance being caused by the submarine's speed and not by the movement of the fishes. With the lens being too close to the glass window and the submarine at a fast rate of speed, my camera did not work well leaving us with not much photo opportunity.

The narrator described what was happening at certain depths of the ocean as the Atlantis was slowly descending. Apparently, some creatures thrive on certain depths of the sea while others prefer other depths. There are depths of the sea where fish do not thrive at all, so the narrator said.

At Kona Submarine Ride, Kona

We descended slightly more than thirty feet below the surface and stopped for a while. We observed ocean creatures including small crabs lazily doing what they normally do as inhabitants of the ocean floor. Worm-like creatures were creeping from rocks to rocks. After an hour or so watching other unknown creatures on the seafloor and listening to the narrations about the oceans, the submarine proceeded back to port and surfaced.

Passengers were safely and carefully let out of the submarine. We had to let other passengers out first so that we would not be obstructing the exit. Amelia climbed the stairs very slowly naturally recanting her agreement to go on the submarine ride; she did not appreciate the ride at all, I could tell from her looks. We went back to the ship and spent the rest of the day resting and relaxing.

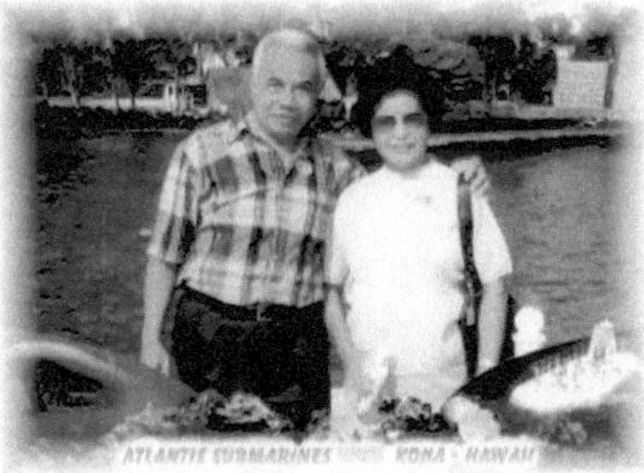

Up to this time, all of our excursions - we made a few already - were on land and above the surface of the water. The submarine ride took us down below the surface of the ocean, a different experience that added a new perspective to my view about the environment. The ride was an absolute success as far as I was concerned, and I recommend it without hesitation to marine lovers.

At the Thurston Lava Tube, Kilauea

The trip to the rim of the Kilauea volcano, Hawaii, took us through different, suddenly changing weather conditions. At one point on the same highway, the weather was cold and in just seconds it became humid followed by a stretch of cold weather again; it was a humid-to-cold and vice versa weather condition repeated a few times. Such was the case for a few miles through lush green rainforests.

Thanks to our guide, as his way of promoting Hawaiian products, he handed plenty of sweet local bananas - not the kind normally seen on the mainland - to the passengers to eat. Though some were still unripe, the bananas tasted so much sweeter and different from those we buy at the grocery stores. The bananas served as a replacement for the fruits I brought along from the ship for Amelia. She ate some of them in time when she felt that the bothersome hunger syndrome was starting to make its presence known.

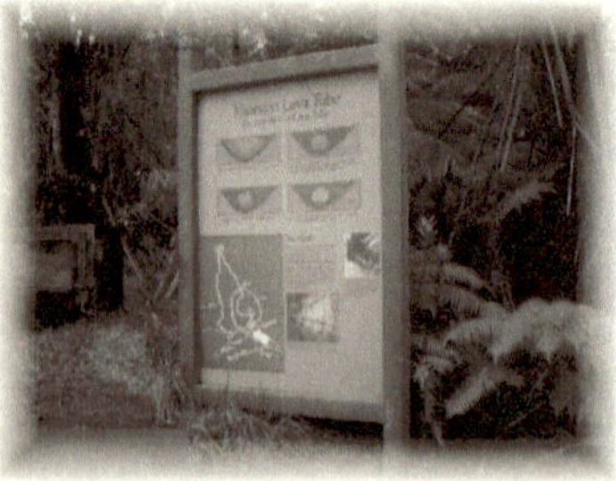

The Kilauea Volcano has been erupting on and off since 1983, but the lava from the volcano does not necessarily reach up to the rim all the time. We had a panoramic view of the lava bed which is vast and wide as the eyes can see from the Kilauea volcano viewing site. Plumes of light smoke could be seen from some spots on the bed. Curious at the presence of rescue equipment at the site, we were told by the guide that some people do fall over the rim and the equipment is used to retrieve them.

At the Thurston Lava Tube, Kilauea

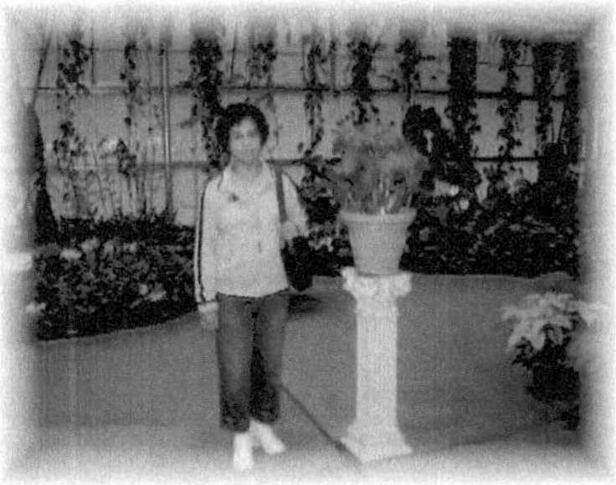

The main prize of our excursion was the Thurston Lava Tube which was formed more than four hundred years ago from the eruption of the nearby Kilauea Volcano. The tube wall was formed when the lava flow hardened on the outside while the inside was still flowing. When the last muckle of the inside lava left the tube, the hardened wall was left intact creating the large tube. There are other lava tubes in Hawaii, but the Thurston Lava Tube is the biggest and most frequently visited by tourists.

The tube is about six hundred feet long and averages eight to ten feet high from floor to ceiling, and is wide enough for three people to walk side by side comfortably. It is lighted but some areas are damp, so care must be exercised when walking inside the tube.

Due to the steep descent and ascent to and from the tube, Amelia was unable to join me in the walk through the Lava Tube. She, nevertheless, enjoyed the sight of people disappearing into the gaping hole of the tube on one end and surfacing later on the far end. We spent more than an hour at the Kilauea Volcano viewing site and the Thurston Lava Tube.

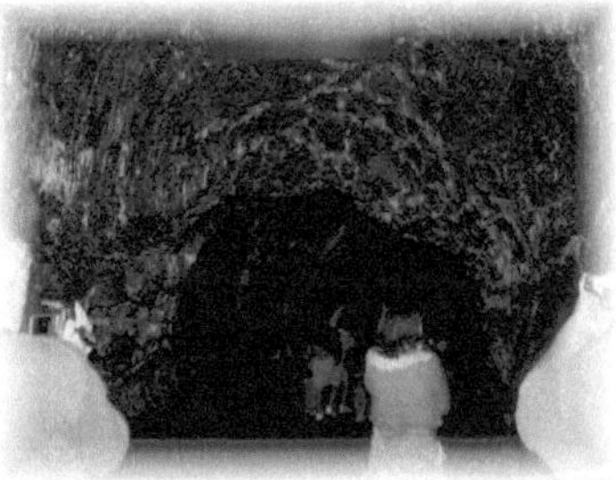

Coming back from the excursion, we took a different route and stopped at a nursery which exports orchids to clients all over the world. Orchids grow lushly in tropical weather like Hawaii's than in any other condition, an additional knowledge I learned from this

At the Thurston Lava Tube, Kilauea

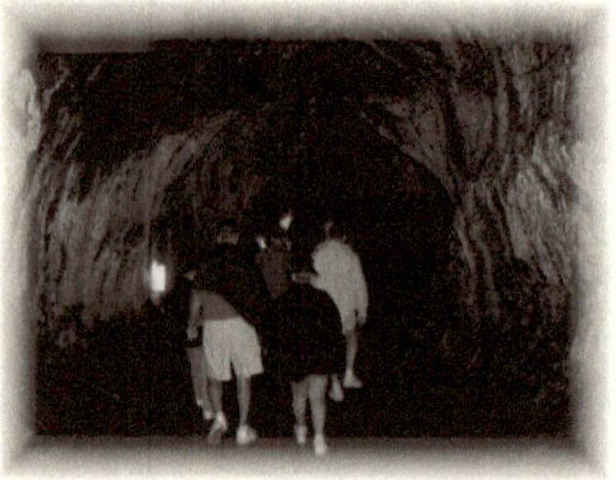

particular excursion. Farther down the route through more rainforests, we were treated to a demonstration of how hard it is to crack a macadamia nut.

Finally, the bus took us back to the ship where we spent the rest of the day resting and relaxing, waiting for the nightly entertainments, and pondering over the day's activities related to the just concluded excursion.

Through sheer force, nature can create wonders like the Thurston Lava Tube, for people to see and admire. The Kilauea Volcano with its unharnessed lava flow during eruptions in particular, helps to create the Hawaiian Islands a nature lover's paradise. From the simple nut cracking demonstration to the cataclysmic volcano eruptions, one will find Hawaii the most sought after vacation place in the world.

At Hilo, Hilo

At Hilo, Hilo

Owing to Amelia's difficulty in walking, we did not sign up for an excursion at Hilo, but we decided to get off the cruise ship to look over the town at the pier area. Amelia was limping slightly and was not ready to do too much walking except when we joined a group we knew from the ship, to walk to the bus stop. But the group left when the sports utility vehicle they contracted to take them to a volcano crater appeared and picked them up.

Another couple from the ship also came along and asked us if we would like to join them in a trip to the volcano crater, first by car to the assembly point, thence to the crater itself in a sports utility vehicle. We gladly accepted.

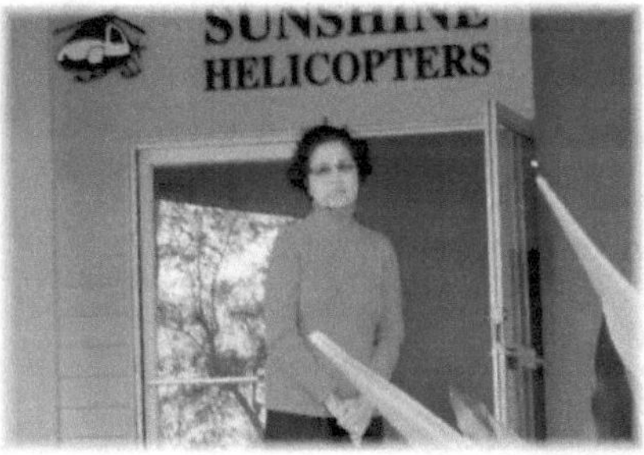

Obviously with some experience or training as a tourist guide, the driver purposely took the round about ways along some green scenery before reaching and dropping us at a marketplace, the assembly point for the tour. We wondered why she refused to take the gratuity we offered and found out later that our deal with her was not yet over; we would be seeing her again.

The marketplace appeared as not actively busy for some days. Some stores were closed while some were just lazily kept open, not earnestly soliciting business notwithstanding the presence of a cruise ship at the harbor.

Where we were dropped off, there were four or five other tourists from the ship, who were waiting to join the tour to the volcano crater. We were supposed to be part of their group filling a big

At Hilo, Hilo

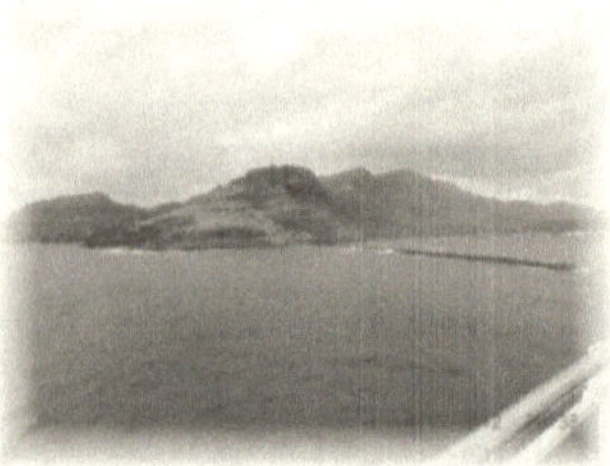

sports utility vehicle - about fifteen passengers - which would take us to the crater.

The driver of the car who initially brought us to the marketplace drove back to the pier area to solicit more would-be passengers, then coming back with three. On her third trip, we abandoned the excursion to the volcano crater and asked her to take us back to the pier area. She obliged and again refused to take the gratuity we offered.

We stayed at the pier area shopping for some souvenir presents for our small grandchildren. Not finding ones appropriate for them, we decided to take a taxicab to the main stores about twenty minutes away. Sharing the taxi fare with us to avoid the long wait for a taxicab, we were joined by yet another couple who turned out to be staying just three doors from our cabin on the cruise ship.

We separated from our couple friends and ate lunch at Starbucks. There was not much to see in the stores that were different from what the stores in Los Angeles carry; the trip only left Amelia exhausted and visibly limping.

She had difficulty negotiating the wide street from the store to the parking lot where we would be hailing a taxicab. We did not know that a regular bus was picking up passengers from the pier area and letting them off at the shopping center, and then picking up the returning passengers and dropping them off at the pier area.

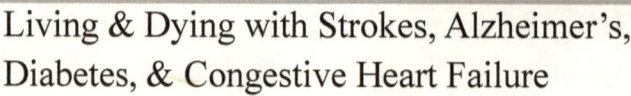

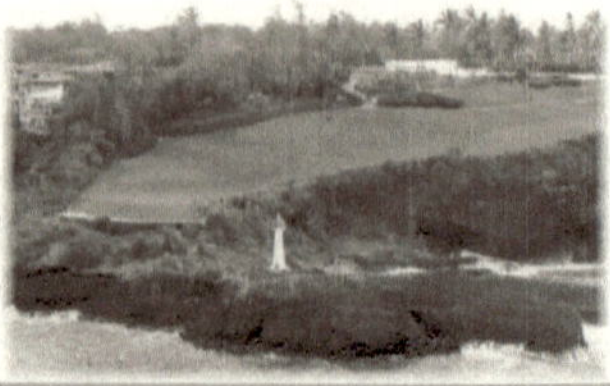

At Hilo, Hilo

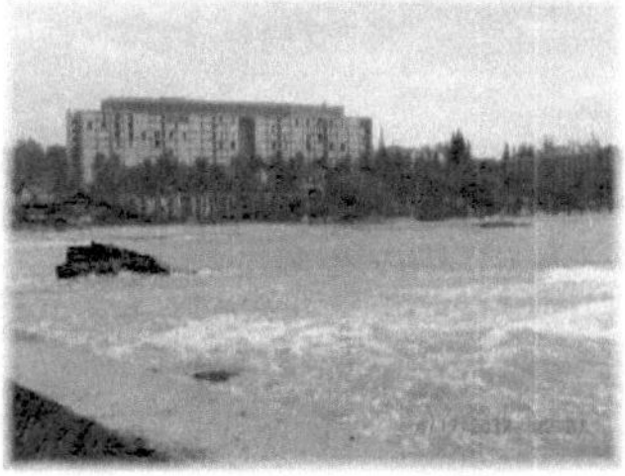

Hardly able to walk, Amelia indicated to take the bus presently waiting at the bus stop, but it left before we could make the crossing to the stores front. We were still crossing the street when another bus appeared which took us back to the pier area.

Exhausted and tired, Amelia demanded that we go back to the ship where we rested until late afternoon when we prepared for dinner. By then the ship was picking up anchor and getting ready to leave for the next stop in the itinerary. Following dinner, we got ready for the nightly shows and entertainments.

A disappointing experience like we had at Hilo is not a broad picture of cruising. On the contrary, it is an encouragement to regroup and make up for it on the next port. The disappointment was attributed to our lack of energy than it is to Hilo's lack of attractions. The reason why Hilo is in the itinerary is because of its appeals to tourists beyond the pier area.

The comfortable accommodation at the cruise ship diminishes the effects of temporary bodily aches related to travels, and gets one ready and energized again for the next excursion.

At the Buddhist Temple, Hawaii

After a few hours of a tour bus drive on the freeways at Oahu, our first full stop on our way to the North Shore was at the Buddhist Temple. I was unable to tell on which side of the island is the temple located because I lost my sense of direction and being unfamiliar with the state. Comparing the complex ways of negotiating through unfamiliar state highways, driving on the Southern California freeways seems less confusing than driving in Oahu.

We were kept on the bus for a few minutes while apparent negotiation between our tour guide and members of the staff at the gate was going on. We did not know what the matter was but after a while and a body count of the passengers, the bus was allowed to park at a designated place. Then the tourists were allowed to step down and proceed towards the temple. From where the bus was parked the temple already appeared imposing.

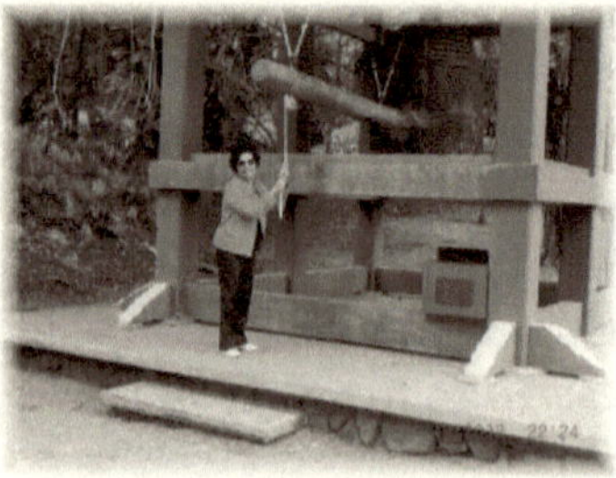

It was quite a long walk from the parking lot to the temple, and Amelia would not have a part of it because of her disability. She would rather stay on the bus than struggle walking on the smooth but slightly inclined up and down path towards the temple. I encouraged her a few times to join the tourists at the temple, each time she refused.

I supposed that I would have to stay with her if she preferred to be left alone in the bus, completely missing the opportunity to closely see the temple in more details. So we opened a few windows to

At the Buddhist Temple, Hawaii

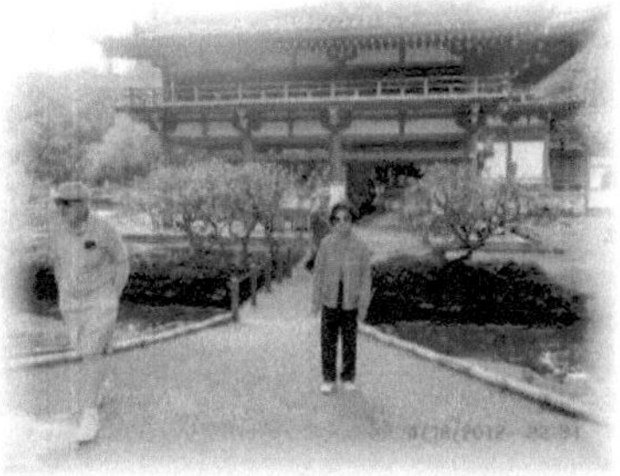

make us feel as comfortable as possible because the motor and the air conditioner were turned off.

While we were conversing, I mentioned to her that the cemetery - she did not immediately notice it when we drove in - across the parking lot is where some famous people in the island were buried, according to the guide. It did not take me more to encourage Amelia to come down from the bus and walk to the temple; on her own, she stepped down and started walking. Apparently not comfortable looking at the cemetery across, she in fact, was the one who hastened me to walk faster.

Amelia painstakingly walked to the temple with a little bit of struggle, but when she got there, her pain of walking appeared to have dissipated. Beautiful displays relating to the faith are evident outside the temple, and taking pictures is allowed. Even more interesting displays are inside the temple, but due to Amelia's difficulty in removing her shoes and later putting them back on, we did not enter it. As an act of reverence, wearing shoes inside the temple is not allowed.

We had enough time to walk around the temple and take pictures of the surrounding area which is well maintained, with the grass well-trimmed. The area is teeming, the fish ponds with goldfish, and the bamboo groves with hundreds of small chirping birds. What caught my attention most is the construction of the temple itself, with massive beams used for support as well as for the

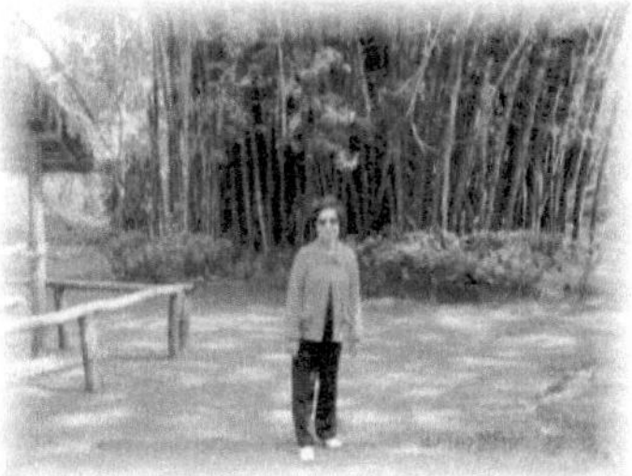

At the Buddhist Temple, Hawaii

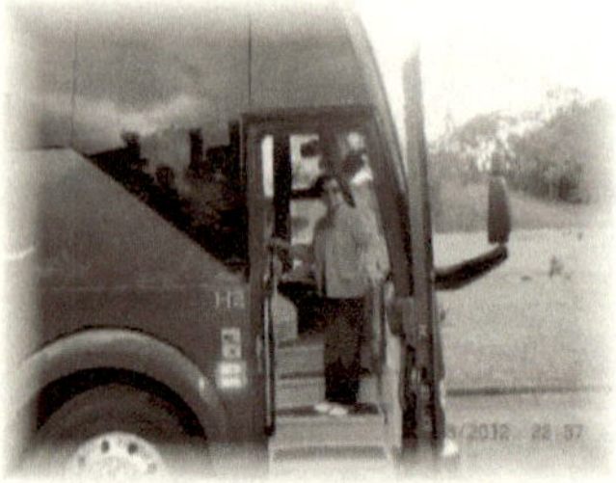

distinguishing artistic display of the faith and other symbols.

No longer feeling the pain of walking, Amelia walked towards the huge bell, and when it was her turn, swung at it with the wooden ringer creating a bellow that was heard around the temple. She did it twice and wanted to do more, but she was not allowed because other tourists - more were coming from other groups - were waiting for their turns to ring the bell.

We stayed at the temple for about an hour. Confronting us next was the problem of getting back to the tour bus which required going by a small bridge from where a slight uphill incline had to be negotiated. Again with my help and progressing slowly, Amelia was able to get back to the bus nonetheless, though we were the last ones to get on. The bus proceeded to the main destination, the North Shore.

The Buddhist Temple is just one of the many Hawaiian displays of its diversity regarding population makeup. With a history of diverse ethnic groups settling in Hawaii during the later part of the eighteenth century and early part of the nineteenth century, other faiths are represented in ways other than by temples. The Buddhist Temple being the most popular and one of the biggest is the one visited more often.

At the Thomas Jaggar Museum, Kilauea

At the Thomas Jaggar Museum, Kilauea

Our trip to the Kilauea volcano was not considered complete unless a visit to the Thomas Jaggar Museum was made as well. That was the case when Amelia did not want to go because she was exhausted, although we were almost there watching tourists coming to the museum. Fearing that she might feel ill while I was gone, I did not want to go alone either and leave her in the tour bus. We completely missed visiting the museum, an utter disappointment.

But our desappointment would turn into an opportunity somehow. Tourists loved to recount their shore experiences, particularly in the food deck during casual gatherings and conversations. When a young couple who were studying the subject of volcano in school mentioned about not leaving Hawaii without visiting the Thomas Jaggar Museum, we offered to join them. They confirmed their car rental arrangement and accepted our offer to share the cost of the trip to the museum.

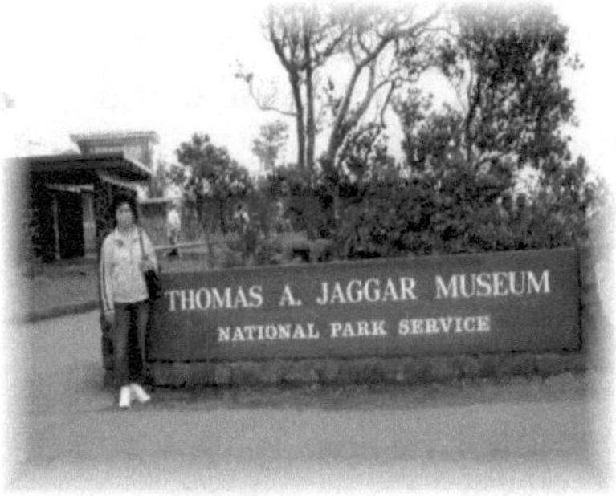

We retraced the route that the tour bus took us through during our previous visit to the Kilauea Visitors Center. Driving directly without interruptions as was the case in the tour bus, we reached the museum in very short period.

The museum was built in honor of volcanologist Thomas Jaggar who moved to Hawaii from the United States mainland to dedicate his life studying volcanoes. Located at the

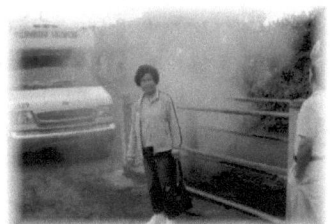

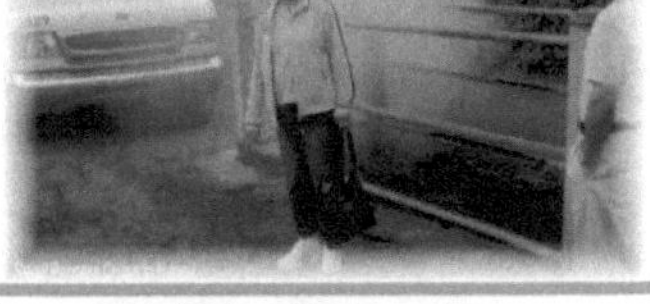

At the Thomas Jaggar Museum, Kilauea

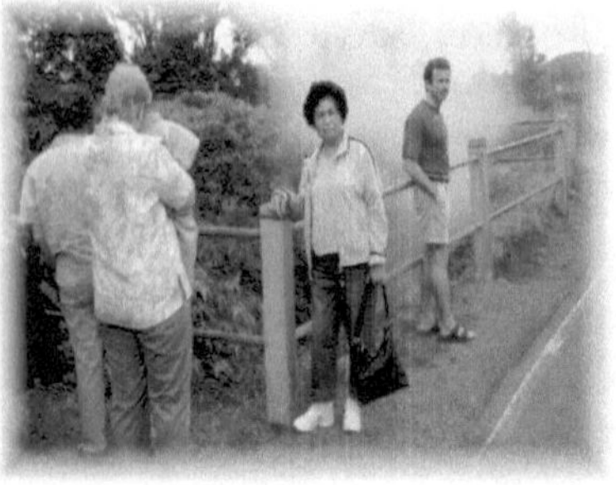

highest elevation of the Kilauea crater rim, the museum has an excellent view of the Kilauea crater. We learned that the view is even more spectacular at night especially when glowing lava is cascading. Administered by the National Park Service, park rangers show their presence at the museum to keep it and its surroundings safe and clean.

The museum has a store selling compact discs, maps, books, and other souvenir items mostly relating to volcanoes and the earth's movements. On display as well, are seismographs and other earthquake recording gadgets of the old kind. A scientist of world renown, Thomas Jaggar, the founder of the museum, has a short history and a mural of his own in the museum. For the convenience of visitors, the museum is equipped with amenities to keep them comfortable.

Additionally, stationary telescopes are available to guests who wish to view the crater of the Kilauea volcano clearly. Also visible by telescopes, and by the naked eyes only on clear days, are smaller volcanoes in the area besides Kilauea. Being the biggest however, Kilauea is the designation of the area known all over the world.

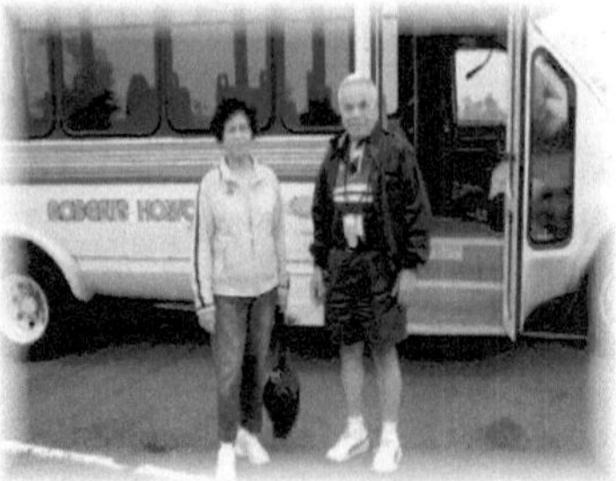

Done with the tour of the Thomas Jaggar Museum, we headed back to the ship in time for dinner and the departure spectacle when the cruise ship prepared to leave for the next port. Like everybody else, Amelia and I liked to stay on the open deck and watched the ship departed

At the Thomas Jaggar Museum, Kilauea

passing by landmarks, waving crowds, and heading towards the open ocean.

With our trip to the Thomas Jaggar Museum, our sightseeing tour of volcanoes was considered significant. Though our cruise was principally leisure and vacation in nature, education and scientific knowledge was gained as well. The Thomas Jaggar Museum is one I recommend to visitors who happen to be in Hawaii in the Kilauea area.

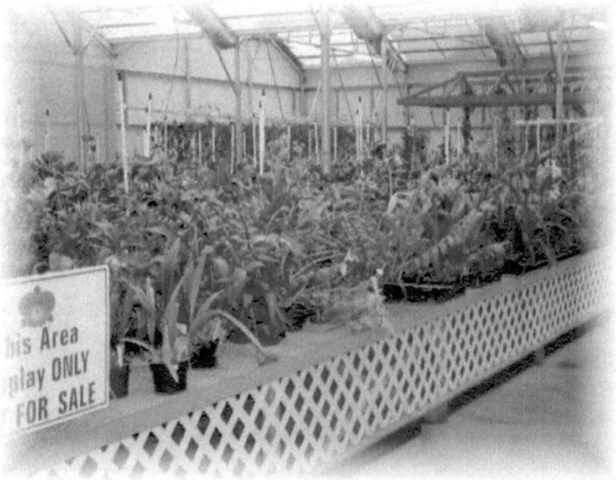

At the Thomas Jaggar Museum, Kilauea

Chapter 14 – Destination Italy

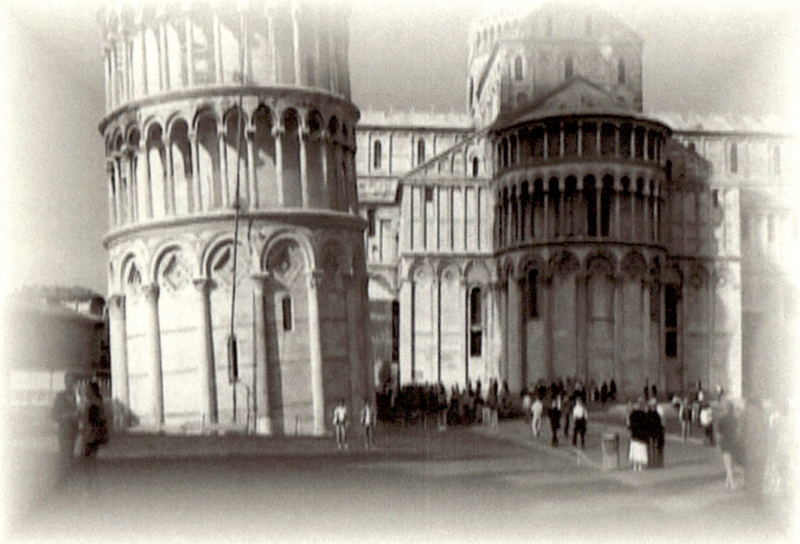

At the Ruins of Pompeii, Naples

At the City of Pompeii, our tour bus was one of the many in the queue waiting to discharge their passengers. It did not surprise us that we were let off the bus much farther away from the entrance to the ruins. To match Amelia's pace, Dolly, Dennis, and I had to slacken ours going to the assembly point of our guided tour. The slow pace allowed us to initially look around the walls surrounding the ruins.

Without first being inside the city, one could tell how significantly big the City of Pompeii was by visually surveying the still standing peripheral walls. Some walls had grown shrubs and trees indicating that the ash that devastated the city from the eruption of Mt. Vesuvius covered the walls and provided the nutrients necessary for their growth.

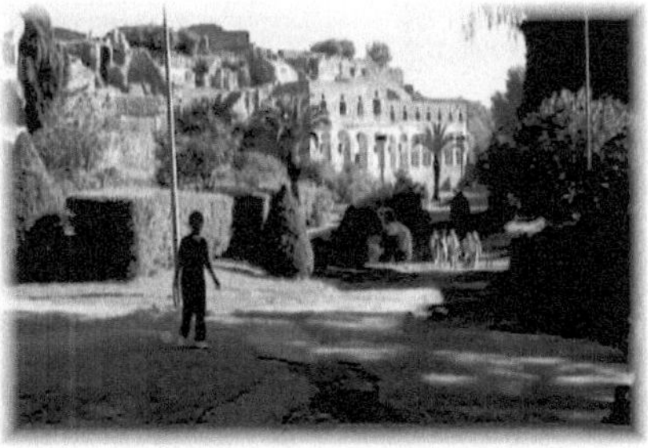

When we caught up with our group, it was just breaking up and was on its way after some informational details about the ruins. Surveying the terrain and path through which the tour was being guided, I concluded that it was not suited for Amelia because of her disability.

We broke up from the group and without a guide, toured the ruins on our own, focusing and concentrating only on areas that appeared attractive. Because many tourists came in smaller disorganized groups not necessarily requiring guides, we knew which spots were popular by the number of tourists gawking and ringing around them.

At the Ruins of Pompeii, Naples

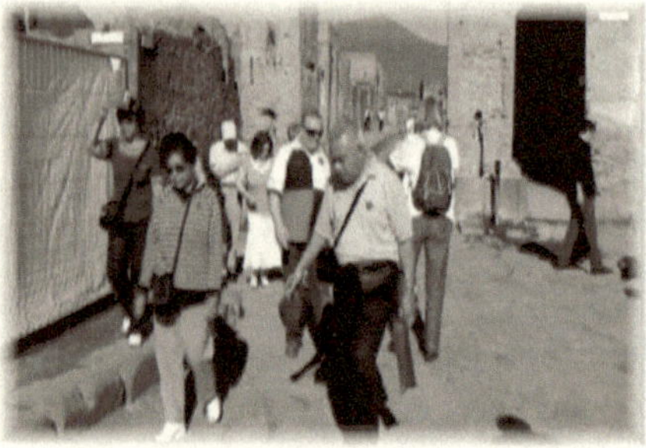

What immediately caught our attention are the mosaics that adorn some walls and the floors of the city; they are as modern and up to date if not more so, than those anyone would find in the present day building materials store. Pillars that withstood the force of the volcanic eruption are still upright, perpendicular, and intact. The architectures, obviously without the aid of modern gadgets, are as contemporary as anyone would find in any city today, making me wonder how early engineers grappled in their designs with only crude tools and equipment.

We witnessed the remains of humans preserved in ash, some of them appearing to cower into whatever available space there was seeking refuge from the deadly residue. Apparently suffering from suffocation, some remains seemed to breathe through their mouths, making me wonder how long they remained painfully conscious before they succumbed to their deaths. The sight of the remains is very disturbing even with hardened ashes replacing the flesh.

The yard that was the venue for public entertainment in those

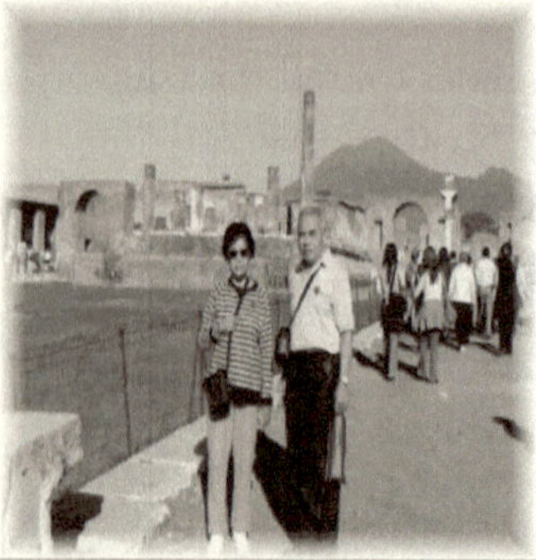

ancient times is still in excellent condition. It is big enough to accommodate chariot battles and races that in those days would usually end in deaths to one or more of the participants. It is easy to imagine the gladiators evidently being the focus of attention in the arena as they entertained the crowd in mortal

At the Ruins of Pompeii, Naples

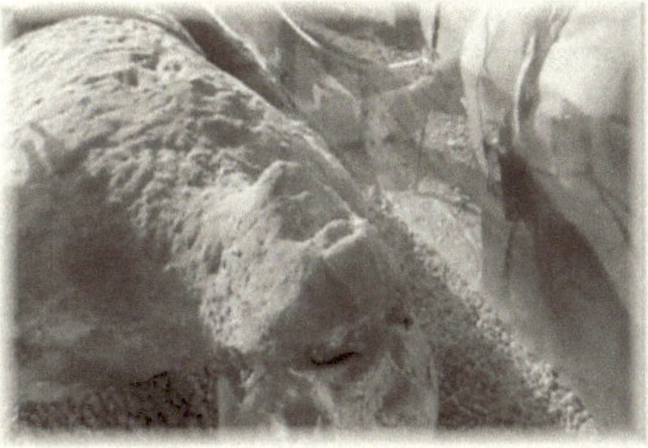

combats. Just a few doors away from the yard, are the cells that housed the gladiators.

Many obstacles are on the way for touring the rest of the ruins especially for one with a physical disability like Amelia. Tired, exhausted, and badly needing rest, we ate at a restaurant just to have a place to sit before directing our attention to more locations in the ruins. The crowd was growing quite rapidly making the place look like a festival. After the much-needed rest, we only proceeded to areas in the ruins where there was a growing crowd to indicate their tourism value.

Having done all the sightseeing in the near area of the ruins, we decided to go back to the main entrance and waited for our group to finish the tour. The group did not appear until about two hours later, a measure in time of how big Pompeii used to be, before it was devastated by the eruption of Mt. Vesuvius in 79 AD. Mt. Vesuvius still sleeps and ominously looms at a visible distance from Pompeii.

Appearing uneasy and fearing that hunger syndrome might start to bother Amelia, I bought some food, fruits, and drinks for us from the market near the entrance to the ruins. Unable to find seats and not allowed to get on the bus till later, we were forced to eat while standing. Later in the bus, almost every passenger looked haggard and

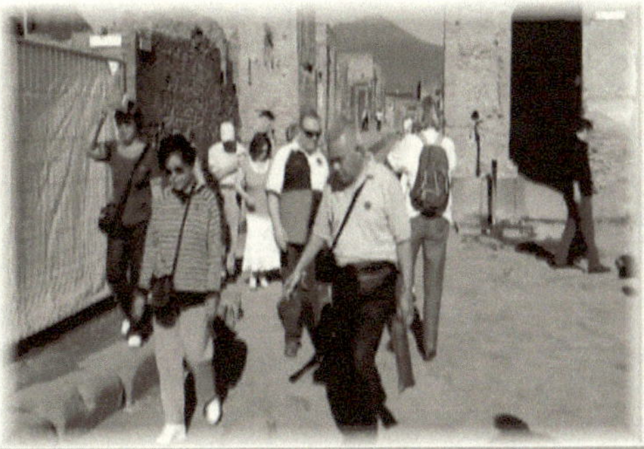

At the Ruins of Pompeii, Naples

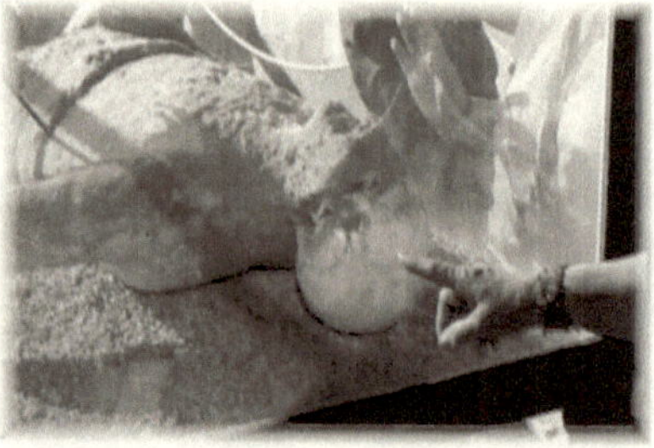

careworn. The tour bus headed back to the ship where food was always waiting for us at any time. We rested and relaxed on the ship, waiting for the nightly entertainments.

Despite our decision not to complete the tour as planned because of Amelia's physical condition, the tour was an absolute success. We were physically at the ruins to witness the remains of the City of Pompeii after the cataclysmic eruption of Mt. Vesuvius, whereas some people only know about Pompeii from watching movies, reading books, and listening to history teachers.

By some accounts, the city was completely submerged in ash, and its excavation was not completed until a few years ago. It is a compliment to the City of Naples for managing the location and in effect, preserving history.

At the Leaning Tower of Pisa, Pisa

The trip to Pisa, the site of the Leaning Tower, took a few hours through the Tuscany area of Italy, along beautiful rural open fields still in their natural contours. What easily came to my mind about Tuscany was Andrea Bocelli who hails from the place and is one of the most famous artists whose songs I will not get tired of listening. The trip through the open green fields took a different atmosphere from pleasant to unpleasant, upon arrival at Pisa on account of the enormous crowd of tourists and the moderately warmer weather.

Dismissive of the fact that our tour bus was made to park at the very far end of the parking lot, Amelia immediately discounted the trip as unnecessary and not worth going. But she no longer had any choice; we had to pick our way through streets with vendors aggressively pushing their wares and products. Our attention being focused on the leaning tower, we did not dare gawk at the souvenir shops lining the streets. Painstakingly and with my assistance, Amelia and I made it to the tower of which a short history follows.

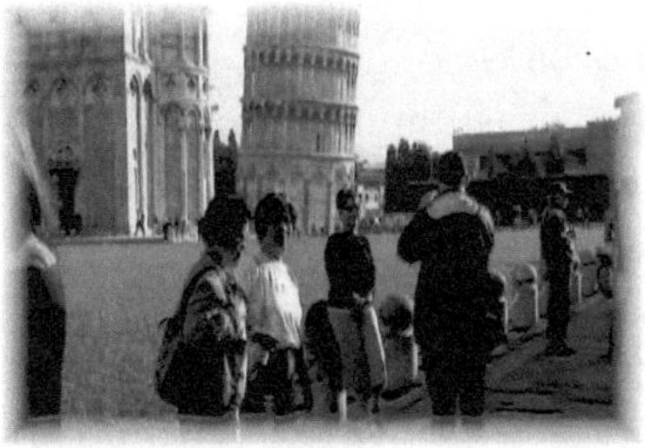

Construction of the tower started some eight hundred years ago. After just a few levels of construction, the tower started leaning; the foundation on one side of the tower was on a loose ground causing it to sink slowly. The construction was halted but not completely abandoned.

At the Leaning Tower of Pisa, Pisa

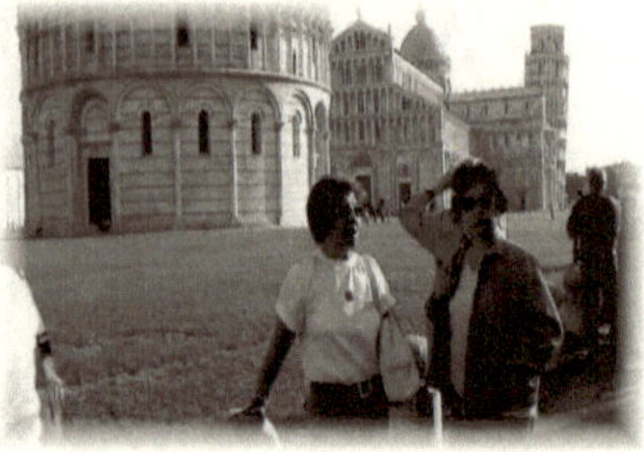

When construction was resumed, one side of the tower was made higher than the other to compensate for the lean. The compensation made the tower uprightly crooked, and it did not help correct the flaw either. Even though construction was favored on one side of the tower, the lean has been continuing. The corrective measures were no match against the law of gravity; but gravity on the other hand, has not managed to topple the tower up to this time. The tower's base had been shored up to prevent it from toppling over, or at least slow down the inevitable gravitational triumph.

Thousands of tourists visit the tower not because of its architectural design, but because of its lean - it is leaning precariously for a structure of its size. The tower forms a good background in a picture of one with extended arms and hands appearing to push and straighten it. I understood that a limited number of visitors are allowed to climb the tower up to certain levels.

Souvenir shops numbering in the few tens had brisk business in the area with shoppers having a field day. Fearing the incidence of Amelia's glucose level getting low and causing her to be uneasy and dehydrated, we ate at one of the restaurants which appeared popular from the number of customers waiting to be served. Although the food was not to her liking, it energized Amelia until it was time to leave and bid goodbye to the Leaning Tower of Pisa.

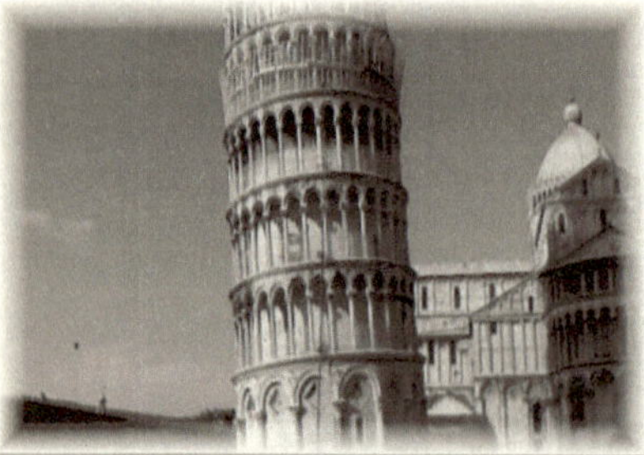

At the Leaning Tower of Pisa, Pisa

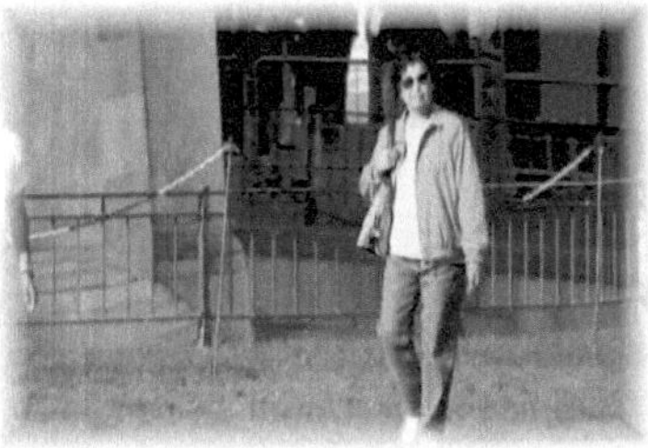

Personally, I think the restrooms were more profitable than most other businesses. For $0.50 per visit and capitalizing on the call of nature, the restrooms were a natural business model providing income for financing the maintenance of the tower and the surrounding areas, if indeed that is the case.

We stayed at the tower area for approximately four hours before we boarded the bus which took us back to the cruise ship. We rested and relaxed to get ready for the nightly shows and entertainments.

I considered the trip to the Leaning Tower of Pisa a success. The object of mesmerizing curiosity, the tower is historical in the sense that it has been precariously leaning for more than eight hundred years. Despite its lean the tower is a national landmark which invites people from different cultures.; hence the tower is also a cultural symbol from my point of view.

At the Vatican, Rome

Although the cruise ship was still being eased into port at Civitavecchia, Italy, passengers who signed up for the excursion to the Holy City were already in the process of being cleared for disembarkation in anticipation of the two- to three-hour trip. One of the biggest ports in the Mediterranean, Civitavecchia, handles container, ferry, as well as cruise ships, so it was not surprising to see plenty of activities at the port.

Our cruise ship was not alone at the port; there were few others. More than three bus loads of passengers from our cruise ship alone departed for the Holy City, each bus of roughly fifty passengers, assigned with a driver and a tour guide. All the buses looked the same, evidently from the same company. Owing to Amelia's handicap and difficulty of movement, we ended up sitting at the rear of the bus.

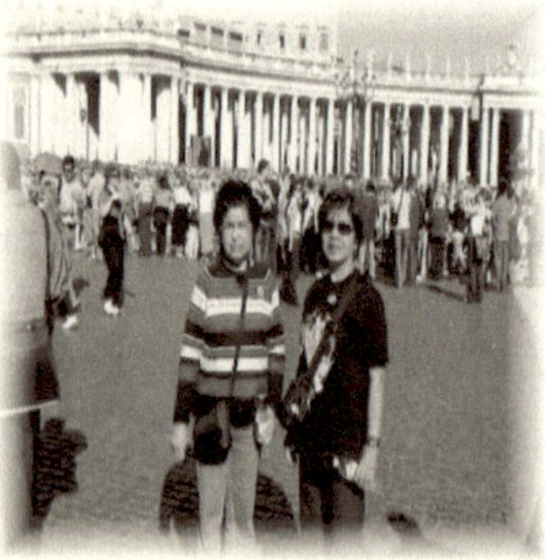

Unfortunately, the buses were not equipped to handle personal necessities, a common complaint among passengers; they kept on going nonstop for more than two hours. As if to taunt the passengers further our tour guide devoted a long part of his historical account of a Roman Emperor, Vespasian, whose project included a requirement of installing toilets in homes and public places for the people's convenience.

Arriving in Rome after more than two hours on the highway, our first order of business naturally and urgently was to find restrooms. We did find four locations but hampered by Amelia's slow pace, we always ended up at the rear of the lines. We had no excuse but to

At the Vatican, Rome

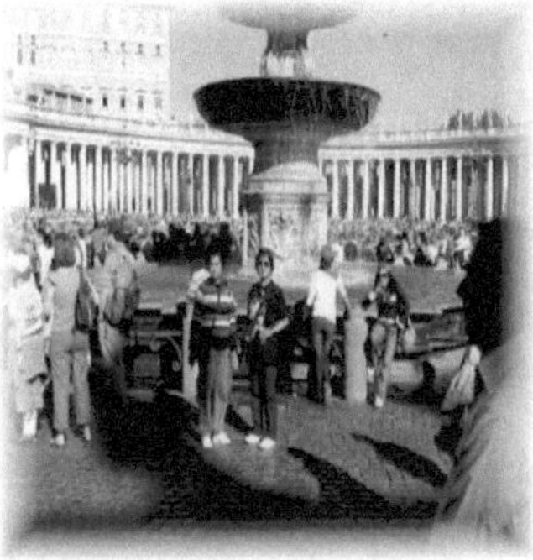

patiently wait for our turns, presuming that other tourists were in similar situations as we were.

We witnessed the Pope saying mass only from a distance due to the huge crowd at St. Peters Square. Not wanting to squeeze ourselves amidst the crowd in a moderately warm and slightly humid day because of Amelia's inability to move quickly, we took pictures of the Pope only from such distance. The mass was being played on a giant screen, making the Pope appear bigger than his figure while sitting down.

After the mass, it was time to explore St. Peters Square. Recalling the song "Three Coins in the Fountain," we figured that one of the fountains in the square was the prop used in the movie, so we took pictures of all of them unsure which one was the recipient of the coin tosses. It was time to walk out and avoid the growing crowd, having covered as much ground as we could of the square.

Though she was not complaining, Amelia was moving ever so slowly and stuttering slightly, a sign of an impending attack from hunger syndrome, a characteristic she was inflicted with after the massive strokes. We picked a small corner outside the square but facing the Pope's residence, and the four of us, Dolly, Dennis, Amelia, and I ate the bread, fruits, and candies I brought along from the ship. The arrangement paid off and saved us precious time from having to

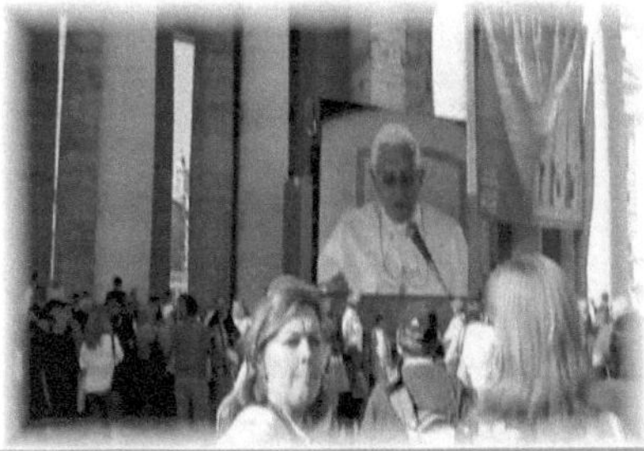

At the Vatican, Rome

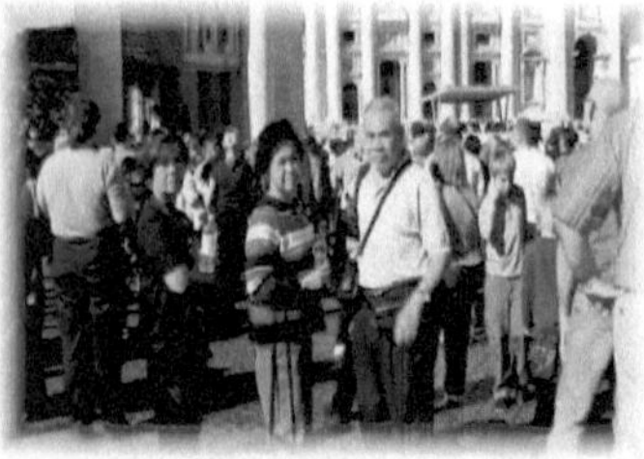

follow long lines at the eating places.

After the improvised lunch, we explored the area some more, looking for souvenirs to buy and bring home. One particular item that caught my attention was a Chinese made rosary bead ridiculously priced at $350.00. I did not know what it was made of, but I surmised that there was no way a rosary bead as expensive as that, could save my soul even if my sins are of the light type.

Not having enough time to tour the area without us getting exhausted in a very short period especially Amelia, we stopped exploring much farther. We went to the assembly area of our group and waited for our tour bus. This time we went earlier than the rest of the passengers allowing us to pick better seats. We were ready to go back to the cruise ship, except that the excursion included a tour of the city, the City of Rome.

The tour bus took us around the areas of the city frequented by tourists, both on foot and on vehicles. We drove by the Colosseum which is pockmarked with holes all around due to pilferage for metals which are smuggled and sold profitably, according to the tour guide.

Apart from the Colosseum many other magnificent structures were pointed out to us by the guide, as critical in the administration and history of the city, ultimately in the expansion of the Roman Empire. Tourists appeared to be pouring into the city from every conceivable direction.

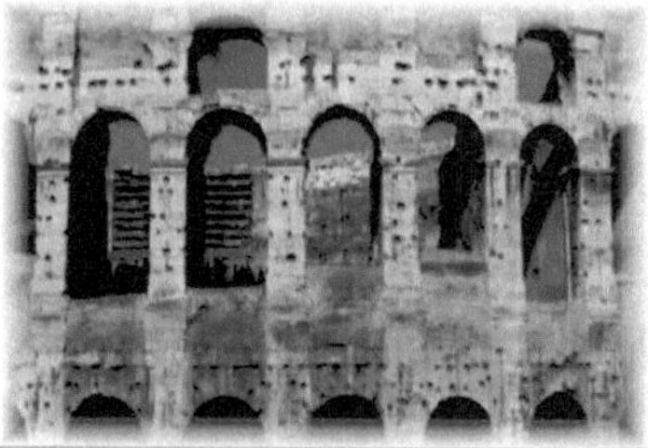

At the Vatican, Rome

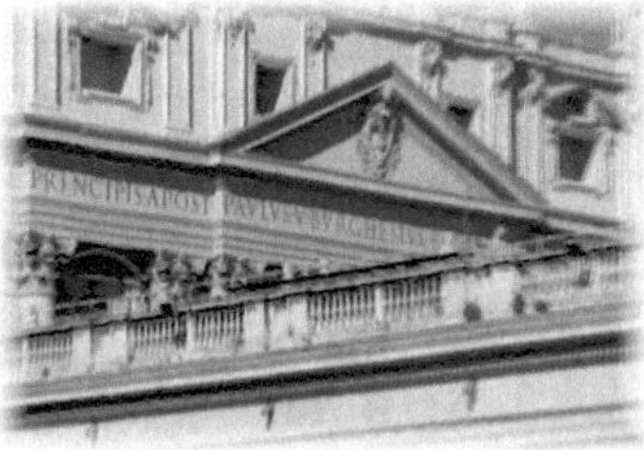

We departed from the city very tired and could not wait to catch a much needed nap in the tour bus during the two-hour drive back to the ship. Arriving at Civitavecchia at sundown, Amelia and I chose to rest after dinner instead of going to the night shows and other entertainments.

Despite the hectic day of our visit to the Holy City, I rated the excursion very successful, accomplished in a single day from a distant port. We have had a few excursions to our credit, but this one to Rome was of a religious nature allowing us especially Amelia who is afflicted with multiple bodily disorders, to renew our faith as a Catholic even for just a short time.

At the Vatican, Rome

Chapter 15 – Destination London

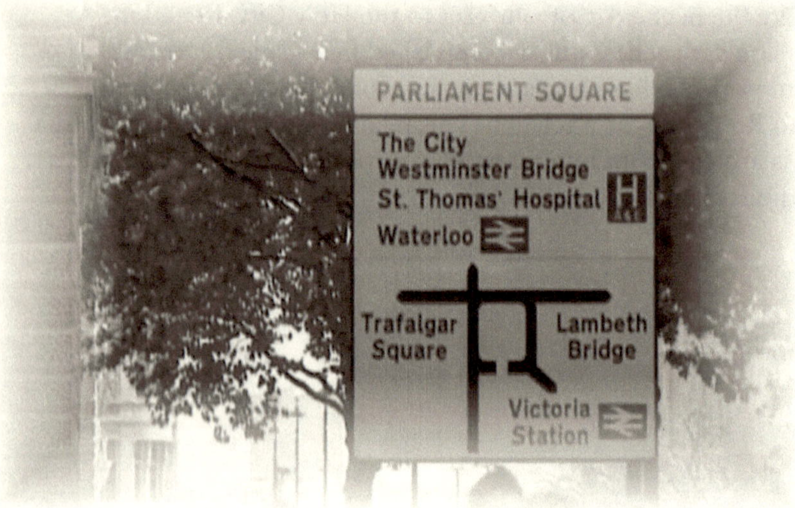

At the Buckingham Palace Parade, London

The idea of watching the changing of the guards at Buckingham Palace did not occur to us until we were already on the train and contemplating what to do with our day when we arrived in London from Paris. Glancing at our watches, we appeared to be on time for the spectacle if indeed there was one, and if the train arrived on schedule.

Without knowing whether the changing of the guards ceremony is held every day or only on certain days, we decided that our first order of business in London was to go to Buckingham Palace. The Palace after all, is a tourist attraction by itself even without ongoing activities.

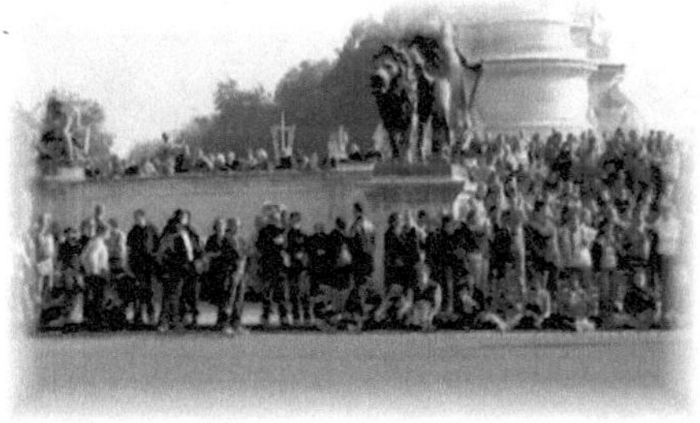

To our surprise the taxicab driver would not be accepting Euros, the currency we had, at the end of the ride at Buckingham Palace. We had to find a currency changer first to exchange the Euros for the English currency before we could pay him.

While waiting for the change, the driver told us that there was no changing of the guards ceremony on this day. What we could expect to witness was a simple parade which would fill our time after all, considering that we did not have definite plans for the day.

The taxicab dropped us on an ideal spot for watching the parade. Since we arrived early we positioned ourselves in front of the parade route, with two or three rows of people pressing behind us later on.

At the Buckingham Palace Parade, London

The parade was just turning towards us but not quite within a clear camera shot yet, when Amelia started feeling sick, an indication that hunger syndrome was poised to make its presence known. I knew we had to leave, so I tried to take as many pictures as I could of the parading soldiers on foot and on horseback, but waving hands were getting in the way and spoiling my shots.

We left our ideal position in the parade route and crossed the street towards a statue which was also teeming with parade watchers. Picking a tiny spot under the statue, I opened my carrying bag and fed Amelia with fruits and bread which I always carried for her on long trips.

We all ate at the same time, I continuously coaxing Amelia to eat faster so we could resume watching the parade even from a distance. She tried, but by the time she finished eating, the parade was already in the foreground with the crowd completely blocking our view and depriving us of taking pictures.

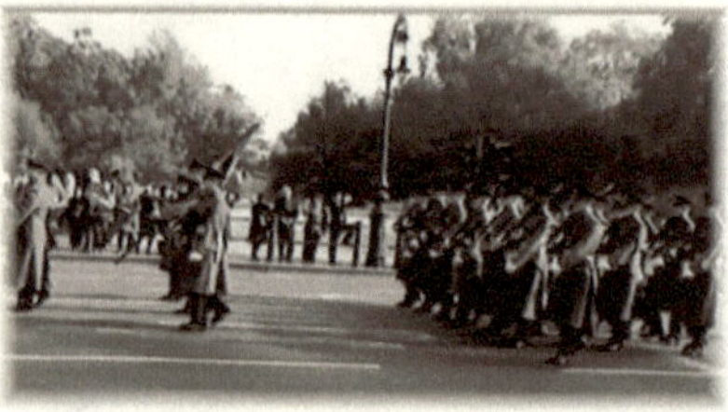

This day was the only opportunity for us while in Europe to witness parading soldiers in front of Buckingham Palace, so we pursued the parade until it disappeared in its final turn. Due to its small contingent, it disappeared quickly leaving us with not much photo opportunity.

Insignificant as the parade was though, we did our best to take as many pictures of it as we could for appreciation later. Most of the pictures I took were of the tail end of the parade when the parading soldiers had their backs turned to the camera.

At the Buckingham Palace Parade, London

Amelia had recovered slightly and showed signs of energy again, but I was still worried that she was already tired from the train ride between Paris and London. We were ready, I suspected, to compound the problem by walking away from Buckingham Palace to some place we did not know.

We left on speculation and instinct that there are other tourist attractions in the area besides Buckingham Palace. We could have hailed a taxicab of course, but to where we did not know. We had to adjust our pace to match Amelia's, hers being measured and slow making me conclude that her glucose level was down. She was struggling with every step.

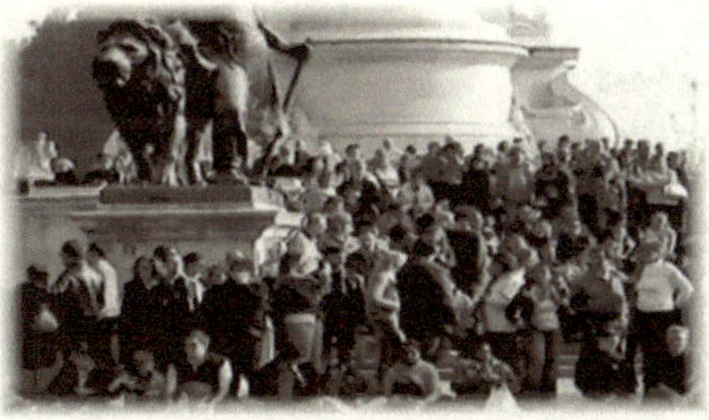

The iconic Big Ben clock, known all over the world, finally loomed ahead indicating that we were still in a populated tourist area of London notwithstanding the rows of buildings with a rare glimpse of ongoing human activities. We walked towards the clock, took pictures of it, and proceeded until we reached a queue of hop-on-hop-off buses. Boarding one of them, we started the bus tour of London.

In the past we had regularly watched parades like the Annual Hollywood Christmas Parade and the Annual Tournament of Roses Parade. Both famous parades are themed to principally entertain the parade watchers

On the other hand and in addition to entertaining the parade watchers, the Buckingham Palace Parade honors the head of state. Other than the cadenced steps of the soldiers and the parade horses, not much fanfare was evident similar to the two previously

At the Buckingham Palace Parade, London

mentioned parades. The parade was all military in the very strict sense.

Disappointed as we were for not being in the front row along the parade route and because of Amelia's slight emergency, we still relished the experience. For us who did not have a definite plan for the day, the spontaneous selection of the Buckingham Palace parade was an absolute and perfect utilization of our time.

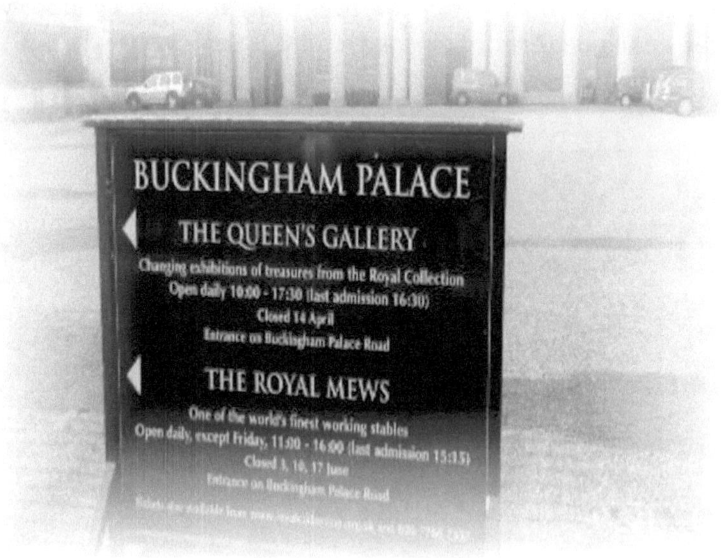
BUCKINGHAM PALACE
THE QUEEN'S GALLERY
Changing exhibitions of treasures from the Royal Collection
Open daily 10:00 - 17:30 (last admission 16:30)
Closed 14 April
Entrance on Buckingham Palace Road
THE ROYAL MEWS
One of the world's finest working stables
Open daily, except Friday, 11:00 - 16:00 (last admission 15:15)
Closed 3, 10, 17 June
Entrance on Buckingham Palace Road

At a London Bus Tour, London

Done watching the short Buckingham Palace parade and with Amelia showing signs of fatigue and struggling with every step, we kept walking in the direction of Big Ben, the iconic clock known the world over. Amelia was visibly getting tired.

We reached an area past Big Ben where tour buses were picking up passengers, and not knowing where to go, boarded one of them. Told by the bus driver that the bus tour would be ending at exactly this same area where it would be starting, we were relieved that at least we would have Big Ben as a reference point in case we got lost. The hop-on-hop-off bus tour is a convenient way to look at some limited tourist areas of the city.

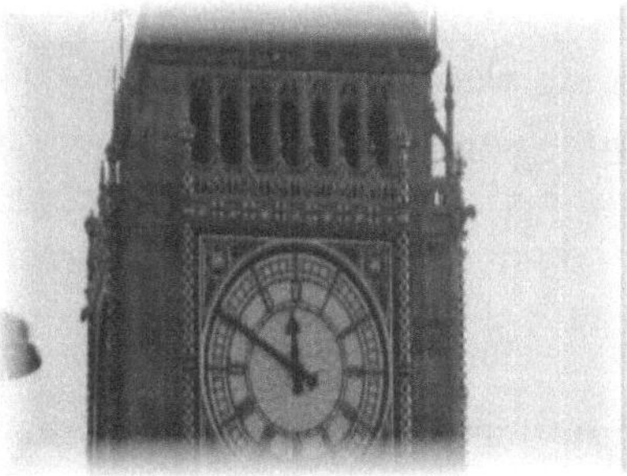

The weather was slightly chilly and cold leaving the upper deck of the tour bus with plenty of empty seats. Braving the wind and the cold weather, Dolly, Dennis, and I ended up at the upper deck to have an unobstructed view of the route the bus was traveling through. I left Amelia comfortably sitting just below the steps to the upper deck where she could also watch what was going on outside the bus while I would be watching her from time to time to be sure she was safe.

Less than an hour into the tour while listening to the descriptions of the scenes around, I noticed Amelia hardly able to keep her eyes open; she was drooping and looking exhausted, yet she was not complaining as I had eye contact with her. Abandoning my seat at the upper deck and completely ignoring photo opportunities that were coming along, I went down to check on her.

At a London Bus Tour, London

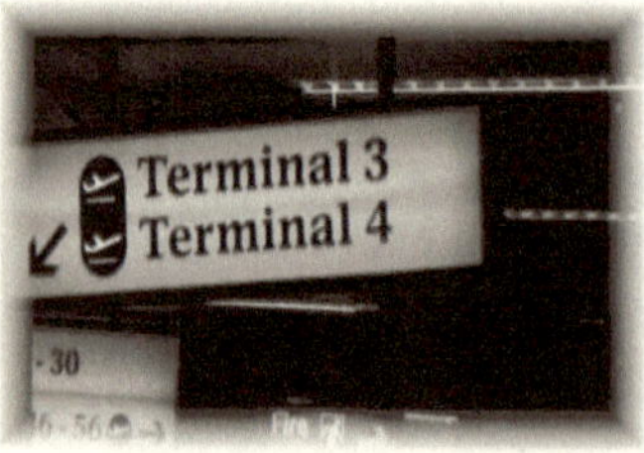

Even with her jacket on she was cold and almost shivering as I felt her body, but she would not say if anything was the matter despite that her looks and expression were saying differently. I was ready to tell Dolly and Dennis that we would be getting off the bus to take care of Amelia's emergency. Before I could do so however, the bus driver announced that the next stop would be at the famous Trafalgar Square where most tourists would be departing for a longer stay in the area.

The four of us alighted from the bus and immediately looked for an eating place, knowing that Amelia needed food and hot coffee or some liquid. The Square was crowded, and I concluded that if Amelia had a real emergency, I could quickly summon help. Luckily that did not happen; we ended up at a small crowded restaurant less than a block from where the bus stopped.

With restrained anxiety, I asked one of the servers to courteously bypass customers in front of us and serve Amelia with food and liquid ahead of them because Amelia was looking dazed and slightly shivering. The server obliged and immediately served Amelia with hot tea and snacks while Dolly, Dennis, and I waited for our turn in the queue of customers.

Gradually Amelia's complexion returned to normal as she consumed her food and drank hot tea, relieving us from worry that she might be having an emergency. We stayed at the restaurant for half an hour after eating to rest and to be sure that Amelia was in a position to

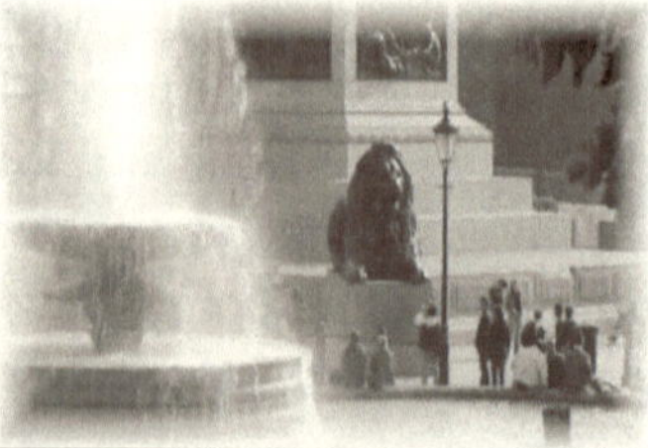

At a London Bus Tour, London

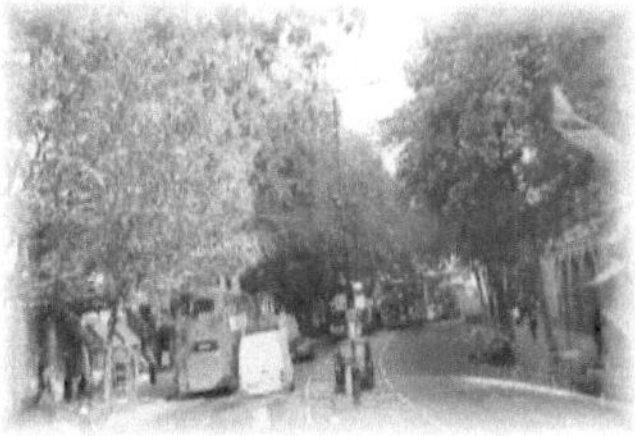

move out safely without further discomfort.

We stayed at the Square for about two hours to look around some more, with me always checking Amelia's status. Then taking a taxicab to the train station, we boarded the last train to Paris, arriving there early evening, Paris time.

What we accomplished in one day - round trip travel between Paris and London, watching the Buckingham Palace parade, and taking a short tour of London - was short of astonishing given that we were only visiting London for a short time with no itinerary and definite plans. The trip alone from a vast metropolis - that was Paris - to another metropolis - that was London - and back across an ocean on a single day was a major feat I thought was impossible to accomplish. By Southern California standards, that was equivalent to a shopping trip in San Diego from Los Angeles.

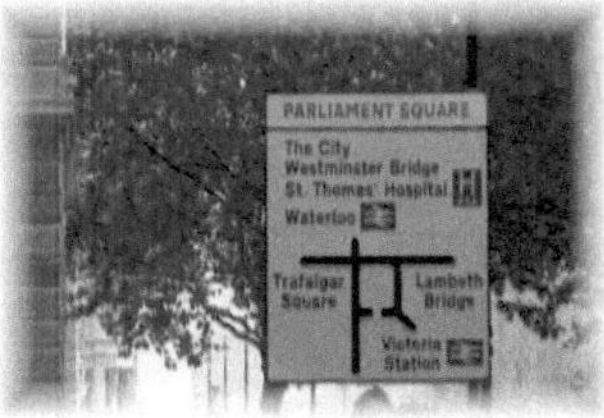

Freelance travelers might duplicate what we did, but I am not recommending it. A city as big as London has many tourist attractions to offer than those viewed from the deck of a tour bus.

At a London Bus Tour, London

Chapter 16 – Destination Mexico

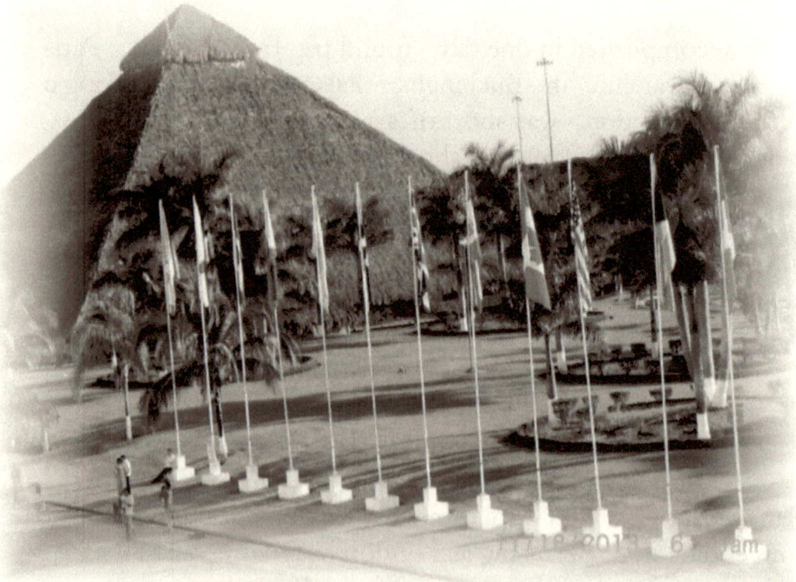

At Ensenada, Mexico

Coastal Cruises is a relatively short cruise schedule, only four days, in this case plying the Pacific coast covering California and part of Mexico. Ensenada was the last stop on the itinerary before we headed for the home port of San Pedro, Los Angeles.

The port area of Ensenada is immaculate with the buildings uniquely Mexican in design, mostly painted with bright red. It being in Mexico, Ensenada was the last international port on this cruise, and passengers were made aware that the next day will be disembarkation day and that meant having passports and other travel documentations ready at the immigration screening area.

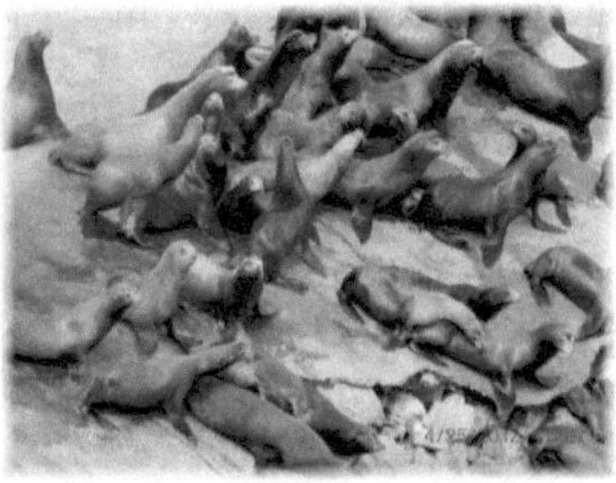

Owing to Amelia's disability and having been there previously, we waived our chance to join an excursion to La Bufadora, a natural attraction very popular among tourists. La Bufadora is a natural phenomenon where the air is trapped in a cave and forced out at a blowhole creating a geyser and a roaring sound.

We figured that on this gorgeous day, La Bufadora would be so crowded that Amelia was already indisposed to make the trip. In the first place, Amelia was not comfortable walking the length of the pier to the port buildings and out to where the tour buses were picking up the passengers.

I did not regret missing the excursion however, because on the ship, entertainments were non-stop. As we got closer to the end of the cruise, shows became more intense and livelier. With three birthday celebrants in the family all of whom were on the cruise

At Ensenada, Mexico

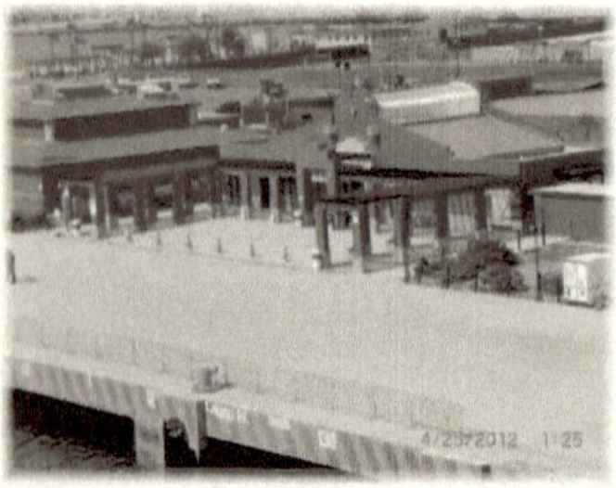

ship, this cruise was occasioned to provide plenty of entertainments and food without being burdened with preparation worries and post celebration cleanup.

Staying on the ship allowed us to move around and have a 270-degree view of the city including a large area of the harbor, from one side. On the other side we had a 180-degree view of the area across the canal from Ensenada.

As we did not come ashore however, we only had photo opportunities from the ship, of the city's skyline dotted with high-rise buildings, and a section of the harbor full of pleasure boats. How the residents of the city are getting along in their economies is profiled by the sheer number of pleasure crafts in the marina which was just a few hundred feet away from the cruise ship.

Ensenada is home to different kinds of sports, hang gliding being one of them. But sports fishing is more popular. The many yachts moored in the harbor indicate how much free times the residents of the city have been enjoying. Because of its proximity to the United States, some of the pleasure yachts and boats are owned by U.S. residents. With its port shielded from the huge Pacific Ocean waves especially during storms, Ensenada is a haven for fun crafts.

The port of Ensenada generates substantial commerce for Mexico. Some cargoes destined for the United States are unloaded in Ensenada and subsequently trucked across the border.

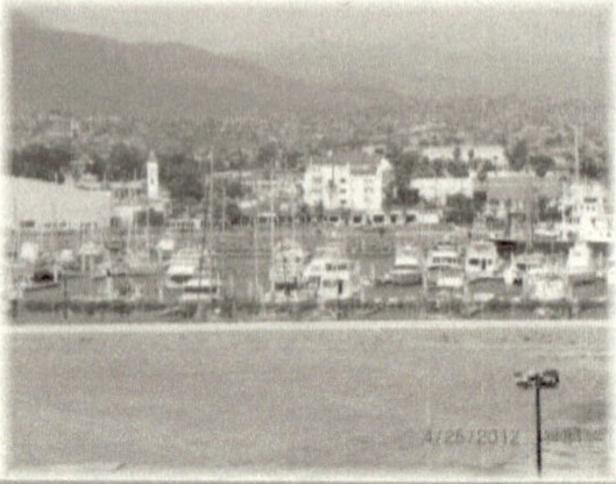

At Ensenada, Mexico

Because of its depth our cruise ship and a couple of large cargo ships were able to dock at just a single pier at the same time with room for two or three more. Of course, the sight of few cargo ships in the inward direction from the harbor entrance indicates that there are more piers of even larger capacities, deducing from the number of containers each ship carries. On this day that our cruise ship was docked at the port few massive cargo ships had been coming in and out of the harbor.

Passengers on the cruise ship were fascinated by a large number of sea lions basking in the sun on the slopes along the pier. Unmindful of the presence of humans, the animals appeared to like their pictures being taken, and the tourists were equally excited, but when they got too close to the animals, the sea lions slid into the water in unison.

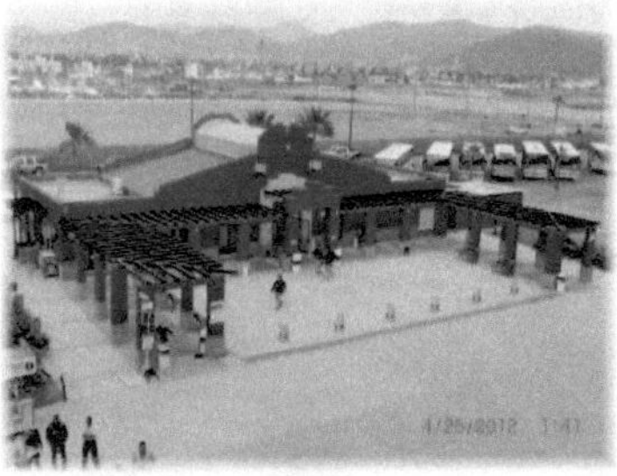

Final entertainments were being prepared for the last night of cruising. On every cruise we have been to, the last night is the most colorful and entertaining with all sorts of tricks, dances, loud music, uncorking wine bottles, and other festive activities, lasting up to midnight and early morning in some cases. This final night was not an exception.

Having been on land in Ensenada previously, the inability to join an excursion due to Amelia's disability was not a major failing. The object of this particular cruise was food and entertainment to coincide with multiple birthday celebrations in the family, after all.

For a short cruise vacation, a strip to Ensenada, Mexico, is as exciting as a longer one. It is inexpensive and does not need much preparation. Although entertainments are not as extensive and

At Ensenada, Mexico

broad as in longer cruises, they soothe the body and mind just as well, especially of ones who want to get a break from the 24/7 work schedules. The cruise usually includes one or two other ports in California, making it more diverse with respect to port features.

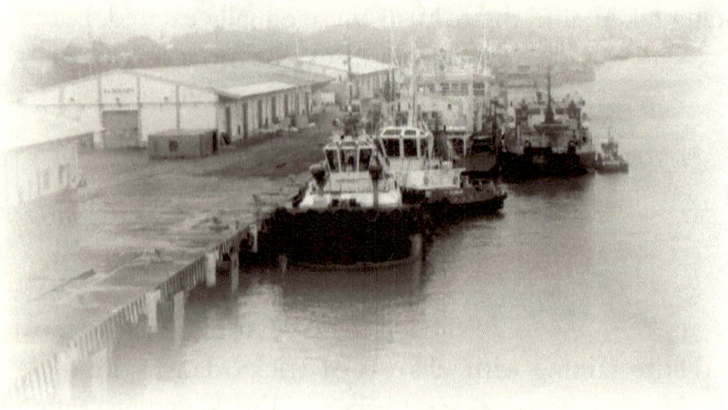

At El Eden Jungle, Puerto Vallarta, Mexico

The excursion to El Eden Jungle was recommended to us by the members of the staff on the cruise ship and some people who had been there before. A glowing description of the jungle on the flyers finally won us over that it, among many, was the excursion we would like to join in. When enough tourists to fill one bus signed in for the excursion, we left for El Eden Jungle.

The first half hour of the excursion was to showcase some of the beautiful beaches of Puerto Vallarta. We did not start the ascent to the mountains until we reached Mismaloya where some very wealthy people in Mexico reside, according to our tour guide. In fact, he compared Mismaloya to Beverly Hills, he having lived in Los Angeles and made few trips to both cities many times.

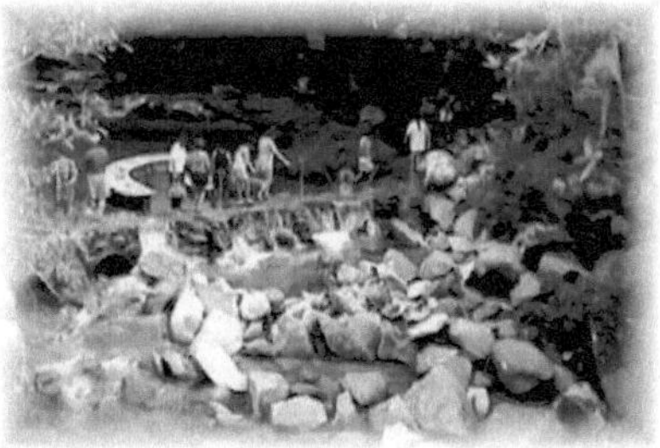

El Eden Jungle is located in the mountains over Puerto Vallarta reachable by a mostly graveled road which provoked fear among passengers when the tires of the bus were just a couple or so feet away from the edge overlooking very deep gorges. Some segments of the road are so narrow that vehicles coming from the opposite direction had to stop to give us the right of way. Nevertheless, some not-so-careful drivers were making pinpoint passes just inches shy of the side of the tour bus.

Driving along the deep ravines made us feel like we were on top of huge and tall trees which appeared miniature due to the depth of the canyons. More than once we witnessed full grown coconut trees growing on top of tall trees of a different variety, somewhat a natural way of grafting. The account has it that the coconut fruits

At El Eden Jungle, Puerto Vallarta, Mexico

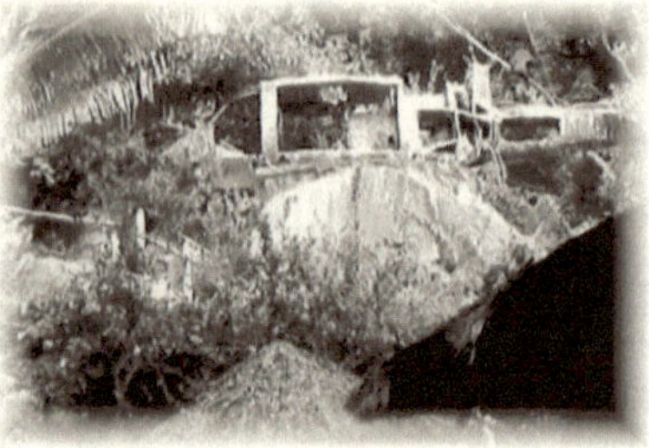

got caught on the trunk of the other tree type when they fell and started growing to full maturity.

Restrictions on how far out one can venture into the jungle from the roadway and the picnic areas preserve the surroundings of El Eden Jungle. Although the area of possible exploration is limited, the place attracts hundreds and hundreds of tourists solely lured by its unmolested and undisturbed pristine state.

A likely place to harbor some predators if any exist at all, due to its dense forest, El Eden Jungle was where some of the scenes in the movie 'The Predator' were filmed. The helicopter is still left intact near the brook where some of the slugfest scenes occurred.

Where the stream forms a deep pool, boulders that create waterfalls are used as slides by people who wanted to swim. Few ropes strung from a cottage overlooking the water are used to swing outward to plunge and splash into the clear water below.

At El Eden Jungle there is no shortage of food, it having a big fully equipped restaurant capable of seating a huge crowd and serving mostly Mexican food. In addition to the indoor furniture, benches and tables are also located outside the cottage where tourists can mingle and meet new friends.

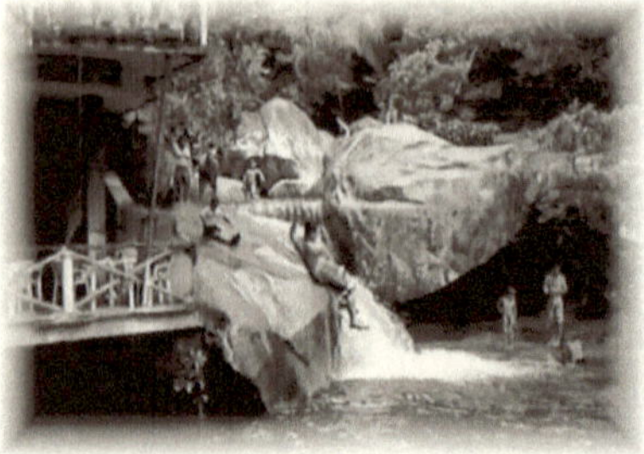

Done with lunch and after spending about two hours at El Eden Jungle, we proceeded back to the city, relieved that the tour bus was now being driven on the side of the road closer to the

At El Eden Jungle, Puerto Vallarta, Mexico

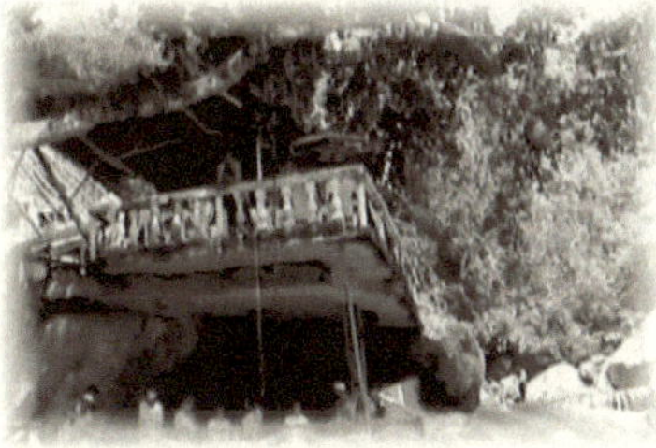

mountain. The route back took us through downtown Puerto Vallarta with a stop at the church where Elizabeth Taylor and Richard Burton solemnized their wedding.

The excursion took a good part of the day leaving Amelia exhausted and not in a condition to explore the downtown area of Puerto Vallarta further. While other tourists decided to get off and walk around, we stayed on the bus which took us to the beach area closer to the cruise ship where we strolled for a few minutes before boarding. We spent the rest of the day resting and relaxing waiting for the night time entertainments.

Although the trip to El Eden Jungle was somewhat rough, it was worth it for it illustrated the beauty of the land that is untouched and unmodified by humans. Leaving the jungle alone assures that many generations to come will have the same chance as we now do, to witness nature's ability to replenish its natural attributes. .

At the Mayan Ruins, Chiapas, Mexico

My chance to explore the ruins of the Mayans who disappeared without written history was at hand at Chiapas, Mexico. It was the Mayan calendar's prediction of the world's end in December 2012 that aroused my interest even more.

On this particular morning, we found our cruise ship maneuvering for position along the pier at Chiapas, Mexico, one of the scheduled stops in our Panama Canal cruise itinerary. The port with well-trimmed grass and hedges and a backdrop of three imposing giant pyramid-like structures is one of the most beautiful I've ever seen. Because of its beauty and its pursuit to share in the economy generated by tourism, it is already a popular destination for cruise lines.

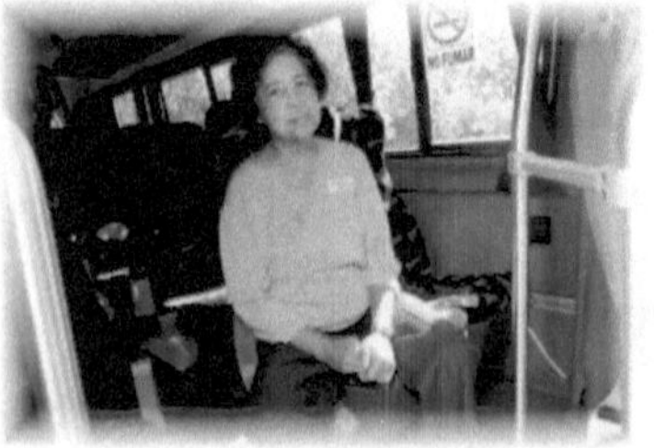

Flag-waving groups of Mexican-clad men and women playing Mexican songs accompanied by mariachi band were on hand to welcome the tourists from the cruise ship. As the cruise ship permanently moored, the welcoming activities got even more intense creating an atmosphere of glee and celebration.

One of the excursions promoted on the ship was the Mayan ruins of Chiapas. To break the monotony on the ship after being on it for a few days and assured that the tour bus was air conditioned and that there were seats for passengers with disability, I signed up for the excursion.

Amelia, whose recent stroke was only three months ago, had to walk slowly using her walker and with me assisting her, the entire length of the pier to the tourists' assembly area. Obstructed by

At the Mayan Ruins, Chiapas, Mexico

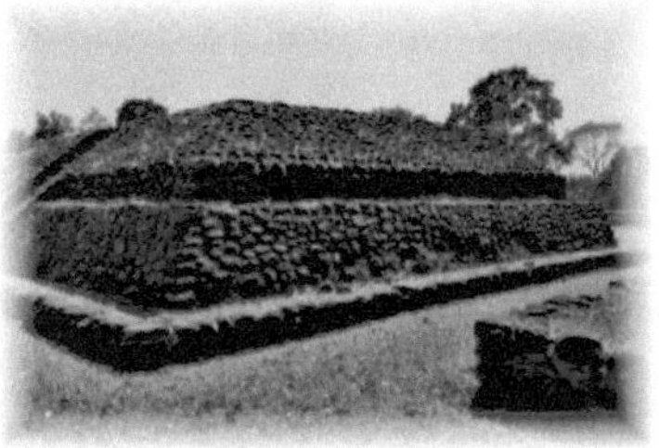

ongoing exhibitions and entertainments on a hall leading to the bus stop, our progress was further hampered, that by the time we reached the assembly area, all the seats on the tour bus were taken.

We were offered seats at a sports utility vehicle which we reluctantly accepted. At first, the trip was comfortable, the vehicle being able to provide enough cold air for all the passengers. As we traveled farther and farther away towards the mountains however, the heat started to intensify, and humidity was getting miserable particularly at the back of the vehicle where we were seated.

Amelia was perspiring profusely asking me if we could go back to the ship. Unfortunately, despite our dislike of the condition inside the vehicle, there was no turning back; we were committed to complete the excursion before we could turn back.

We reached the Mayan ruins at Chiapas with Amelia very exhausted and with diminished energy. She could not get off the sports utility vehicle because of extreme humidity on top of the heat - about hundred plus degrees - even though the vehicle was kept on running to keep its interior cool. She moved to the front seats of the vehicle with not much relief from the extreme temperature.

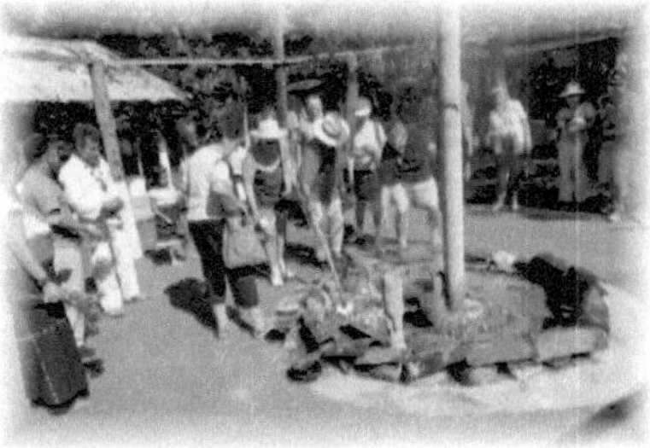

I could not leave Amelia in the vehicle for an extended period, so while I was exploring the ruins I kept coming back to check on her and to inform her of what was going on outside the vehicle. She was more

At the Mayan Ruins, Chiapas, Mexico

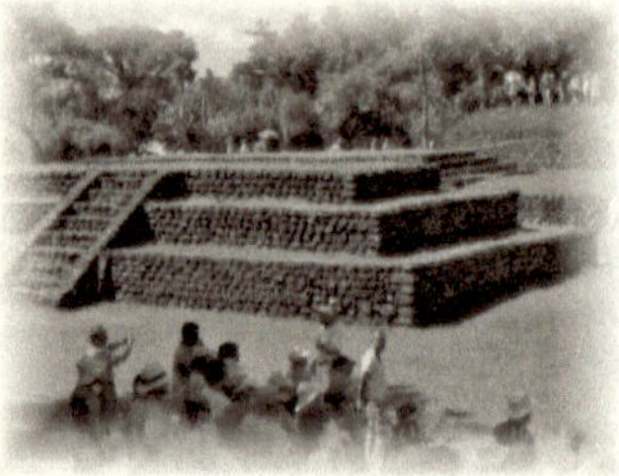

interested in getting back to the ship than contemptuously knowing what was happening outside the vehicle. Even the supposed Mayan priest went to the vehicle with me to check on Amelia, whispering words which I could hardly hear and understand.

I witnessed and participated in the offering ceremony - Mayan style - to the Mayan gods. I made some offerings myself, silently praying that Amelia would be healthy enough to get back to the ship without incident.

Cocoa-making from abundant cocoa plants in the area is a big local industry. I witnessed how locals produce cocoa which earned them some prestigious international awards.

After more than two hours exploring the ruins, we headed back to the ship. I rated the excursion not very successful only because of the condition in the vehicle. Otherwise, it was fascinating and informative. The Mayans and their ruins remain a mystery to me.

The ruins are small in comparison with other sites, I understand, but it is big enough to represent the Mayans' advance culture. When one considers that the Mayans existed several hundred years if not thousands before the birth of Christ, they were pretty savvy; they were builders, astronomers, and agriculturists among other skills. Perhaps other Mayan ruins are more intricate and able to provide more details about their culture and disappearance. I felt though that the Mayan ruins at Chiapas more than filled my curiosity about the Mayans.

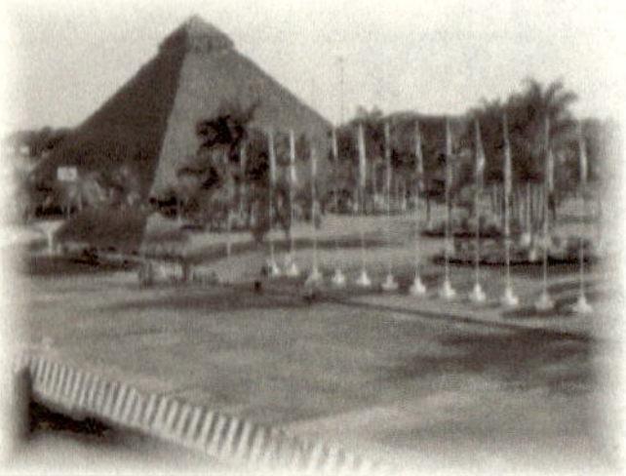

At Huatulco, Mexico

Done twice a day and having an unopened bottle of fifty test strips before the start of a 15-day Panama Canal cruise, I did not expect to run out of them for testing Amelia's glucose level. At that frequency of testing, I would still have test strips for ten more days when we would already be at home by then. Then Amelia's glucose level started to behave erratically.

I did not know what was causing it, perhaps it was the food or the weather. Amelia was only four months in her recovery from a recent stroke, so it was easy for me to associate the stroke with the unusual changes in her glucose level. All I had to do was to give her the prescribed medications that ought to normalize her glucose level. It had been working before; there was no reason it should not be working this time. The assumption was wrong; her glucose level which I kept between 80 and 165, was registering higher than 240 even after taking her prescribed medications.

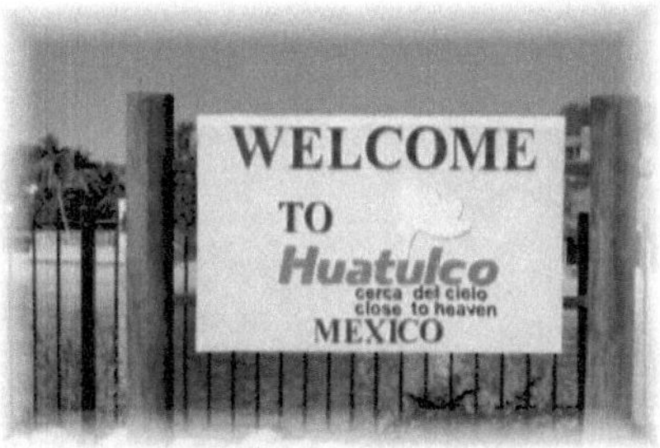
WELCOME
TO
Huatulco
cerca del cielo
close to heaven
MEXICO

Concerned and horrified, I tested her glucose level more frequently until the supply of test strips was down to zero, when we were still three days from the end of the cruise; by then we were already on the Pacific Ocean side of the itinerary. I was frightened and nervous; Amelia's condition became my primary concentration over the onboard entertainments.

I asked for test strips from the ship's dispensary, but theirs were not the kind that fits into Amelia's test meter. Considering that glucose level testing was not an emergency, the clinic would not offer to do

At Huatulco, Mexico

the testing either. However, a member in the medical staff suggested that I get off the ship at Huatulco which was the next scheduled stop on the cruise itinerary, and buy the strips from a drug store at the pier area. She even gave me the address of the store.

Finding the ship docked at Huatulco in the morning, I urgently prepared to disembark to purchase the test strips, but the passengers were not allowed to disembark until final clearance was announced. I used the extra time before disembarkation, to half-heartedly admire the city from the ship.

The city looks immaculate with residences and apartments overlooking the ocean from the cliffs not too far from the dock. Close by where the cruise ship was docked, is a marina with plenty of pleasure crafts unfurling their sails getting ready for whatever activities they had to do, mostly leisure sailing, I assumed. The water along the cliffs looked bluish or greenish suggesting to me that even at that close to the shore the water is very deep. The pier itself is not very far from the cliffs.

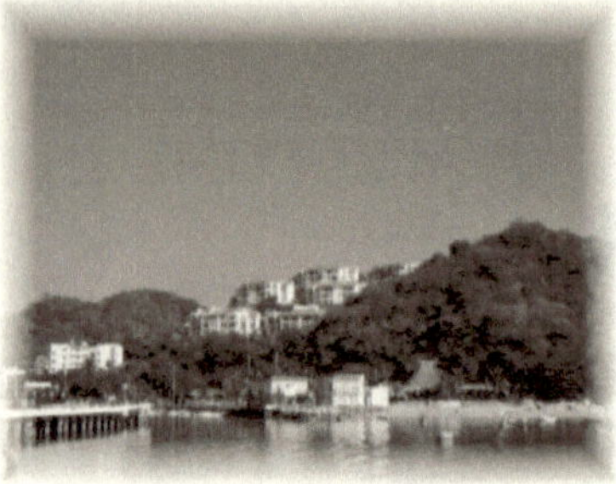

I contemplated whether or not to take Amelia with me to the stores at the pier area. She tried a few steps at the pier, but because of the heat and the distance to cover, she decided to stay on the ship and let me buy the test strips alone. We were right, the walk from the ship to the stores looked short, but in reality, it was exhausting, long, and not appropriate for one with a disability.

The drugstore did not carry the type of test strips that fits Amelia's test meter. The pharmacist suggested to me to place an order for

At Huatulco, Mexico

pickup the following morning in the same pharmacy, or buy it from the downtown drugstore. I asked the pharmacist to call the downtown store to have the test strips ready for me for pick up in just a few minutes.

The taxicab took twenty minutes or so to the address of the drugstore at downtown Huatulco, where an unopened bottle of fifty test strips was waiting for me. I had the taxicab wait for me, and after paying for the test strips, I took the same taxicab back to the pier area.

Back at the ship, I was relieved that I was able to check Amelia's glucose level again even though it was still behaving erratically. I was still bewildered by what was causing it to fluctuate. Shortly after disembarkation at the end of the cruise, I took her to the doctor for examination. The result did not reveal anything wrong with Amelia overall, not to mention her glucose level.

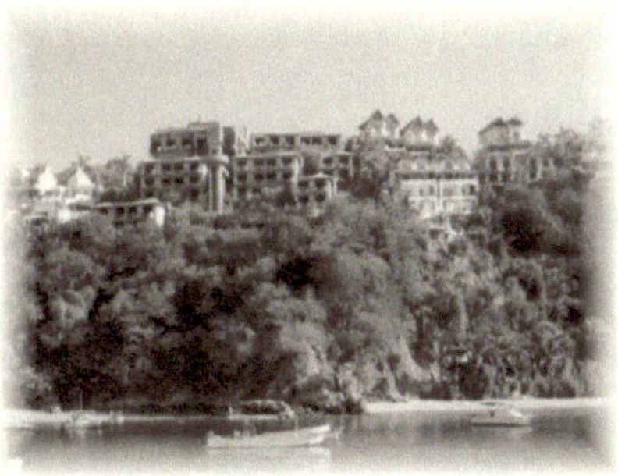

We were lucky that nothing serious was the matter with Amelia despite the erratic glucose level readings. Unsure at the time though, the readings did not absolve me from worrying and thinking that our cruise vacation might be for naught instead of leisure. The fact that Amelia had a stroke just three months ago did not help calm me. Fortunately, the incident occurred on the last three days of the cruise, almost home port bound.

At Huatulco, Mexico

Notwithstanding the extremely distressing incident, the cruise ended successfully; we were issued certificates of completion of the Panama Canal transit from the Caribbean Ocean to the Pacific Ocean.

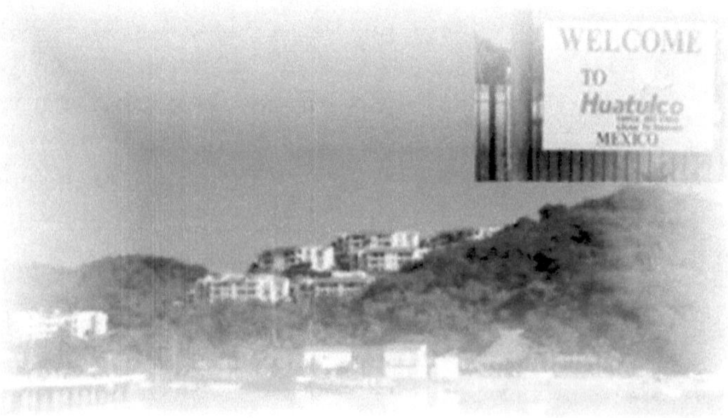

At Cabo San Lucas, Mexico

We cruised to the Mexican Riviera a couple of times before, but only once did we go ashore and then only on the pier area. This time I was more motivated to look around the downtown area of the city despite Amelia's discomfort on boarding the tenders. The cruise ship was anchored a couple or so miles out in the harbor, and the ocean was very choppy making the tenders sway wildly. It took an impassioned plea on my part to make Amelia agree to go ashore.

We chanced upon a couple from the ship - it is very easy to make friends on the cruise ship - who wanted to explore the downtown area of Cabo San Lucas as well. Sharing the taxicab fare, we accepted their offer to take us along for the ride. Though not fluent in English, on our request the driver drove us around few of the popular destinations in the city, describing why such places are considered landmarks and traditional.

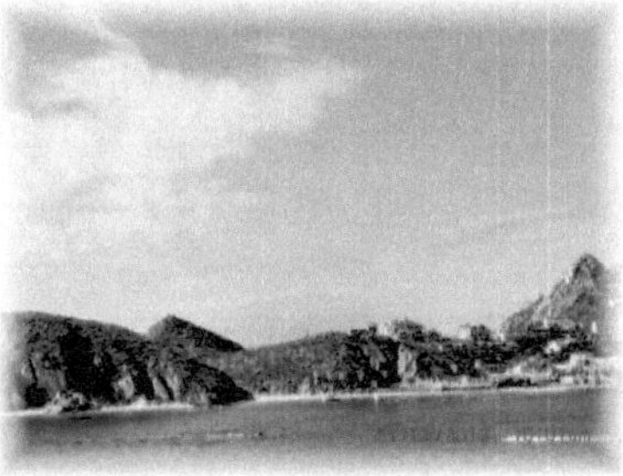

Indicating to him that we did not have a particular location to visit, the taxicab driver suggested that we go to the Town Square and spend some time there. That was agreeable and to our liking because we did not want to stray too far off the main downtown area. Amelia and I preferred to get back to the ship should the short trip cause her some hardships. The driver dropped us off in front of a big Mexican restaurant just across the Town Square.

At Cabo San Lucas, Mexico

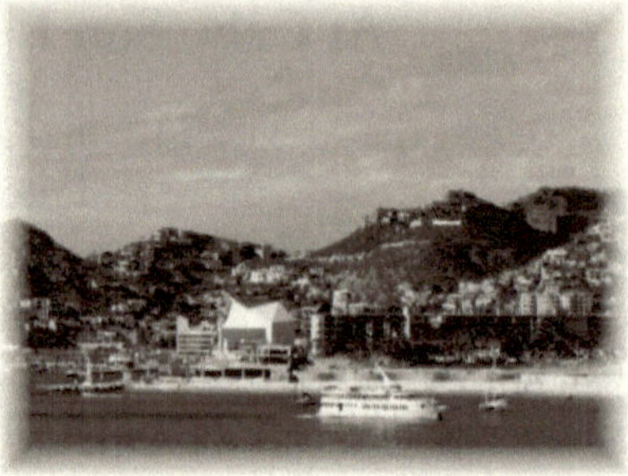

Amelia is not fond of Mexican food, so I ordered some pastries and soda instead to ease her looming hunger while the other couple ordered some Mexican food for themselves. Apparently taking time, it took them a little longer to eat their food while we finished ours in a few minutes with plenty of leftovers because Amelia did not like them.

We courteously told the couple that we would be eating lunch at the cruise ship and that we would be walking out to the square on our own before proceeding by taxicab to the pier area. After a short walk around Town Square and seeing that Amelia was limping quite noticeably, we rested for more than five minutes before I hailed a taxicab to take us to the pier area.

The tenders were coming and going every fifteen to thirty minutes, unloading tourists just coming off the cruise ship and picking up returning ones. The water was still quite rough, and tenders were still swaying wildly. We waited for the water to smoothen somewhat for a comfortable ride.

Souvenir shopping at the pier area was fun with seemingly non-stop price haggling. Thus, while waiting for the tenders to come, we tested our negotiating skills to get the best price for souvenirs we did not seriously want. We ended up buying a couple of throw blankets made from what appeared to be alpaca. I purchased a replica of the Rolex watch for myself which started falling apart after wearing it for a couple of weeks at home.

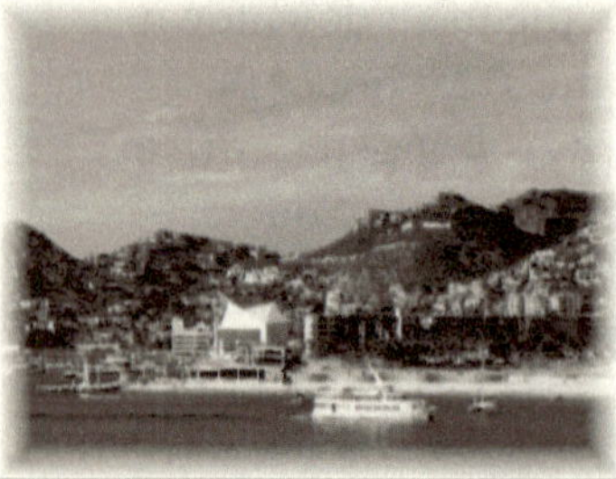

At Cabo San Lucas, Mexico

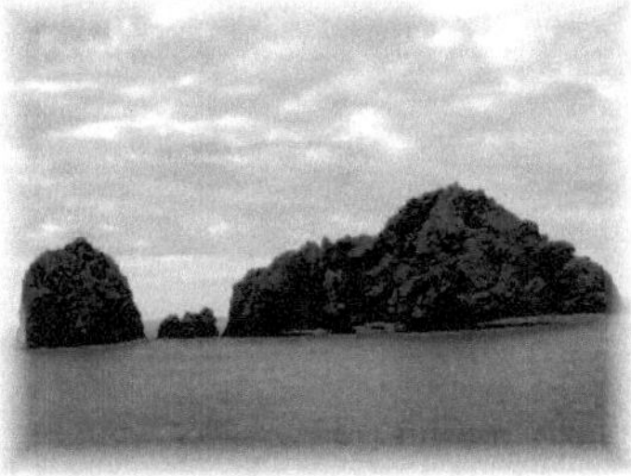

Evidently, the temperature and the humidity were causing Amelia to dehydrate. Visibly uneasy and needing something to drink, she asked that we take the next tender to the cruise ship where she had one. We spent the rest of the day relaxing and waiting for the night entertainments.

Cabo San Lucas is one of the most popular tourist destinations in the Mexican Riviera. Its skyline attests to its affluence and share of the economy in the region. On the previous cruises we had when the weather was calmer, we observed pleasure boats dotting the harbor, beachgoers flocking to the beaches, and some kayakers displaying their skills.

When the arch on the signature island landmark appears it tells one that Cabo San Lucas is near. It is the most photographed landmark of the city. I considered the short tour of the city a success and I recommend it for further exploration to other tourists.

At Cabo San Lucas, Mexico

Chapter 17 – Destination Niagara Falls

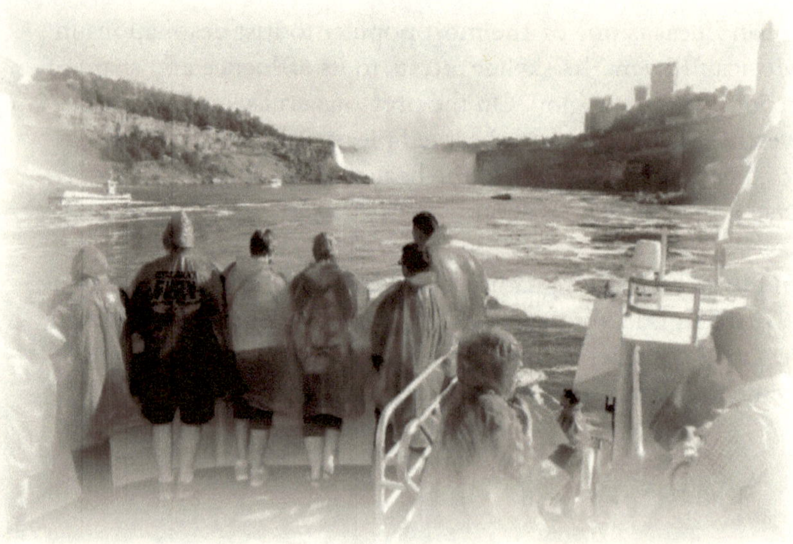

The Fury, Niagara Falls

The Fury, one of Niagara Falls favorite tourist attractions, was included in the hotel accommodation package I purchased online. I had no idea what the attraction was, but having experienced sustained hurricane force winds when living in a region known as typhoon belt many years ago, I rightly guessed that the title was about the fury of nature.

The furies I expected to watch were the sustained 75-mile-per-hour ferocious wind that blew homes and toppled trees, the furious 15-foot high waves that pounded the cliffs along the shores, the unrelenting rains that blew horizontally instead of falling vertically, and other violent and destructive forces related to climate change.

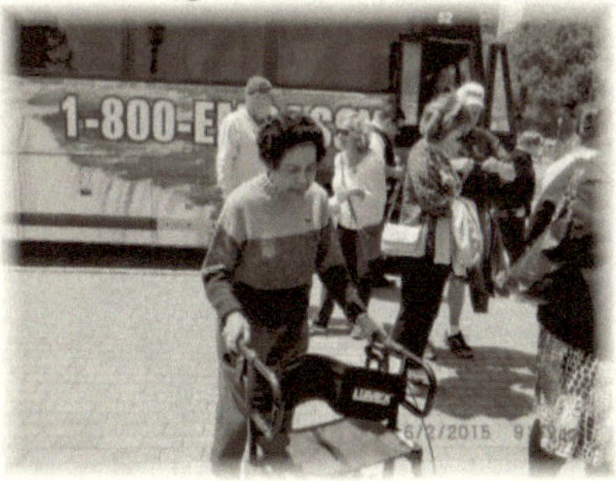

The tour bus did not travel very far from the hotel to the site of The Fury. After assembling the passengers and giving each a casual look for later identification, the bus driver who doubled as our tour guide separated the wheelchair bound tourists including Amelia and me from the rest of the group. The wheelchair bound tourists were taken down to the show site, two guests at a time due to the limited elevator space. We rejoined the main group by negotiating pathways through souvenir shops.

Our group of about fifty tourists was eased and merged in the crowded room with more groups from different tours resulting in Amelia on her walker and me being separated by three visitors from a different group.

The Fury, Niagara Falls

We were handed plastic ponchos before the show started. Before I could put my poncho on after I did Amelia's, the lights were turned off; I heard Amelia's faint scream to complain of darkness. Realizing Amelia's disability, the people between us stepped aside to let me join her. I felt her discomfort in the darkened room.

The show featured animations of how Niagara Falls was created during the Ice Age. With a beaver as the main character, the movie appeared to be more appealing to a child than to an adult. The movie depicted the different stages of upheavals and down thrusts of glaciers on the earth's surface, leaving scenes and beautiful landscapes that only violent force of nature can create. The depiction oriented the minds of the tourists in preparation for the second segment of the show.

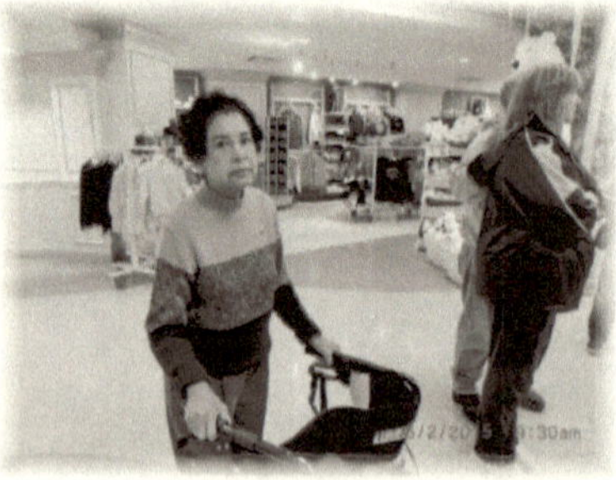

I felt that the show was very informative for one who was interested in the geological history of the earth. Amelia did not like it, momentarily relieved when the show ended in less than fifteen minutes. To her disappointment however, The Fury was only done with the first of two segments.

We were asked to move to another room that has a moving platform, grab bars, and surrounding movie screens from about eye level to the ceiling. When the visitors were secured on their footings, and were firmly holding on to grab bars, the lights were turned off, and The Fury started the second segment of the show

The Fury, Niagara Falls

The movie screens mimicked the scenes from the first segment, and the platform began to shake violently. The rumbling sound started at a low level increasingly becoming intense and deafening, at the same time that icicles and sprays of water were dropping, getting us wet and making us feel as if we were participants in the actual geological disturbance. As the scenes on the screens changed a few times, The Fury repeated and changed accordingly. Different scenes to make the show more realistic simultaneously appeared on the screens triggering varying levels of ground, shaking, and rumbling sounds.

The second segment of the show, like the first, lasted less than fifteen minutes. I would have preferred zero minute of animation and more minutes in the depiction of the actual fury which is sustained, violent, and destructive. That was what I would have liked to watch in the simulation.

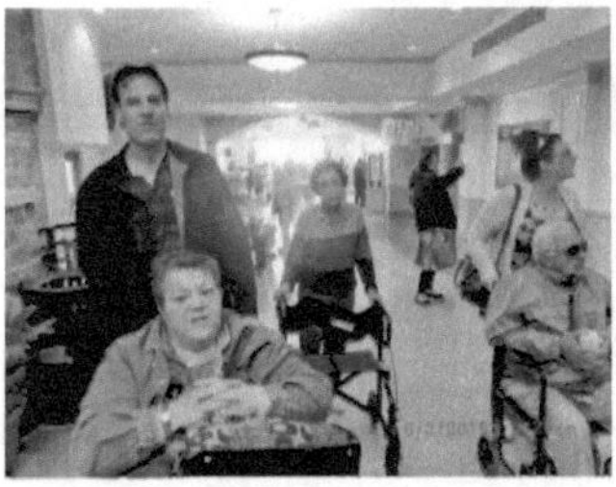

Considering that The Fury was a bonus offer from the hotel, I felt it was good, worthwhile, informative, and educational in a non-classroom setting. I recommend it to tourists who happened to be in the area especially those interested in the geological history of our planet; it is one of a kind simulation of actual events that happened millions of years ago.

Behind the Falls Tour, Niagara Falls

"It's not fun for one who visits Niagara Falls not getting wet," said the bus driver who doubled as a tour guide, and one way of getting wet was to join the Behind the Falls Tour that was part of the hotel package I purchased online.

Before the tunnel tour, I asked the tour guide why each time he loaded and unloaded Amelia's walker he appeared to examine and feel it. His response was that he wanted to see if the walker was sturdy enough for negotiating the tunnel with Amelia sitting on it; otherwise, we would have to use a wheelchair. Assuring me that it was, I did not think much about the eventual hazard that we would be encountering during the tour.

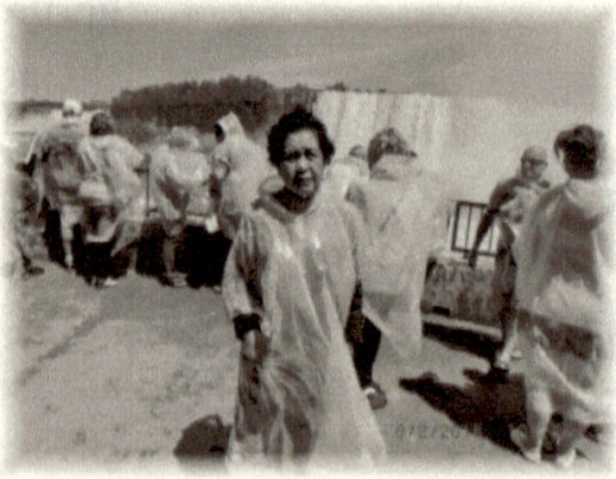

We descended to the staging area of the tour by taking an old elevator with just a space for one passenger on a wheelchair and an assistant. The rest of the group reached the staging area by way of a ramp through souvenir shops. After we had regrouped, we were handed yellow plastic ponchos, yellow to distinguish our group from other groups of different colors. Within our group certain guests were designated as leaders whose only function was to walk ahead of us; they did not even have to look back or adjust their paces.

We started the tour on a slight downward incline, with me pushing Amelia on her walker. The degree of the slope gradually increased making the travel more treacherous on the wet path. While I picked the spots to maneuver the walker, Amelia was pointing out to me which designated leader to follow – all guests in our group were wearing yellow ponchos.

Behind the Falls Tour, Niagara Falls

We reached the first viewing platform of the falls with slight struggles but with awesome feelings. Amelia assured me that the guest in front of us was the leader of our group. We followed him all the way down to the viewing platform only to find out that he was the leader of a different group. Amelia got off from the walker which we temporarily set aside, and we descended a flight of stairs to get very close to the edge of the viewing platform. And there the falls was – 1,000,000's of gallons of fresh water in front of us!

The spectacle of one-fifth of the world's fresh water flowing sixty-five kilometers per hour was there for us to appreciate and admire. Close to 2,800 cubic meters of fresh water was flowing from the 13-story high brink of the falls every second; that was 622,000 gallons per second or 37,000,000 gallons per minute, of precious water right in front of us.

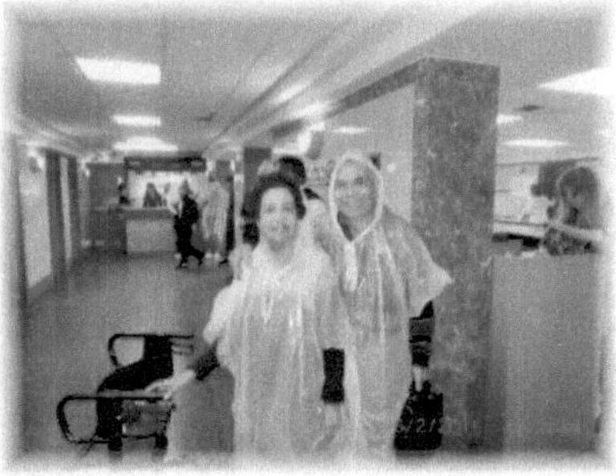

The falls creates its own turbulence that splashes mists on the viewers, disabling us from taking pictures lest the water ruins the camera's electronics. The ponchos helped us from getting wet throughout, but were not enough to stop Amelia from shivering. Because Amelia was not comfortable being wet and cold, we did not stay on the platform for longer than five minutes, five significant minutes of witnessing one of the wonders of the world.

We climbed back up the stairs, located Amelia's walker, and proceeded to retrace the tunnel towards the exit. On the walls are pictures depicting the history of the falls, and the people who skillfully engineered the intricate tunnel and its surroundings.

Behind the Falls Tour, Niagara Falls

We were concerned that we might be completely separated from our group and not be able to find our way out on time. But when we caught up with a wheelchair bound guest with her assistant, we eased our anxiety – they were part of our tour but of a different group. They too were retracing the tunnel on the way out.

When we reached the next viewing platform and disguising my desire, I asked Amelia if she wanted to take another look at the falls. Wet and shivering, her response was an emphatic 'no'; she did not want any part of the falls anymore. She was eager to get out of the tunnel so she could take off the poncho and have something hot to drink.

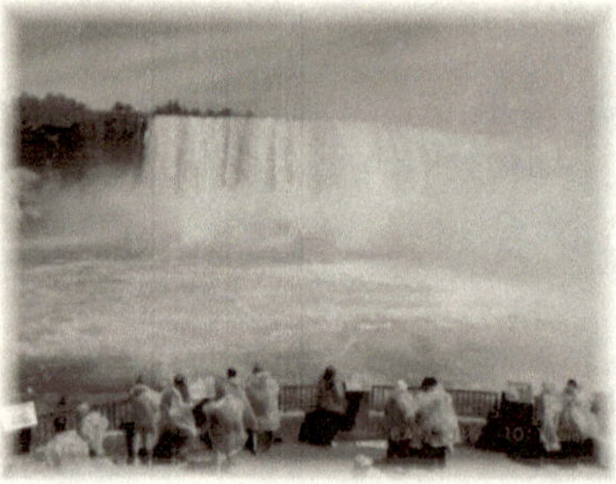

We came out of the tunnel, took our ponchos off, and hurried for a cup of hot chocolate which Amelia urgently needed. Disappointed only by my inability to take pictures where the falls was most awesome, we earned the bragging right to say that we watched the falls close at the base level despite Amelia's physical disability.

The journey was exciting, albeit challenging for one with a disability like Amelia. We came at the right time of the year when the weather was very favorable, and tourists were just arriving for the season. If I am in the area, I will not hesitate to join the Behind the Falls Tour again but with a waterproofed camera. I unequivocally recommend the tour to anyone who comes within a few hours to Niagara Falls.

The Maid of the Mist Boat Ride, Niagara Falls

The boat ride was part of the package that the hotel offered for sale online. Without knowing the physical exertion demanded by the ride, I booked the hotel package for a sizeable discount. I did not regret including the ride, considering that it was a once-in-a-lifetime experience for Amelia and me.

The Maids of the Mist – I counted two – were the boats that were taking the guests back and forth between the American and the Canadian sides of Niagara Falls. From the water level to the street level where we were dropped off by our tour bus, I roughly estimated the vertical height to be more than 150 feet. That was how much height I had to push the walker with Amelia sitting on it, in a zigzagging pattern.

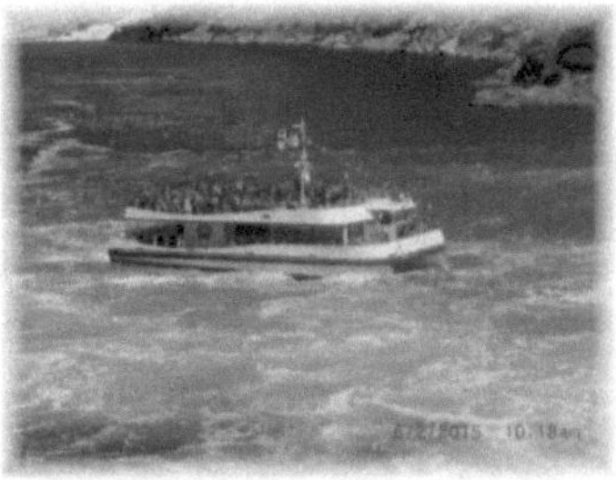

Because of Amelia's physical condition, we were initially directed to follow a path for people with disabilities, which rejoined the main path after a few hundred feet. Then we were again directed to follow another path which rejoined the main path ending at the gate. A couple of other guests in wheelchairs and we were appreciative of the arrangement. Nevertheless, it was exhausting for me having to control the speed of the walker with Amelia on board.

Past the boarding gate, we were handed plastic ponchos, a hint of a wet and watery adventure ahead. There appeared to be more than two hundred excited guests forming a queue. When one guest strayed away from the line to take a picture of his friend, everybody with their ponchos on, seemed to follow and dispersed to take pictures of friends and relatives. To my chagrin, I could not even

The Maid of the Mist Boat Ride, Niagara Falls

unhook my camera because I had to put Amelia's poncho and mine on before reaching the ramp leading to the Maid of the Mist.

The ride started on the American side of the falls with the Maid of the Mist getting as close as possible to the rim so that the guests could feel the enormous energy generated by the falling water. True to its name, the Maid of the Mist was immediately engulfed by the cold mists from the falls sending some guests including Amelia to the inside rooms for protection. The braver ones stayed on deck taking pictures of the natural spectacle that was dropping one-fifth of the world's fresh water, in one place

I had to move back and forth between the deck and Amelia's location to be sure that she was comfortable with the wet poncho on and the mists hitting her face. Despite her very low tolerance for wintery weather, she was enjoying the ride but with repeated questions of when it would end.

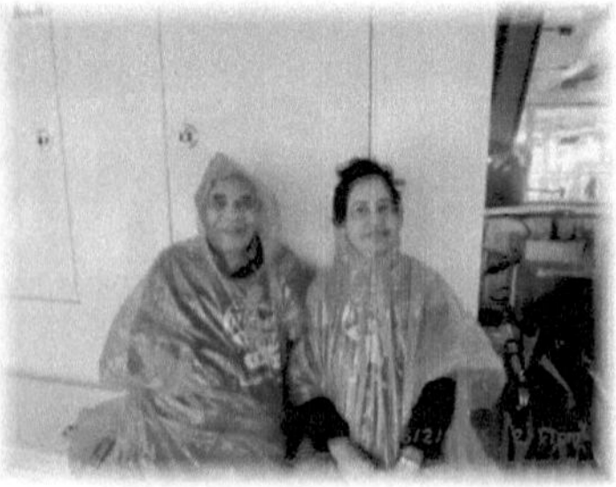

Whereas the tunnel tour provided eye-level views of the falls from the viewing platforms, the boat ride provided upward angle views of the same. With care, I was able to take some pictures only possible from the boat. Rainbows and thousands of birds were some of the objects I was able to capture in my camera. The real excitement though was the suspense, anticipation, feeling, and sensation of the power of nature being displayed in a single impressive package known as the Niagara Falls.

The Maid of the Mist Boat Ride, Niagara Falls

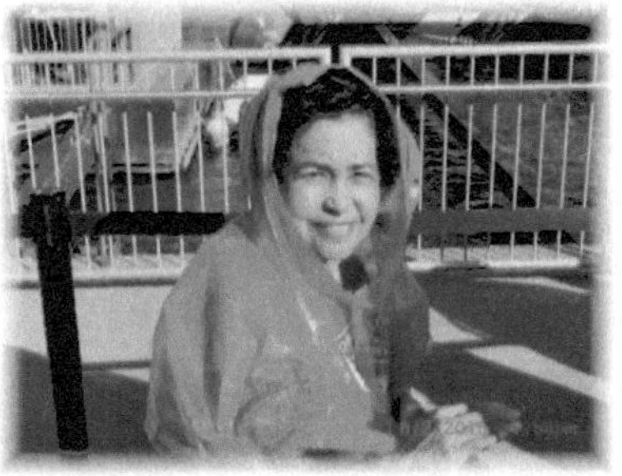

At the Canadian Horseshoe Falls, the Maid of the Mist turned around to head back to port. I saw Amelia's pleased reaction when I told her that we were heading home. She could not wait to take off the wet poncho only to be dissuaded when a burst of mists would blow in her face. Asked if she enjoyed the ride, her response was positive.

The challenge left for me after the boat ride was the uphill push of the walker with Amelia on board. As I was still eager to stay around and take pictures, I did not care if the tour bus left us behind, I was ready to hail a taxicab if needed, to save myself from being overly exhausted. The tour bus did wait for us, though, taking us back to the hotel in time for dinner.

As I mentioned earlier, the boat ride was a once-in-a-lifetime experience specially for us who live far away from Niagara Falls.; I would like to take it again if I have the chance. The ride was an unbelievable experience we can relate to friends and relatives, despite Amelia's disability due to strokes, Alzheimer's, diabetes, and congestive heart failure. I wholeheartedly recommend the ride to anyone who has the chance to visit Niagara Falls.

The Skylon Tower, Niagara Falls

Skylon Tower, one of the structures that dominate the skyline of Niagara Falls, was not included in the hotel package I purchased online, but because of an extra hour to spare before the Behind the Falls Tour, our tour stopped by the tower. I surmised that with the summer season just in the offing and the crowd just starting to arrive, the hotel was in its full promotional drive, offering tourists extra activities that hold their attention and earn their goodwill.

After more than three hours in the bus touring the city of Niagara Falls, Amelia was due to eat something, lest hunger syndrome makes its presence known, making her feel uneasy and sick. We opted for the last batch of passengers to travel up the tower by elevator to allow Amelia to eat snacks. That suited the tour's schedule as the guide could only take ten passengers at a time because there were other guests from other tours.

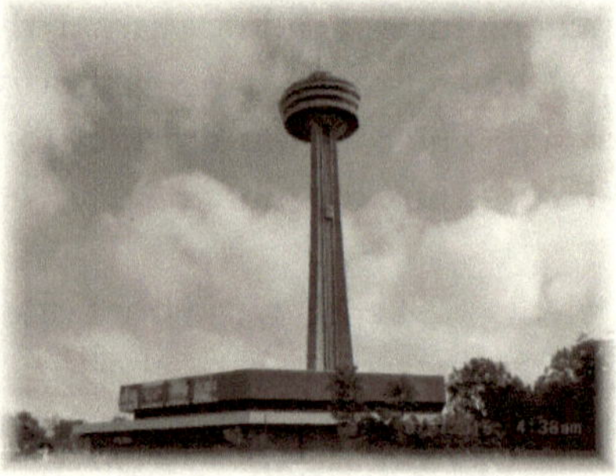

It did not take us long to find a place to eat snacks as there are a few of them at the base of the tower. When the tour guide came back to take us up the tower, Amelia was just done with her snacks.

The outside glass elevator traveled up the tower at a slow rate of speed allowing the passengers more time to look down the streets and up the horizon while appreciating the beauty of Niagara Falls and its surroundings. With the 775-foot vertical height of the tower, the travel made me and some other passengers slightly queasy. Amelia, on the other hand, was not bothered at all by the height. It was somewhat difficult to find a location in the elevator,

The Skylon Tower, Niagara Falls

filled with visitors, where to take pictures of the impressive views in front of our eyes separated only by glass. Perversely, I did not want to be pressed too close to the glass wall of the elevator either.

We did not have the opportunity to eat and dine at any of the eating places at the top of the tower because of the rushed pace of the tour. Due to our short vacation schedule, we were unwilling to postpone the next tour in favor of the sights from the tower. I assumed that those who postponed the next tour for another day by staying longer on the tower, did have fun eating while watching the falls. If there is any place to eat in peace and quiet while enjoying the sights around Niagara Falls, Skylon Tower is, so the tour guide said.

We did have a 360-degree view of the surrounding areas of Niagara Falls. Most impressively, we had spectacular views of the American Falls, the Canadian Horseshoe Falls, The Great Gorge, and the Niagara wine district. The sight of the American Falls and the Canadian Horseshoe Falls in whole is more comprehensive when viewed from the tower than when viewed from the street level.

In most of our travels, I pick a landmark among few as a memory tickler to reminisce about each visit. Although the falls at Niagara Falls is the most coveted attraction, the Skylon Tower is the most visible because of its height, hinting to the travelers that when it comes into view, Niagara Falls is near. With its radiating reflections caused by the sun's rays, the tower is an absolute iconic landmark. I recommend, without reservation, the Skylon Tower tour to anyone visiting Niagara Falls.

Extra Day at Niagara Falls, Niagara Falls

Already done with the original and most exciting schedules in our vacation, we were still left with an extra day to look around the city, for secondary attractions of which there are countless more, based on the handouts at the hotel lobby. The Niagara Parkway was a good starting point because it runs parallel to the falls with Table Rock - I called it passenger transfer hub - being so close to our hotel and separated only by a wall from the Canadian Horseshoe Falls.

Now was our opportunity to use our WEGO passes which were included in the hotel package I purchased online, to board the public transportation bus which initially took us to Table Rock. We could have taken the inclined elevator which is itself a tourist attraction just a few steps from the hotel lobby, but because of Amelia's physical difficulty we took the public transportation bus instead. A short education from the bus driver about the most scenic routes in the city of Niagara Falls helped us choose where to get on and off the bus.

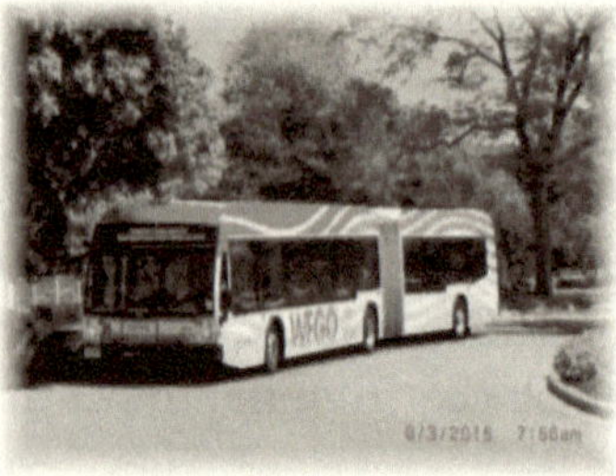

We spent an hour at Table Rock to admire and view the Canadian Horseshoe Falls at different angles without being rushed as was the case with a group tour the day before. Only accessible from the American side of the falls but also nicely seen from the Canadian side, Goat Island was also in perfect view owing to the favorable and clear weather. Unable to stand the cold mists blowing in our faces, Amelia persuaded me to leave as soon as the next bus arrived to go to another tourist location of our choice, in this case, the Queen Victoria Park.

Extra Day at Niagara Falls, Niagara Falls

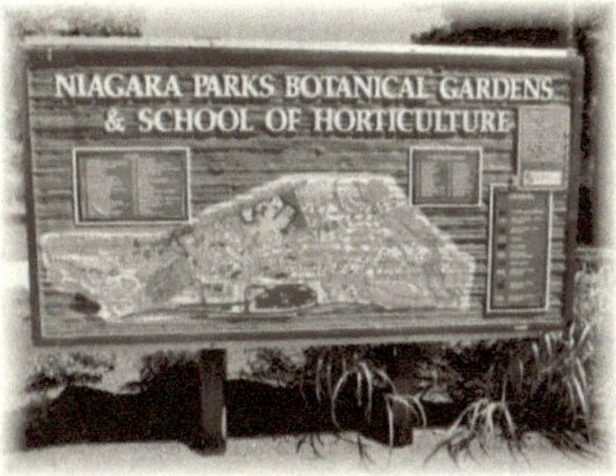

Though the tour bus already took us through Queen Victoria Park the previous day, at the suggestion of the bus driver Amelia and I stopped at a particular location at the Park to view the falls from yet many more angles. Extending from across the Canadian Horseshoe Falls to almost the Rainbow Bridge, the Park offers the most diverse views of both the American Falls and the Canadian Horseshoe Falls; both falls do not stop to amaze me. The Maid of the Mist boat ride which we took a day earlier, started from the Queen Victoria Park, but at that time we were more preoccupied with the boat ride than with viewing the falls.

Our next destination was The Rainbow Bridge which allows crossings between the United States and Niagara Falls, as pedestrians, by bicycle, or by car. The bridge was constructed in 1940-41, is 900 feet long, more than 200 feet above the water which flows approximately 25 miles per hour, and provides yet another location for having a spectacular view of the falls. We stayed about fifteen minutes to have a clear view of the bridge and just enough time before the next WEGO bus came to take us to the next tourist landmark, the Whirlpool Aero Car.

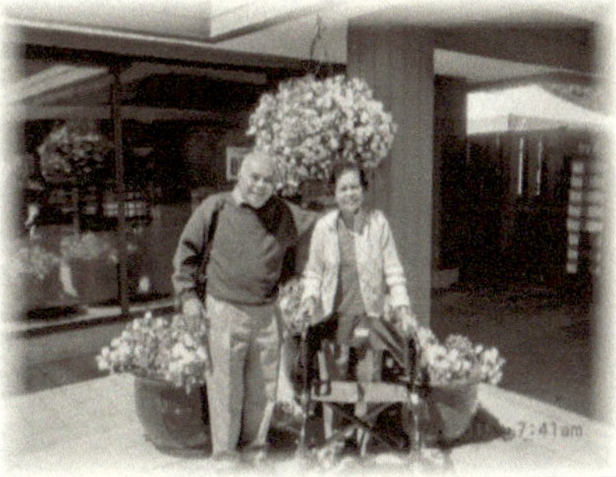

Located along the WEGO route, the Whirlpool Aero Car is a cable car suspended by six cables over the entire approximate half-mile width of the Niagara Gorge. The cable car has been in operation for close to one hundred years. The fact that the car does not allow passengers with a disability like Amelia, did not matter to us because Amelia was not interested in it in the first place, and we were only visiting as many locations as we could to tally the hours of the extra day in Niagara Falls. On to the next destination we went, the Niagara Falls Botanical Gardens

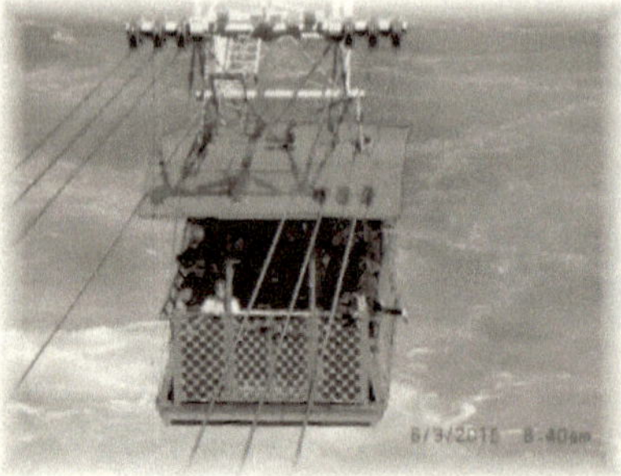

It was lunch time when the WEGO bus conveniently pulled in at the parking lot of the Niagara Falls Botanical Gardens. Having observed in previous travels how gardens are spread out, we decided to eat lunch before we explored the gardens. Hunger syndrome was making its presence known to Amelia after all, with her starting to feel uneasy and slightly tired.

The Niagara Falls Botanical Gardens is a beautifully maintained 40-acre natural attraction established in 1936. Not knowing much about plants and flower seasons, I chose to spend more time enjoying the symmetrical and excessive floral displays along pathways that are crisscrossing the gardens. Even while we were eating lunch, I could not help admiring the plots of flowering plants right in front of the restaurant, and the hanging plants including some orchids from the eaves of the building. Strategically situated are benches along the paths in the gardens for guests who need to rest and take

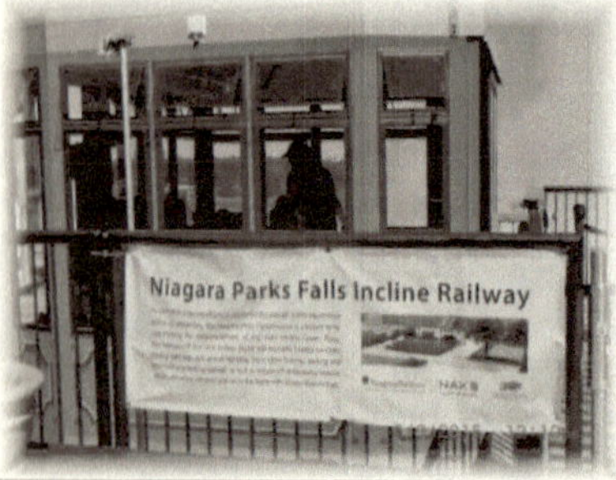

pictures with blooming flowers in the background.

Within the gardens is the Butterfly Conservatory which I imagined, stores every entomological account about butterflies, and which displays countless merchandise promoting knowledge about the alluring insect. Because of Amelia's difficulty, we could not get inside the butterfly enclosure, but we observed thousands of them through the glass wall. It is hard to believe that the glass wall slightly vibrates because of the energy generated by the flights of the butterflies inside.

Staying in the gardens for only forty-five minutes, we missed some of its other impressive displays and features; the vast gardens

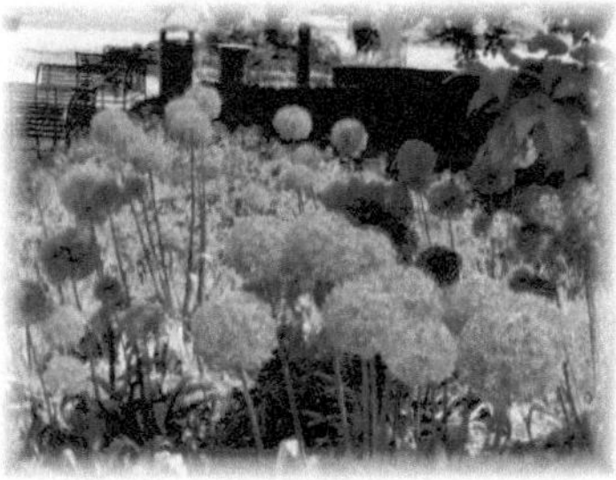

requires longer than a day to be fully appreciated. What we witnessed, though, sufficed me to say that the Niagara Falls Botanical Gardens is one of the prettiest I had ever seen. The gardens made me more curious about the next plant attraction, the Floral Clock along the WEGO bus route.

The Floral Clock was built and maintained in working order by Ontario Hydro, with its designs dating back to 1950. At the time of our visit, the clock was undergoing a biannual replanting and replenishment. Though the area was cordoned off, we could see from a distance, the clock's vastness with more than 15,000 carpet bedding plants on its face – thanks to the service of the Niagara Falls horticultural staff.

We deferred listening to the Westminster chimes as we had to leave with the next WEGO bus which took us back to the vicinity of the hotel in time for the late afternoon brunch. Thereafter we started packing in preparation for the trip back to California early the following morning.

Our vacation days at Niagara Falls were full of memorable experience. For one with strokes, Alzheimer's, diabetes, and congestive heart failure, every minute lived is a minute ought to be enjoyed. That was the case with Amelia with me providing the care. Our Niagara Falls tour was a complete success.

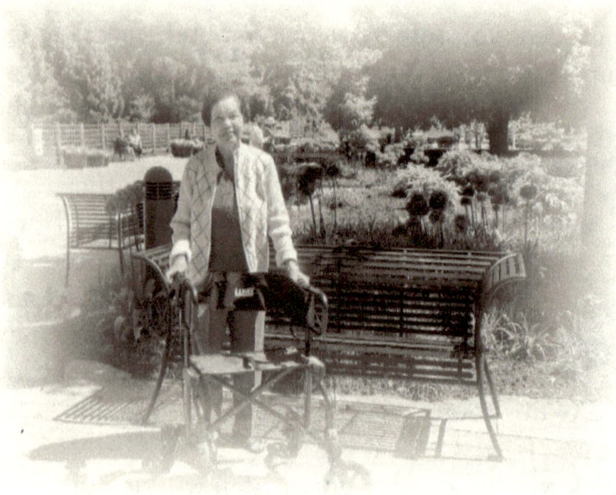

Extra Day at Niagara Falls, Niagara Falls

Chapter 18 – Destination Spain

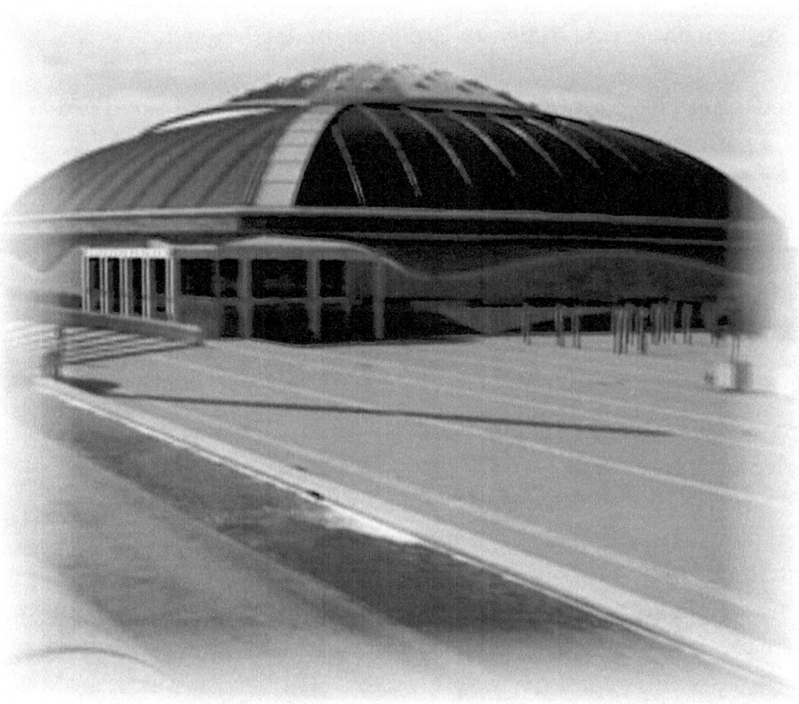

At the Barcelona Olympic Village, Barcelona

After spending a few hours at the Sagrada de Familia cathedral the tour guide offered to take us to more distant tourist attractions in Barcelona, but not having enough sleep during the overnight train ride from Paris to Barcelona, we opted for places close to our hotel. One such place was the Olympic Village, one of the venues of the Summer Olympics of 1992 held in Barcelona, Spain. It is only a short drive from the Sagrada de Familia cathedral

Located where it overlooks a good part of Barcelona, the stadium offers a panoramic view of the city. Accented by several large straight columns, the area surrounding the stadium is as impressive as it is grandiose. Among the columns stands the conspicuous Telefonica grand sign to bestow recognition of the company's role in the economic development of Barcelona, the company being one of the giants of the telephone industry.

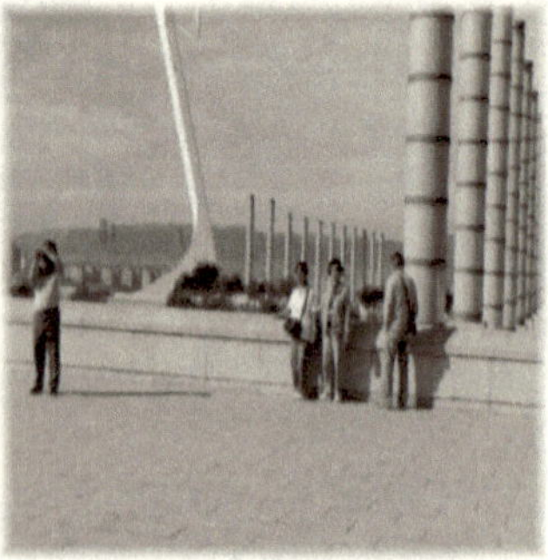

The stadium is immaculate with meticulously trimmed green grass on the track, and a brook is continuously running along the edge creating a clear and distinct rippling sound. With different levels of flat surfaces connected by stairs, tourists can have various compositions and angles of pictures taken. As our visit was at a time when there was no activity of any kind in the stadium, we, together with other tourists and our tour guide, were free to roam around.

The stadium looks impressive and impregnable with doors and walls of shining stones. Our tour guide took us around the different areas of the stadium particularly the viewing platform

At the Barcelona Olympic Village, Barcelona

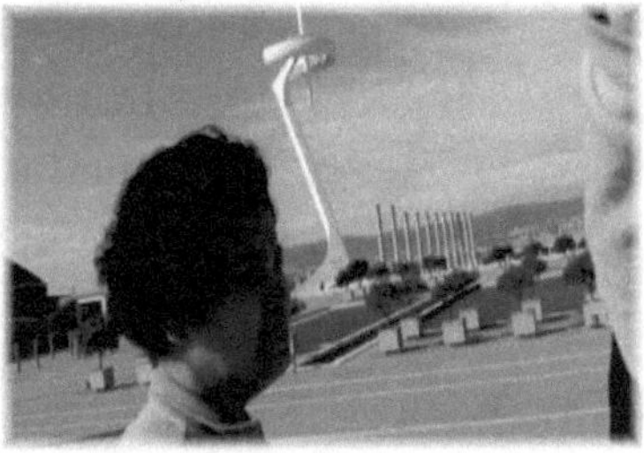

where we had a complete view of the tracks on the field. The stadium with 65,000 seats can accommodate the large type of spectator events.

The stadium is a popular venue for sporting, music, and other activities. Most famous artists from all over the world have held concerts at the Barcelona Olympic Stadium. Soccer, basketball, and other favorite European, as well as American sporting events, have had some appearances at the stadium attesting to Barcelona's claim as a popular sporting destination.

Amelia was showing signs of fatigue for walking and for lack of needed sleep; she too was not well-rested during the train ride. She refused to go farther even though there were more beautiful and inviting sights pointed to by the guide. So we stayed and picked an excellent spot for resting while I let her eat the pastries left over from our breakfast. We were rejoined by our friends and the guide when they came back, but we still had a few hours before check-in time at the hotel.

We drove to Montjuic Park which has a beautiful view of the harbor where the cruise ship we would be boarding the following morning was docked. Because of the park's proximity to the port, it is always crowded with tourists disembarking from the cruise ships; there is always one docked on the pier most of the time, according to the tour guide.

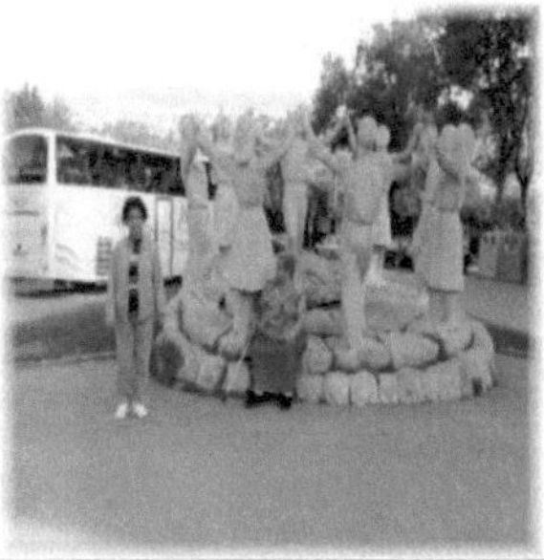

There are areas in the park that attract tourists more so than others. In my case, the attraction was with the vehicle junk

At the Barcelona Olympic Village, Barcelona

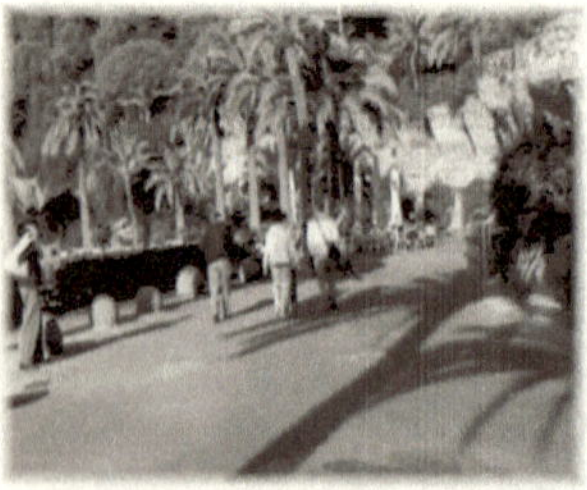

parts being used as paving ornaments. Instead of abandoning them at the junkyards, they are symmetrically arranged in beautiful patterns to pave the streets in the park. The idea helps the economy of the area because tourists likewise attracted by them, spend money at the stores buying souvenirs, and food. Most importantly, it helps in preserving the environment.

By the same token, Amelia was attracted by the rocks lining the streets, each rock a few feet from the other. The rocks invited Amelia because each rock represents a bead in the rosary, as explained by the tour guide. But Amelia was not willing to follow all the rock representations of the rosary bead because of the distance covered, possibly a mile or longer, considering the size of the rocks and the distance between them.

Our tour of the park extended to a passageway under the park, with a cave-like entrance and with the support columns appearing to lean and incapable of holding the weight above. We were now beneath the park at a quiet stage-like area where, the guide explained one could meditate and play musical instruments that trigger a sound that reverberates from the ceiling and the massive pillars supporting the buildings above. As a matter of fact, at the time of our visit one was playing xylophone, unperturbed by our presence.

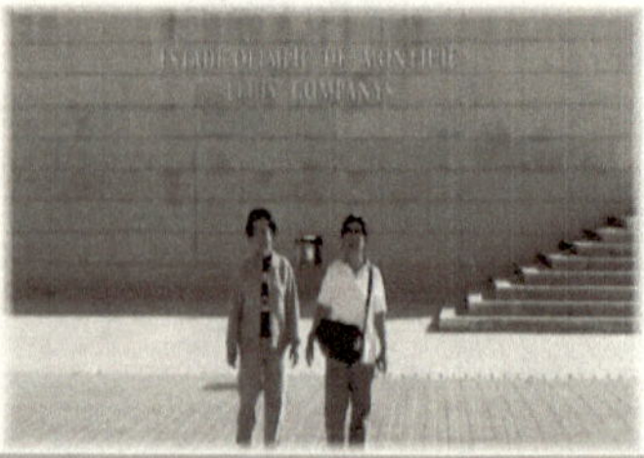

I considered the short tour of Barcelona a success. We finished the good part of the day having gone to the most visited attractions in the pier area of Barcelona. Only waiting to be asked, the tour guide was willing

At the Barcelona Olympic Village, Barcelona

to take us to more distant places in Barcelona, but we were so tired and sleepy owing to the overnight train ride, we could hardly keep our eyes open. Given a chance to visit Barcelona again, I will not miss visiting more exciting places in the city.

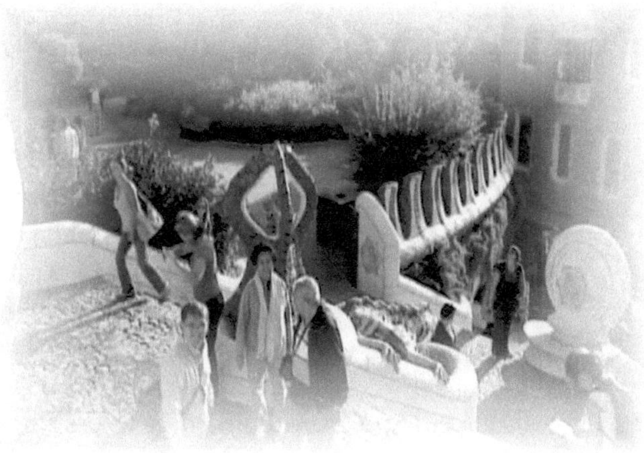

At the Sagrada De Familia, Barcelona

At the Sagrada De Familia, Barcelona

Ending an overnight train ride from Paris, our passports were handed back to us before the train stopped at the Barcelona train station. With just a show of formality by nodding our heads, we were let through the customs gate and past some restriction barriers into the passengers' waiting area where we did not lose time before we saw my name on a sign held up by our expected tour guide.

After a brief introduction among us - passengers, the tour guide, and a driver - the tour guide took us to a small coffee shop where we had breakfast of Spanish pastries and very strong coffee. The place was just opening, but a crowd was already forming. Evidently

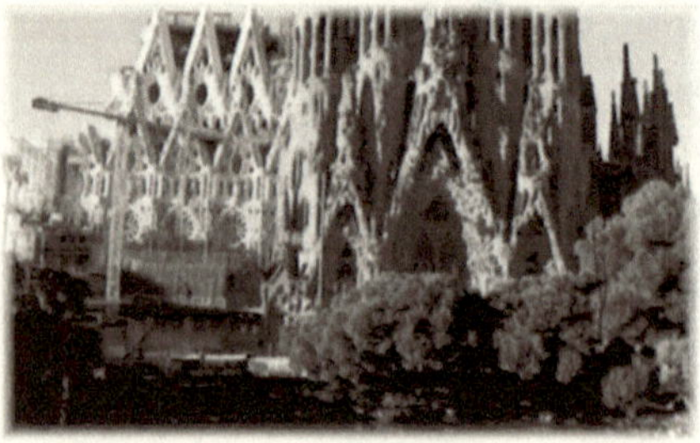

our tour guide had enough experience in his field of work. Observing that Amelia has a physical disability, he felt that we had to stake out a parking space in the attraction he was taking us to so that she would not have to walk very far and cover a long distance. He therefore urged us to eat faster so we could leave early.

The tourist attraction to where the guide took us was the Sagrada de Familia. We got there in time for us to find a street parking space close to the Basilica, thanks to the brilliant foresight of our tour guide. Otherwise, Amelia would have had a problem walking. The guide took us to different locations with the best views of the Basilica. Had we been a little late, he would have a hard time guiding us through the crowd with Amelia having to keep pace with us on uneven pavement and grassy yard.

At the Sagrada De Familia, Barcelona

The guide related the history of the Basilica. Antonio Gaudi, a Spanish architect turned-monk, started construction of the Basilica more than one hundred years ago, but because of lack of funds, the construction was halted, resumed, stopped, and continued again. It has been like this for the Basilica up to this time. Though completion of the Basilica is not yet imminent, it has been attracting thousands and thousands of tourists from all over the world, not only tourists who embrace the Catholic faith but also of other religions.

Funding for the construction of the Basilica depends on private donations. Even with the thousands of tourists visiting the site and donating money for its construction, the Basilica is not expected to be finished soon. The original architect has long been gone yet his project is far from being complete after the foundation was first laid out. Cranes are still atop the spires continuing construction work, and tarps are still covering vast areas of the Basilica, protecting ongoing segments of the undertaking.

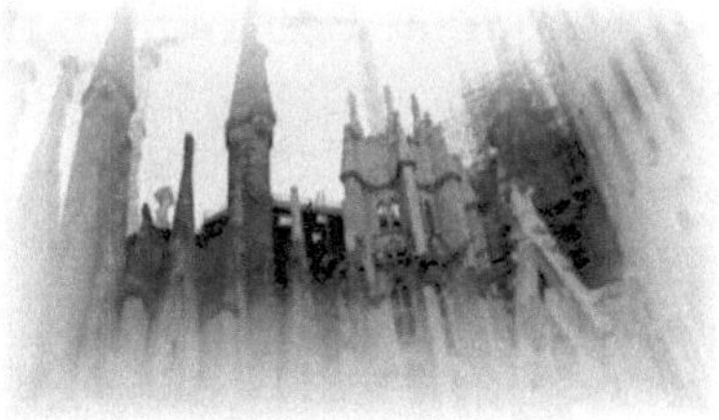

Amelia and Dolly went inside the Basilica to participate in the solemnization of the mass while Dennis and I explored its base, taking pictures and videos where they were allowed. Regarding size and the ground it covers, the Basilica is unbelievably huge requiring a good long walk around to complete. Apparently walking around the base of the Basilica was a disqualifying factor for Amelia notwithstanding our desire to show her and Dolly around.

By the time Amelia and Dolly came out of the Basilica, buses of tourists were already lining up to unload their passengers. Our tour guide was right; we beat everybody else in viewing the Basilica from

At the Sagrada De Familia, Barcelona

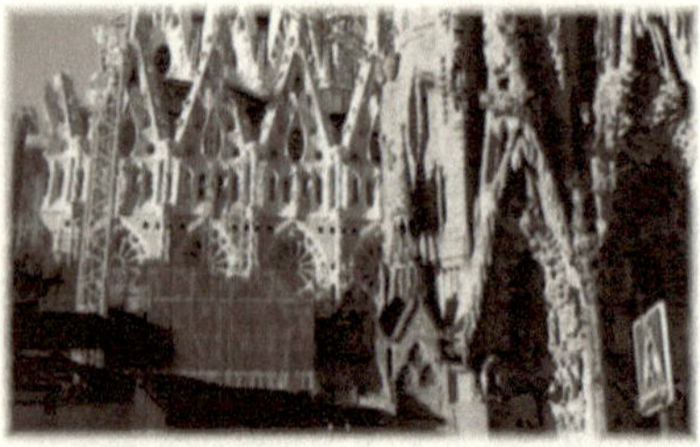

the best locations which were no longer available having been staked out immediately by arriving tourists. At this time one could hardly walk a few feet without bumping into someone, and focusing on a camera shot of the Basilica was becoming tricky without someone passing by and getting into the picture.

The time that we spent at the Sagrada de Familia was well worth it. All of us - Amelia, Dolly, Dennis, and me - being Catholics, had witnessed the influence of Catholicism in practice as well as in architecture. Our visit was a real life experience as opposed to only knowing about the Basilica from reading books and hearing stories about it.

The Sagrada de Familia Basilica is a popular tourist attraction not only because of its strong religious influence but also because of its unique architecture. I think that had the architecture been slightly simpler the number of years for its completion will have been shortened. On the other hand, the fact that the Basilica has not been completed after one hundred years of construction baffles many and creates a following of curious tourists, triggering thousands of visits each year.

Train Ride to Barcelona from Paris

From the comfort of home in the United States, I booked the train ride from Paris to Barcelona apart from the Mediterranean Cruise Tour with a little bit of apprehension that things might go awry. In a separate transaction with the website of what appeared to be an officially sanctioned travel bureau in Barcelona, I arranged for a tour guide to pick us up at the train station to lead us on a tour of the city before check-in at the hotel. All transactions were done online with virtually no authentication of the website that was offering the service.

The Mediterranean cruise we set out on started in Barcelona, but to add more excitement to our tour of Europe without being rushed, we planned ahead and stayed one week in Paris before the final embarkation. On the last day of our stay in Paris, we took a taxicab from our hotel to the train station, almost four hours ahead of departure time.

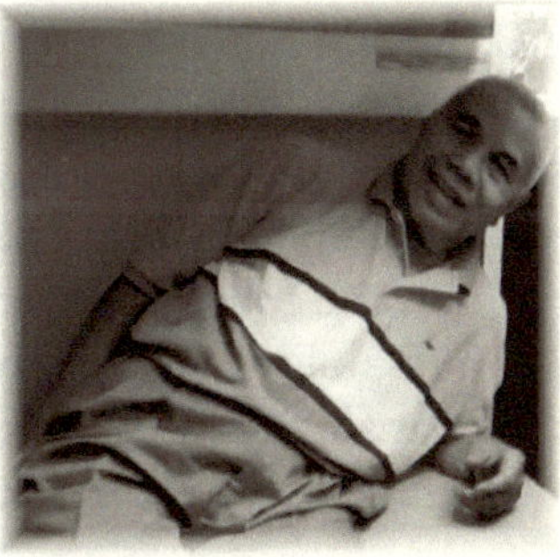

Lest we missed the train in case my scheduling was inaccurate, we ate lunch at the train station never leaving the area at all. It was the moment of truth that uplifted our spirits when without a single question our tickets were validated and stamped with approval for the train ride. The anxiety that the online purchase transactions could potentially be spurious was now dismissed from my mind.

We waited an hour or so for the train to pull in and when the train number was posted on the monitor and the gate to the boarding platform opened shortly thereafter, we proceeded to the car indicated on our tickets. Forced to walk very slowly due to her

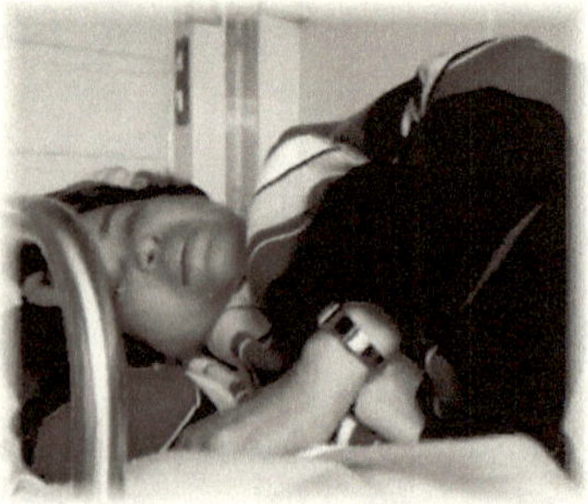

disability, Amelia and I ended up at the tail end of the line leading to the third car, the car where our cabin was located.

When the train car opened, passengers rushed in, turning the hallway into a squeezed mass of humanity and pieces of luggage. Dennis and Dolly each had a piece of luggage while we had two of our own plus a backpack and a purse. Because Amelia was too weak to help push our luggage, I had to struggle with them three-quarters of the way to the end of the car where our cabin was located.

We made it to the cabin though with extreme patience bumping and being bumped by other passengers. My concern was with Amelia, but she fought her way brilliantly as well, unmindful that she has a disability and the other passengers not caring about her condition at all. We settled in our cabin and rested before securing our luggage to make room for ease of movement.

The four of us - Amelia, Dolly, Dennis and I - each had a bunk bed in the cabin, each bed with fresh sheets, pillows, and blanket. Considering that ours was an overnight trip, we could not ask for more, but our cabin was uncomfortably warm, and there was not a

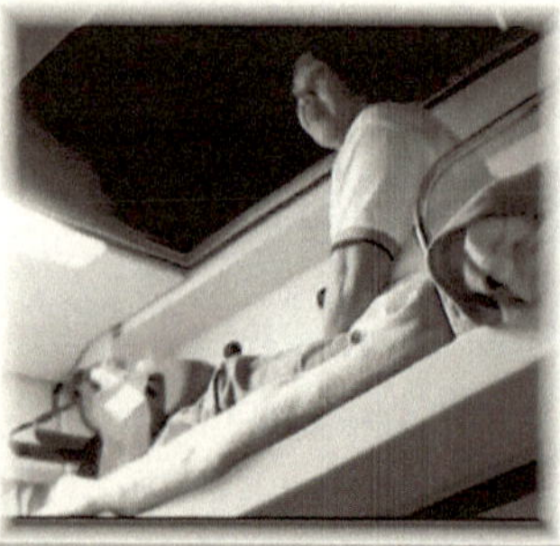

window to open, the cabin being on the interior side of the train. When the train started to move it suddenly got so quiet, and there was no one to complain to about cabin condition. I walked two or three cars up to find someone to help turn our cabin temperature lower, to no avail.

Train Ride to Barcelona from Paris

What I stumbled upon was the train car with the bar filled by a large group of non-English speaking passengers partying, singing, and laughing very loudly. Evidently, they were there earlier even before the train pulled in. Not appearing to be fazed by them, I asked to buy beer. Apparently, the bartender misunderstood me and offered me two cans of malt instead. In a rush to leave the bar, I took the malt thankful that the party was not offended and did not taunt me when I intruded into their space.

Dennis and I slowly boozed on the malt stirring it with whatever little ice was left in a small freezer to make the liquor last longer. With Amelia and Dolly cheering, Dennis and I had such a good time horse playing, joking, telling stories, laughing and hardly sleeping. This was a fun night, it being our first experience sleeping in bunk beds on a train. As always though, I was concerned about Amelia not getting enough rest, but when drowsiness overwhelmed her, she slept soundly.

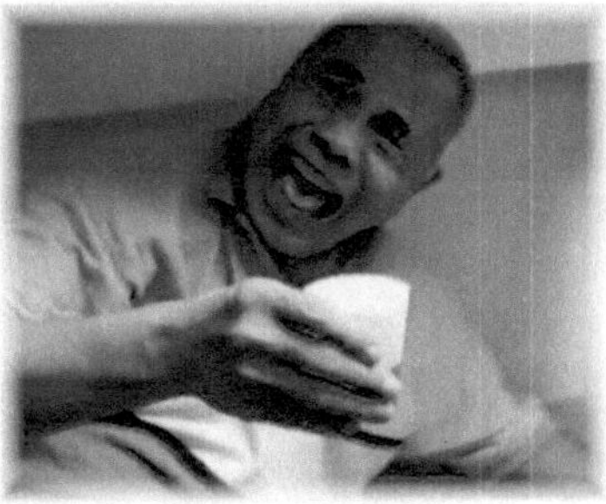

A member of the train staff came around to collect our passports. At first we were reluctant to hand over our identification documents, but seeing that she already had a handful in a basket, we gave ours with no more hesitation; they were returned to us the following morning just before disembarkation in Barcelona.

Not restricted by the rush schedule of a group tour, we had a fun vacation even on the train, the mode of transportation widely publicized as very efficient. The inclusion of a train ride was foremost in our vacation planning to satisfy our curiosity. Honestly, we did not have a way of comparing train efficiencies between that

Train Ride to Barcelona from Paris

in North America and that in Europe, we traveling by cars most of the time in the United States.

However, in Europe, the connections and coordination with timely precision, of hundreds of trains involving several routes to several countries, each train running at an enormous rate of speed and carrying hundreds of passengers, is mind-boggling. I will not hesitate to take another train ride not to mention a bullet train ride again in Europe.

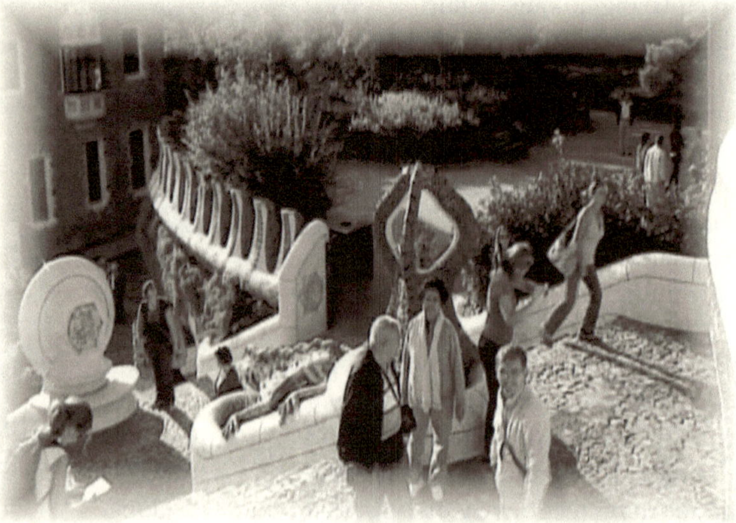

Train Ride to Barcelona from Paris

Chapter 19 – Destination Holland

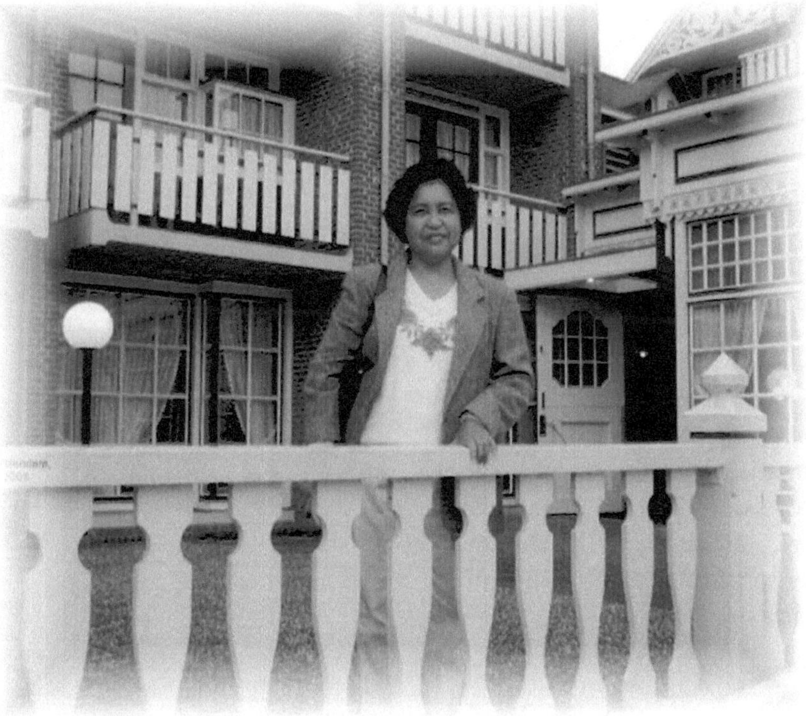

At the Fishing Village of Volendam, Holland

At the Fishing Village of Volendam, Holland

We arrived at Schiphol Airport, Amsterdam, from Seattle, Washington, on time but by the time we cleared through customs, the two tour buses that picked up the passengers from the airport already left for Volendam, Holland. A couple who flew in from Florida also missed the buses leaving them in the same situation as we were.

After a brief introduction and discussion, we joined to take a taxicab and share the cost to Volendam, a ninety-mile drive from the airport. The only known detail about our destination was the name of the hotel; Volendam is a small fishing village that does not have more than one hotel of the same name.

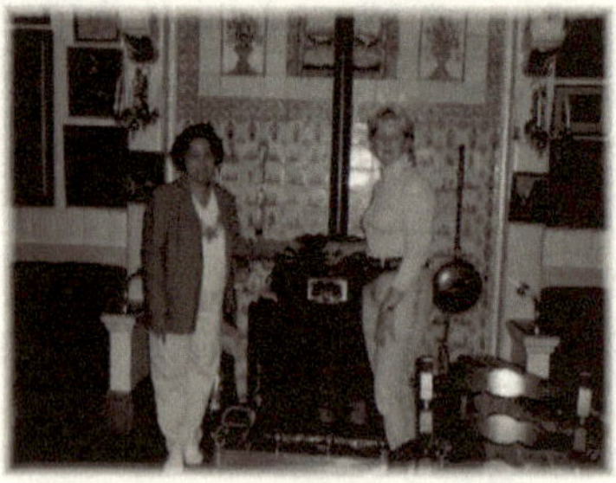

The taxicab ride to Volendam turned out to be a spectacular one with the taxicab driver describing the sceneries and famous landmarks along the route. Neither one of us had seen so many dikes before, that although the day was getting late, we requested the driver to take his time to allow us to appreciate the beautiful landscape.

We reached our hotel at Volendam just slightly later than the group that the buses picked up from the airport. We had an hour or so for the introduction of the bus drivers, the tour guides, and the tourists before dinner was served. Even after dinner we still had enough daylight to look across the ocean which appeared to be almost on the same level as our waistline.

At the Fishing Village of Volendam, Holland

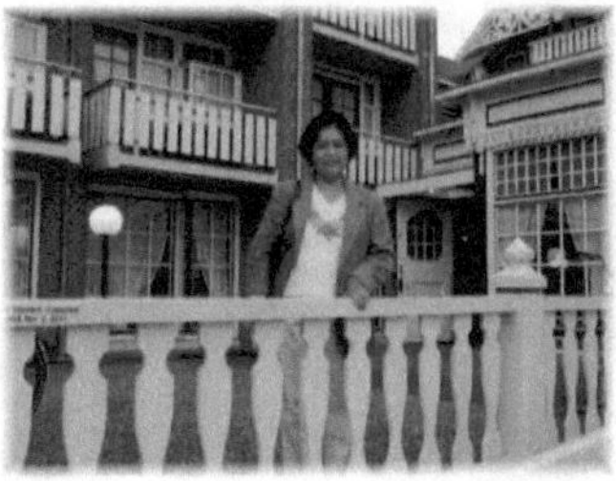

The following morning we explored the area around the hotel, walking on the dikes that are wide enough for regular-sized passenger vehicles to drive on. The hotel is sitting on land that is below sea level, protected only from the ocean by dikes. The fishermen were unloading their cargo of fish from the ocean side of the dikes into crates below the banks of the water on the other side.

Farther away from the hotel and along our way out of Volendam, we stopped at the Ann Frank museum. Ann Frank was the famous Jewish girl who survived the war by being hidden in an attic from the Germans. Time being the essence in this segment of our tour, we did not have the chance to look inside the museum as it was very crowded with tourists.

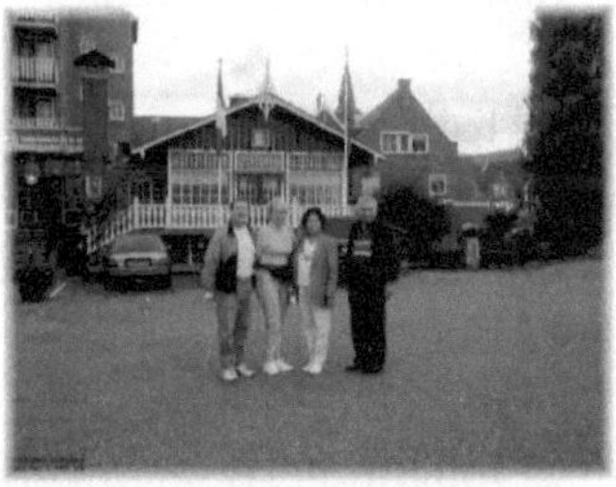

We traveled through flower fields with tulips all around, reminding me of the annual Pasadena Tournament of Roses Parade where some floats are being decorated with fresh flowers imported from Holland. Our tour guide in fact, informed us that tulips from the same route we were driving by are being shipped to places around the world.

Like the tulips, massive windmills are part of the landscape seen in all directions from the bus. Some of them are meant to keep the ocean water from flooding the canals, some are used to generate electricity, and some are used to do both, according to the tour guide.

At the Fishing Village of Volendam, Holland

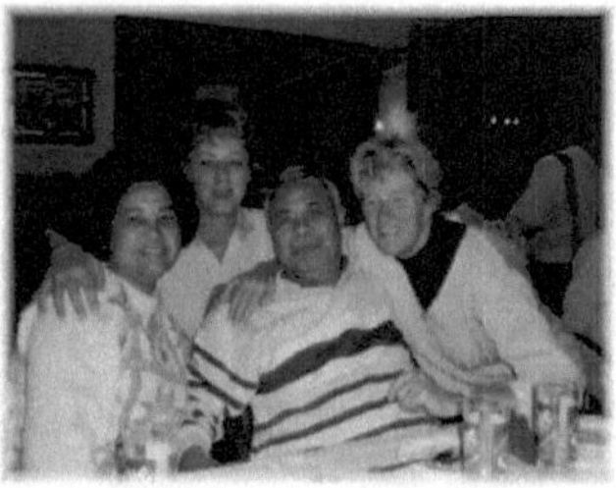

We also stopped by the Heineken beer plant giving Amelia a chance to eat snacks of bread I brought along from the hotel. She did not have to, but as a precaution against hunger syndrome making its presence, we took the 15-minute break from travel to restore her energy for the next leg of our tour.

Coincidentally, during our temporary stop, we got acquainted and developed a friendship with a lovely couple. Knowing Amelia's ailments, the lady who was a registered nurse gave me hints what to do in case Amelia got sick.

We left Holland particularly the fishing village of Volendam, continuing our European tour to Paris, France. What we just left was a one-of-a-kind experience, confirming my knowledge about Holland being below sea level, from the books I read.

I think Holland is an engineering marvel of an enormous expanse, able to fend the ocean from flooding the land by using intricate systems of dikes. I understand that nowhere else in the world so much land exists like Holland does, below sea level.

At the Fishing Village of Volendam, Holland

Chapter 20 – Cruise Incidents and Events

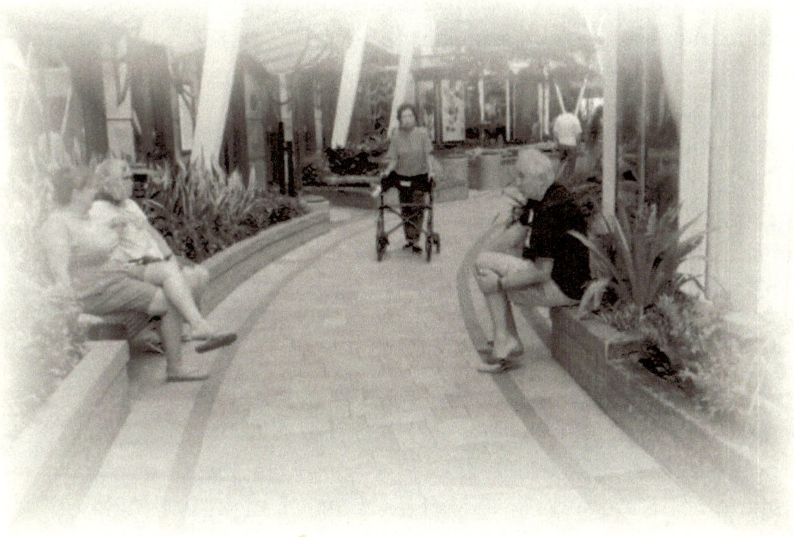

During The Alaskan Cruise

As in all cruises, the cruise ship sails at night, arriving at the target port in the morning, and staying there for a day or longer to allow the cruisers to explore the city, sceneries, and landmarks around it. That was how we, cruisers, found ourselves waking up at Juneau, Alaska, where the cruise ship was docked very close to the main boulevard eliminating the need for tenders.

The cruisers could have chosen to stay on board, enjoy the food, participate in games, listen to music, and watch various forms of entertainment. In our case, we joined the early excursion to the Mendenhall Glacier which is one of the popular destinations in Juneau. The excursion would allow us enough time to enjoy the sight of the glacier and to be back on the ship to relax and prepare for the captain's night or formal night as some cruisers know it.

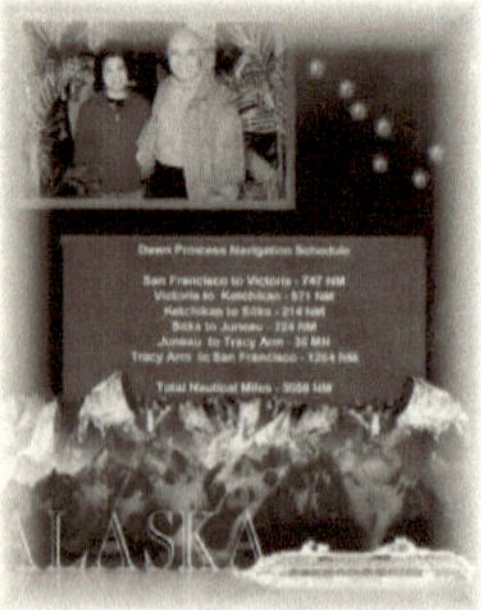

The captain's night was not starting until five o'clock in the evening leaving us enough time to join in the card games, answer some trivia questions, eat snacks, and roam around the ship. The captain's night is a tradition when elegantly dressed cruisers mingled with each other, meet new friends, and carry on conversations with the crews of the ship, particularly the captain and his officers.

Having prepared for and enjoyed captain's nights in previous cruises, Amelia and I did not take very long to get ready for this night's occasion, Amelia in her elegant long dress and me in my tuxedo. We waited for Dolly and Dennis to come out of their cabin which was adjacent to ours. The plan was for us to sit and dine together at one table and enjoy the night, before strolling around

During The Alaskan Cruise

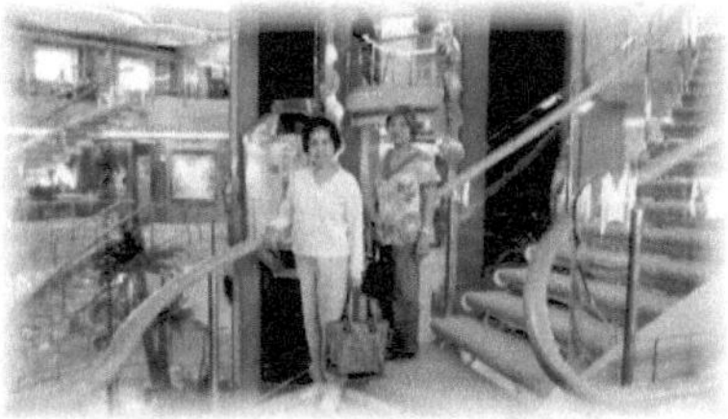

the ship, meeting new friends, taking pictures, and admiring new displays specific for the occasion. There was nothing to indicate that our captain's night would be ruined.

For an unexplained reason, Amelia suddenly felt so much pain in both feet. I was certain the shoes could not have caused the pain because she had been wearing the pair a few times before particularly when going to church. My coaxing her to move only exacerbated the pain, causing her to lean against the wall in the hallway, and slowly sliding to a crouching and writhing position. While contemplating what to do with Amelia, I asked Dolly and Dennis to proceed to the dining room where we hoped to join them later.

Then without warning Amelia vomited on the hallway. Temporarily leaving her, I went inside the cabin to call emergency service for assistance. When I reemerged from the cabin, I noticed that Amelia was still in pain, pale, and begging to be helped back to the cabin. While waiting for the emergency crew to arrive, I directed traffic away from the area in order not to upset other cruisers who by then, were proceeding to the ship's promenade area and dining rooms.

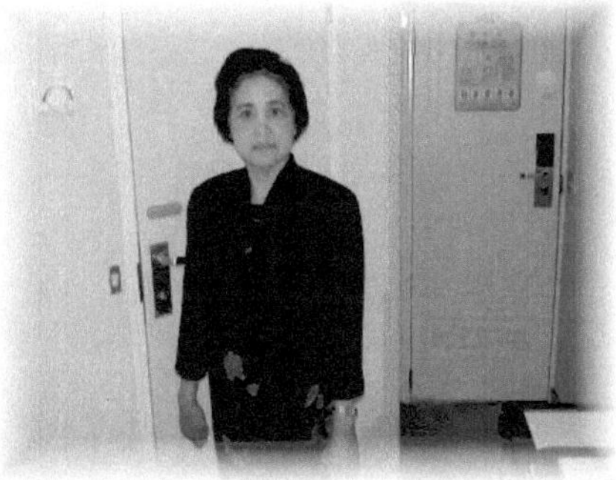

While the area in the hallway was being cleaned, disinfected, and cordoned off by the rapid emergency crew, Amelia was being helped to the dispensary where she was given some medications after examination. In fairness to the

During The Alaskan Cruise

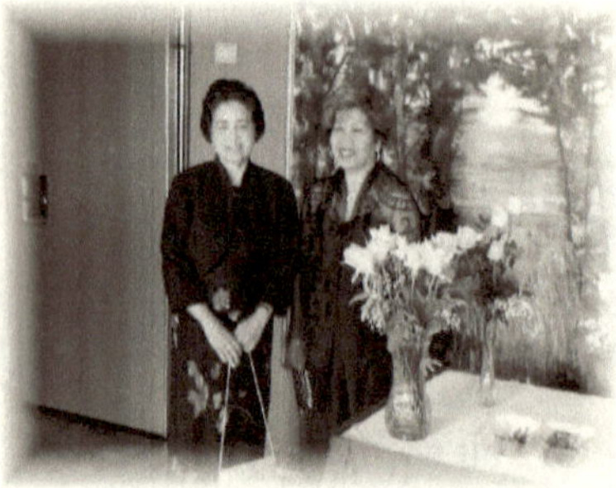

other cruisers, we stayed and spent captain's night in our cabin, never able to explain what caused the pain on Amelia's feet, and whether the pain and vomiting were ailments arising from the same cause. The passage to Juneau was so calm the ship did not seem to be moving, so seasickness could not have been the culprit. Besides, Amelia is not prone to being upset by seasickness.

Tonight's unfortunate event was not a big disappointment though, having attended captain's nights in previous cruises. In fact, we did not miss the next captain's night before termination of the cruise in San Francisco, California. On a seven- to ten-day cruises usually two to three captain's nights are held allowing one to make up for a lost opportunity to participate in the festive activity.

A lesson to be learned on this particular night was that in the midst of a delightful celebration, one must always be prepared for emergencies which can happen spontaneously. We ended the cruise without a further incident.

During the Panama Canal Cruise

Constrained by Amelia's disability, during our 15-day Panama Canal Cruise we developed a routine to enjoy the cruise to the fullest extent. Accordingly, every morning we would go for early breakfast to avoid the crowd at the food deck. And so on this particular morning, I gave Amelia a shower, blew her hair, checked her blood sugar level, and dressed her up before I took a shower myself. The arrangement was working successfully for a few days already; there was no reason that in this particular morning the routine would be interrupted.

I was about done with my shower when I heard a thud accompanied by a short soft scream behind the wall separating the shower from the cabin's living area. The sound emanating from within the cabin was very unfamiliar. The cabins on the cruise ship are sound-proofed; sounds from a cabin cannot be heard in the other cabins.

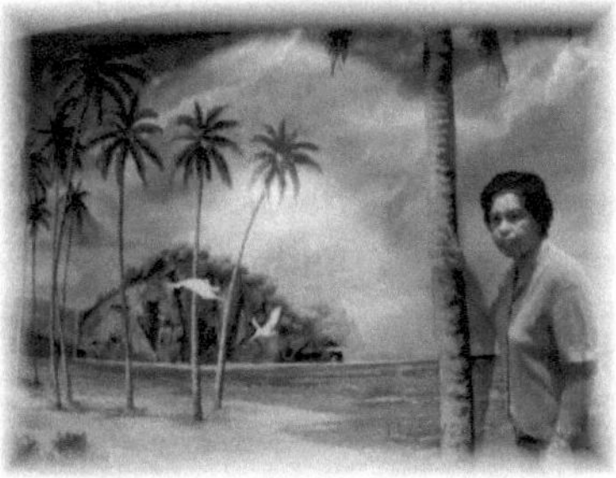

Realizing that only Amelia could possibly make the sound inside the cabin I stepped out of the shower to investigate.

There Amelia was, sprawled on the floor, her head just an inch away from the solid metal door stopper. She was conscious, but her speech sounded slurred to me, an attribute I tend to associate with her even when she is all right, on account of her strokes. Instinctively, I eased her comfortably on the floor without attempting to raise her up.

During the Panama Canal Cruise

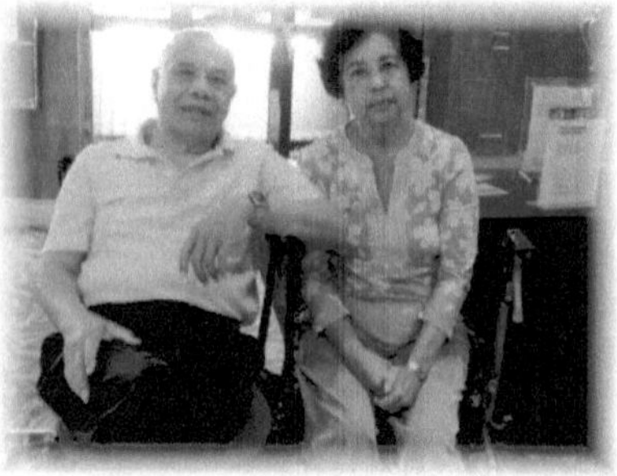

I was considering calling 911 but Amelia dissuaded me because she said she was fine. I kept her lying on the floor for a few minutes, firing question after question at her to get an answer if she hit her head on the door stopper. Assured that she did not and to verify it conclusively, I, watching out for any trace of blood, ran my hand repeatedly on her head to feel for any lump; none was evident. We agreed that the fall did not inflict injury to her, but the incident was not ending yet.

Very light as she was - only 115 pounds at that time- I found it very heavy to raise her up without potentially injuring her and even myself. In the awkward position she was in, and due to her weakened right side, she could not wiggle herself away from the tight space; we could not do it together either. I was afraid to pull her by the arms because they are tiny, I was afraid they might break. There was not enough room for me to maneuver and brace myself to raise her up.

Not wanting to create a commotion, I did not ask assistance from the cruisers passing by in the hallway, but the hallway was the extra space I needed to pull Amelia from her awkward position. Finally, I wrapped myself in a robe, opened the door to the hallway, waited until nobody was passing by, braced myself against the cabin door, and pulled Amelia by the chest. With a sigh of relief, I was able to free and ease her to an upright position allowing her to move and walk slowly.

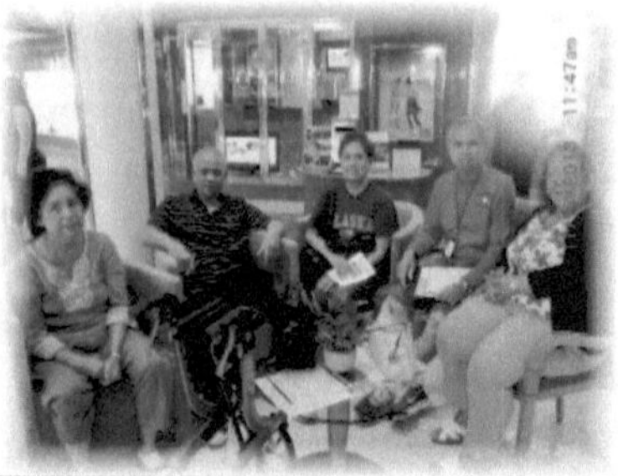

During the Panama Canal Cruise

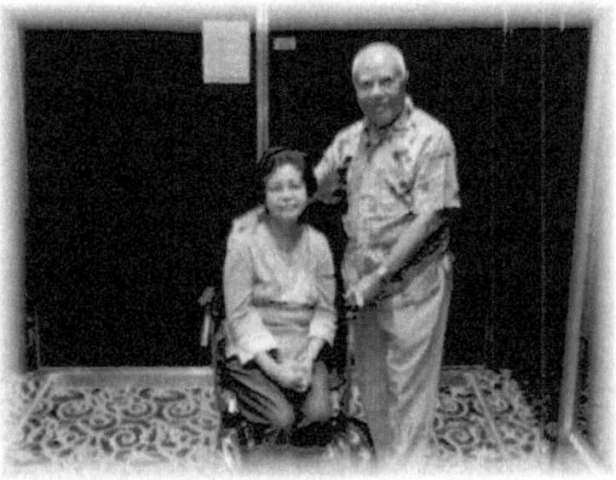

I sat Amelia up on one of the chairs, calmed her down, had her drink orange juice, and measured her glucose level again while still weighing whether to call 911. After five minutes had passed and nothing appeared to be abnormal with her, we proceeded to the food deck for breakfast.

Pressed for an explanation why she fell, Amelia admitted that she was making the bed, a chore already paid for and supposed to be done by the cabin ward, and got off-balance. Amelia has been a stickler for order tending to accomplish multiple work at a time. I see nothing wrong with the trait - in fact, I am happy with it - except that after she had the strokes, she can no longer do what she was accustomed to doing without exposing herself to injury.

Amelia narrowly avoided a serious accident which I attribute to her ailments. Luck, measured in inch literally, was with us. The door stopper on this particular cruise ship – in fact in most cruise ships - is of very heavy solid metal construction installed to absorb enormous repeated bumps daily. That was how close Amelia was from a real emergency away from home to boot.

Struggles with Tenders

Being on the cruise ship is only the beginning of a successful cruise vacation, large part of it being the opportunity to do souvenir shopping, observe different cultures, and visit different places. To go offshore, one has to overcome the inconvenience of embarkation and disembarkation between the ship and the port.

Cruising is fun, but it entails some challenges particularly for one with a physical handicap like Amelia who struggles to get on and off the tenders. Tenders are the life boats of distinct colors that are suspended by cables on the sides of the cruise ship. They facilitate the passengers' essential disembarkation means when the ship is forced to drop anchor away from the shore due to lack of pier space or where the port is not deep enough to handle the depth of the ship's keel.

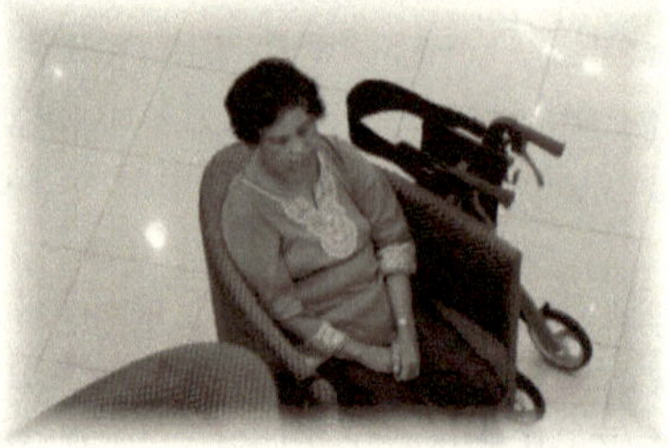

Required by law, just before the ship sets sail, evacuation drills are held to familiarize the passengers of the assembly areas leading to the nearest tenders in case of an emergency. A tender can take as many as three hundred passengers in a real emergency, so its importance cannot be underestimated.

In some ports such as Santa Catalina Island and Santa Barbara both in California, where there are no piers to handle a massive cruise ship, tenders are utilized more exclusively to transport passengers between the ship and the port. Manned by a pilot and at least two crews to assist embarking and disembarking passengers, a tender takes between fifteen and twenty minutes each way to complete a trip. The ocean between the ship and the port can be either very choppy or very calm at certain times. Regardless of the weather

Struggles with Tenders

condition, the intrepid crews have to deliver and pick up the cruisers to keep up with the scheduled sailing times of the cruise ship.

Transferring between the ship's gangway and the tender is where Amelia's problem starts when we do get off the ship to explore the areas around the port and places farther in the localities. Her right side, weakened by multiple strokes, feels heavier and makes her tend to lurch forward and sideward. It will not take much pressure to break her tiny arms, further complicating her transition between the cruise ship and the tender. If the members of the crew manning the tender do not already know, I inform them about Amelia's condition.

Sometimes when Amelia gets on board the tender, she feels dizzy if the ocean is very choppy and the tender rocks and sways. In really inclement weather the tender appears to ride on top of a crest for a brief moment and recovers temporarily then continuing to dip below the ocean level creating splashes that drench the passengers. It is not unusual to find tourists including me enjoying the rough tender rides and cheering the experience and the pilot's navigation skills. Everybody feels the effect of the motion, but more negatively so by Amelia because of her physical and mental condition.

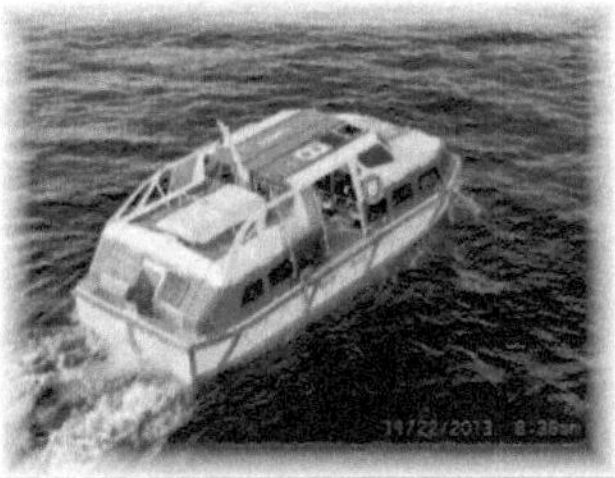

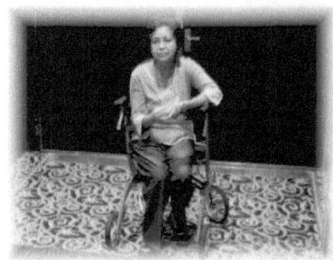

When we return to the cruise ship, the same embarkation procedures on the tenders are repeated in whatever weather condition is prevailing. Amelia enjoys the trip when the weather is calm and suffers the same discomforts when it is choppy. With the return trip

Struggles with Tenders

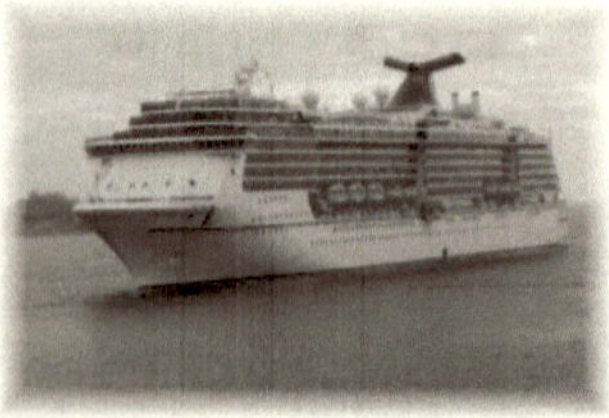

however, we are awaited by plenty of food and drinks on the ship to ease the effects of an unpleasant tender ride.

Despite her problem with the tenders, Amelia looks forward to joining excursions every time we are on a cruise vacation, a desire I do not want to ignore and decline considering her dementedness. Although one may choose to relax on the ship safely, Amelia's choice to go offshore is more like her last wish before any of strokes, Alzheimer's, diabetes, and congestive heart failure takes her life away.

Serenade on Board

At the end of an exhausting day spent on the excursion to the Ruins of Pompeii, we were anxious to go back to the ship to indulge in the free food and drinks while relaxing and waiting for the afternoon entertainments. The long drive back to the ship and the inescapable hunger after having consumed our last supply of snacks were feeding into our quest for anything to suppress our temporary starvation. We wanted to be back on the ship, never mind the inconvenience of enduring hunger a little bit longer.

Like what they did rushing out to join the excursion, upon arrival at the port, the passengers were now rushing back into the ship. Having to match our pace with Amelia's, we ended up boarding the ship later than the rest of the passengers, adding to my anxiety about hunger syndrome making its presence being felt by her.

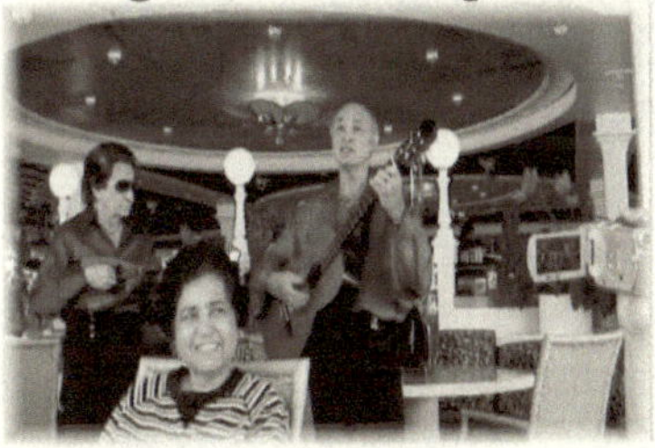

On board the ship I immediately reached for cold orange juice and had Amelia drink it lest she started feeling sick. The long line which formed at the counter prevented us from getting our food immediately, giving us an opportunity to relax first before eating.

Curiously, the ship allowed some entertainers from the port to board the ship, apart from the regular performers. They were conspicuous and distinguishable from the rest of the hungry passengers on board because of their Italian attires and the musical instruments they were carrying.

Serenade on Board

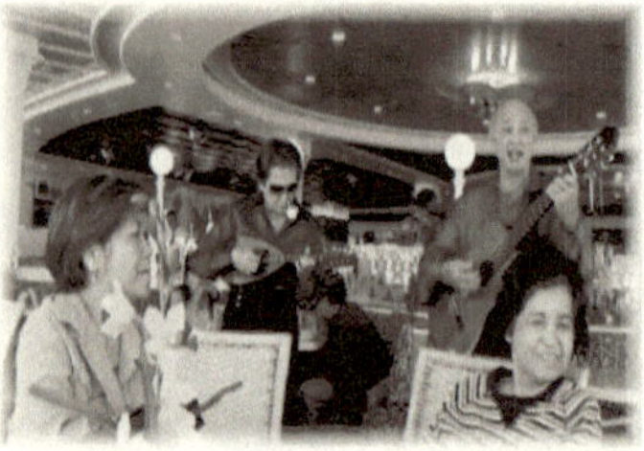

Starting at the table on one corner of the huge dining deck, the Italian entertainers serenaded the tired passengers with Italian songs, naturally. Due to the large number of passengers converging at the food deck at the same time, we did not get serenaded until most of them finished their meals and were already relaxing and leaving. We took this opportunity to get our food and drinks without forcing our way at the food counters.

The entertainers finally reached our table and without a hint from us about what songs we liked, they started playing bait pieces. They asked us what songs we would like them to sing and play. For a small optional donation, we requested them to sing and play songs like Amore, Funiculi Funicula, Sorrento, Ave Maria, and a few others.

The entertainers stayed with us longer and sang more songs than in any other locations, our table being one of the last in the dining area. The fact that Amelia enjoyed the songs and the pieces was an indication that she was feeling well and not suffering much from the just concluded exhausting excursion. Had she had her way, she would like the entertainers to stay even longer and play more songs.

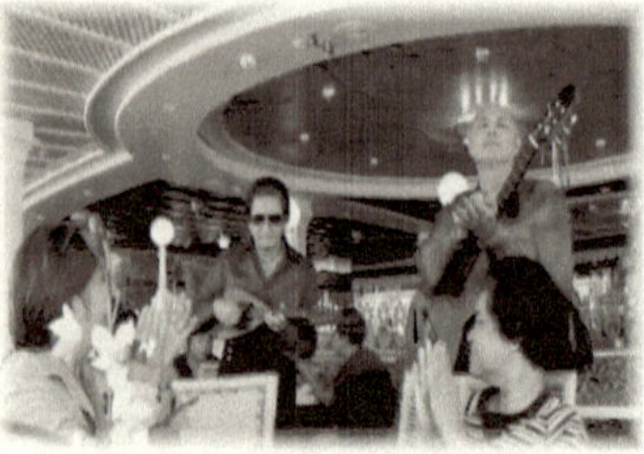

The day ended in an upbeat mode. We had the choice of watching other entertainments on board, but with enough activities already having come to pass earlier, we decided to stay and relax in our cabin until night. Then we came out, ate some

Serenade on Board

snacks, and listened to the music being played on the open deck area by the regular onboard band and performers.

We retired to our cabin after an hour, finally concluding the day filled with so much more activities than we anticipated. We needed enough rest in preparation for the roundtrip travel to Rome the following morning.

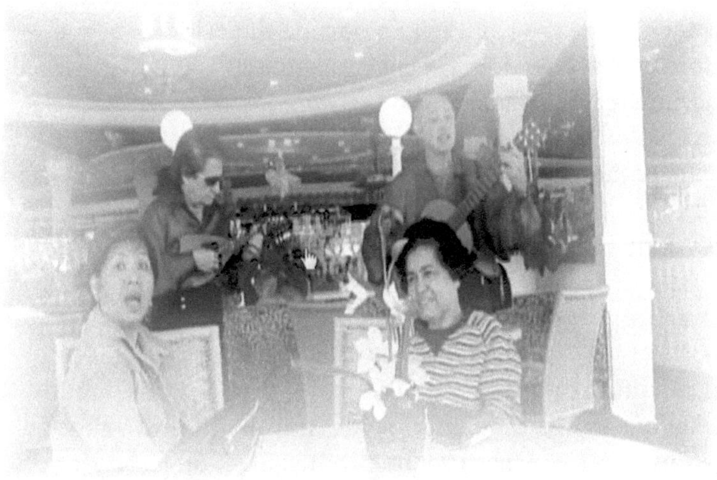

Post Cruise Incident

Having completed a 7-day Caribbean cruise vacation to Haiti, Mexico, and Jamaica from Florida, we were eager to head for home in California, because notwithstanding the comforts in the monster cruise ship, there was no place like home. We were done with the most memorable cruise of our life on the biggest cruise ship in the world, The Allure of the Seas, which can accommodate more than 8,000 passengers and crews

As is the usual procedure in all cruises, we placed our secured pieces of luggage in the hallway just outside the cabin door the night before disembarkation, for pickup and deposit at the marked luggage claim areas. To facilitate light travel, we only had on us the appropriate clothes for the season plus hand carried purses and backpacks containing medications, glasses, cameras, and travel documents.

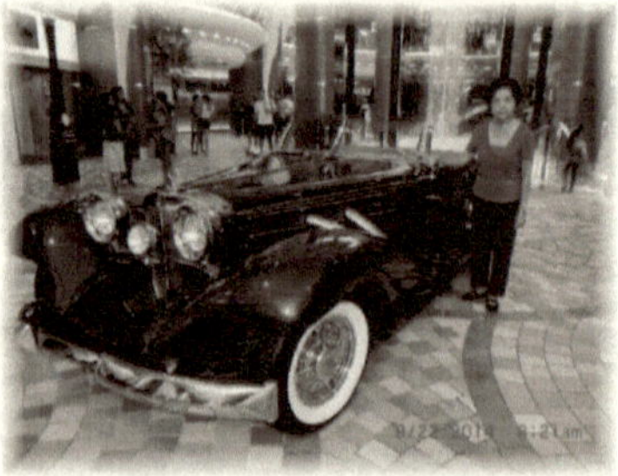

Expecting an intricate disembarkation procedure the following morning, I prearranged a wheelchair pickup for Amelia at the promenade lounge, and we went to sleep early ignoring the boisterous last minute entertainments on the ship.

At 5:00 AM when I woke Amelia up, she was unable to get up due to general weakness of her body. I handed $20 to our cabin ward and asked him to get a glass of orange juice for Amelia. When he came back he informed me that most restaurants would be closing, except the bar on the 15th deck. Because our turn for pickup at the promenade lounge was still an hour away, I was confident that after

Post Cruise Incident

drinking orange juice, Amelia would regain her energy and would be able to walk with her walker.

An hour had gone by, and Amelia still was unable to get up and walk. Every few minutes that I helped her to get up and stand, she would fall back asking to be left alone to rest. Having already finished the glass of orange juice, she was still asking for more, making me nervous and concerned.

To get more orange juice from the bar on the 15th deck, I either had to take the elevator or walk up and down nine decks of stairs with fifteen to thirty steps between decks. I did not want to take the elevator for fear it might be turned off. Neither was I ready to trot up and down the stairs for fear I might get tired and collapse.

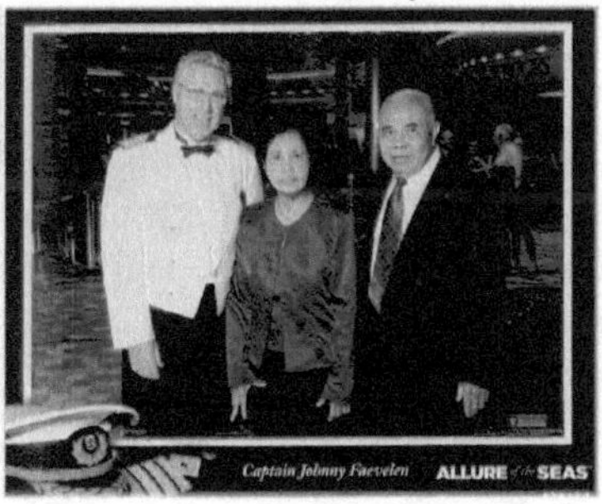

Dreadfully, I did not want to leave Amelia alone in the cabin on the 6th deck as the cruise ship was eerily getting quiet and emptied. The cabin wards were gone assisting in the disembarkation activity. Desperation was setting in on me.

I called the clinic to send someone to examine Amelia. The clinic, now taken over by non-medical personnel, responded that I had to pay $250.00 for someone to get to our cabin and make a determination as to what should be done with Amelia. But since the medical staff already disembarked, it would take two to four hours before someone could get back on board.

Calling the emergency hotline was an option the clinic was willing to do for me, but again with more than 8,000 plus passengers and crews disembarking at the same time, there was no guarantee that

Post Cruise Incident

someone could come and see Amelia in time for the disembarkation. That option was not helpful either.

I explained the terrifying situation we were in to Amelia. She was as cooperative as she could be, asking for just a few more minutes to rest. I was imploring her to summon every ounce of energy so she could get up and walk. In the meantime, a security officer was sent to our cabin to check what was going on. I had the impression that he suspected an ongoing dishonest behavior because he asked to look at every corner of the cabin before he left.

In a flash of sheer determination and like a miracle, Amelia asked to be helped to get up. She was able to stand and slowly started walking with her walker. Hooray was I glad and full of joy! Immediately I called the disembarkation team to dispatch someone with a wheelchair to pick up Amelia.

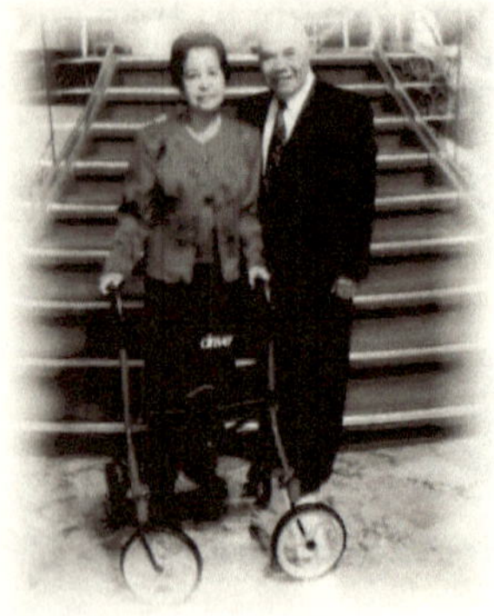

Were it not for the incident, we would have been the first few passengers to disembark owing to the priority accorded to disabled passengers. Out of the ship, we were led through a series of doors and elevators, through an ocean of pieces of luggage to get to ours, and then through security point on to the bus waiting for us for the next tour, Fort Lauderdale Land and Sea.

After the incident at the cruise ship, we were not so ecstatic about the tour of the fort. But we had to take it because the tour would be ending at the Miami International Airport, dismissing the need for us to load and unload our luggage. At the end of the tour, we would be resting at the airport while waiting for our flight to California.

Post Cruise Incident

Despite the post cruise unfortunate experience, I considered the cruise a success. I was always fascinated by the size and amenities of the monster cruise ships, and The Allure of The Seas was not a disappointment; in fact, it was the best cruise vacation we ever had, having been with quite a few previously.

The post cruise incident had nothing to do with the quality of the cruise and the cruise ship itself, leading me to recommend cruising on The Allure of the Seas as an option for enjoying a cruise vacation.

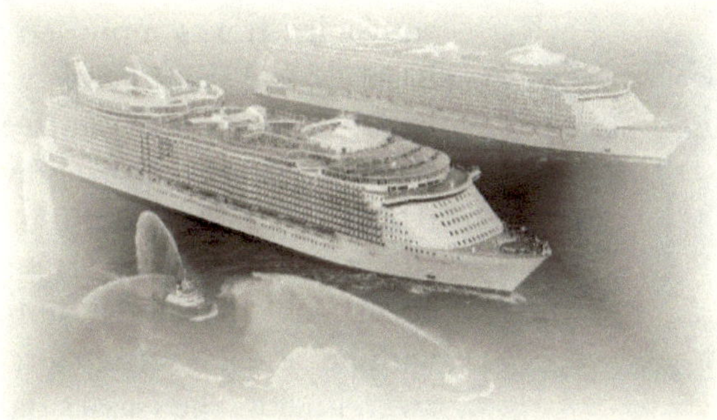

Incident at Lahaina

The excursion to Iao Valley, Maui, Hawaii, was just concluded and the tour bus let the tourists off near the pier area close to the Lahaina Courthouse. Since Amelia moved slower than the rest of the passengers, we waited until most of the passengers cleared the bus before getting off. Finally, when our turn came, it was too late for us to catch the waiting tender with most of the passengers already ahead on the way to the pier. We opted to wait for the next tender in order not to inconvenience the passengers ahead of us by having the tender wait for us.

Meantime we crossed the yard towards the stores to shop for some souvenirs. It was supposed to be a leisurely and short gentle walk under two huge banyan trees on a path paved with coarse gravel, with Amelia holding onto my arms for support. Suddenly she tripped on a small rock and fell flat on her face with her eyeglass flying a few feet away. Luckily the glasses did not break into her eyes; otherwise, they could have caused severe eye injuries.

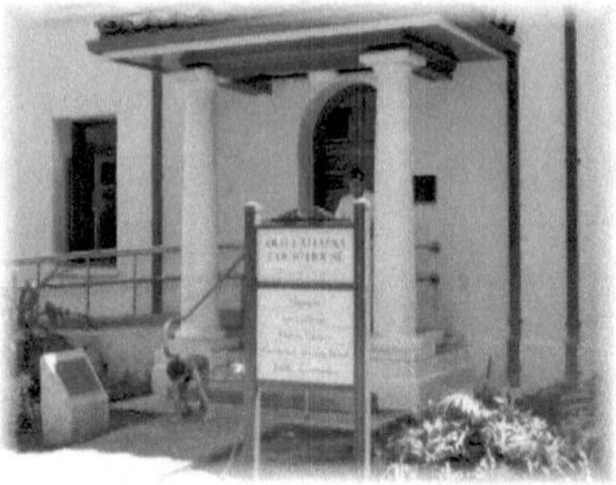

Tenderly I turned her around, and for a moment I was scared she would lose consciousness and stop breathing. With her teeth showing, her mouth was wide open with some gravel inside it. Her face was blue, and some drops of blood were coming off her forehead. She was trying to talk which was a sign that she was conscious.

Incident at Lahaina

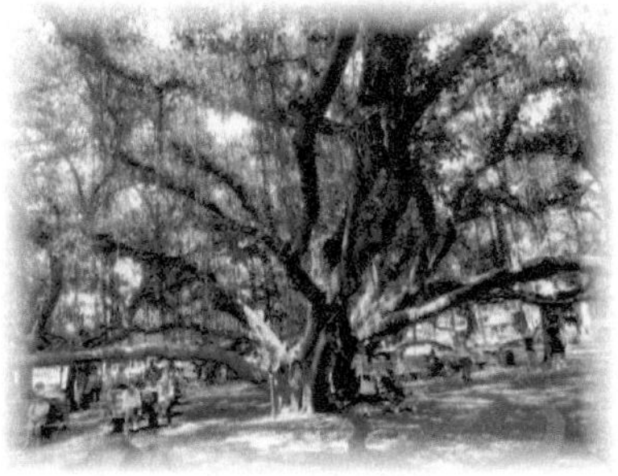

Some bystanders came to help me while I slowly made her sit up. I asked if any part of her body was hurting and her response was negative. Because she always tends to say she is all right even if she is not, I ran my hand over her arms and body to see if any area was hurting or broken; none was, but a bubble about one-fourth the size of a golf ball, was forming on her forehead.

I cleaned her up with water offered by some strangers. She was able to balance herself when I helped her stand up, and I took that as an even better sign. With me supporting her, we walked to a bench where tourists cleared a space for her, and where I continued cleaning her up and making her comfortable.

The nearest medical clinic was on the cruise ship. We had to wait thirty minutes for the next tender to come and take us to the ship. In the meantime, Amelia was asking for a soda or water to ease her heightened emotion resulting from the fall. Not wanting to be left alone if I crossed the street, she settled for ice cream being sold across where she was sitting. The ice cream helped to calm her nerves.

The medical personnel at the cruise ship cleaned Amelia up some more and injected her with antibiotics. After her forehead wound was dressed up, an X-ray was taken of her head as a precaution. The X-Ray returned a negative result. We were advised to consult with Amelia's doctor as soon as the cruise ship

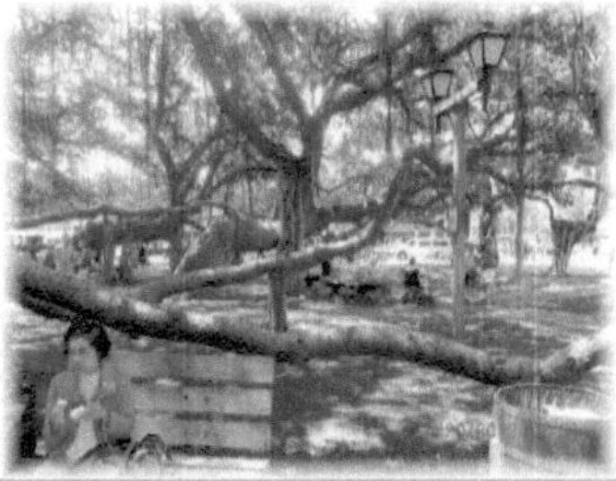

Incident at Lahaina

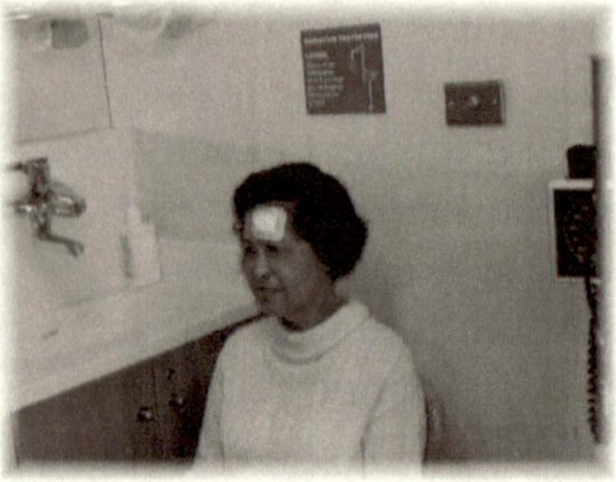

docked at San Pedro, Los Angeles. That was what we did, and all the tests conducted on her returned negative results.

Considering Amelia's physical condition which allows a very narrow margin of error regarding physical agility, I learned a lesson from the incident, namely, being careful in the choice of paths where she needs to walk.

The rock that tripped Amelia was not big, but because of her physical condition, she lost her balance easily. Were a healthy person tripped on the rock instead, an incident of the kind that Amelia had would not have happened.

Chapter 21 - Portents of Sad Ending

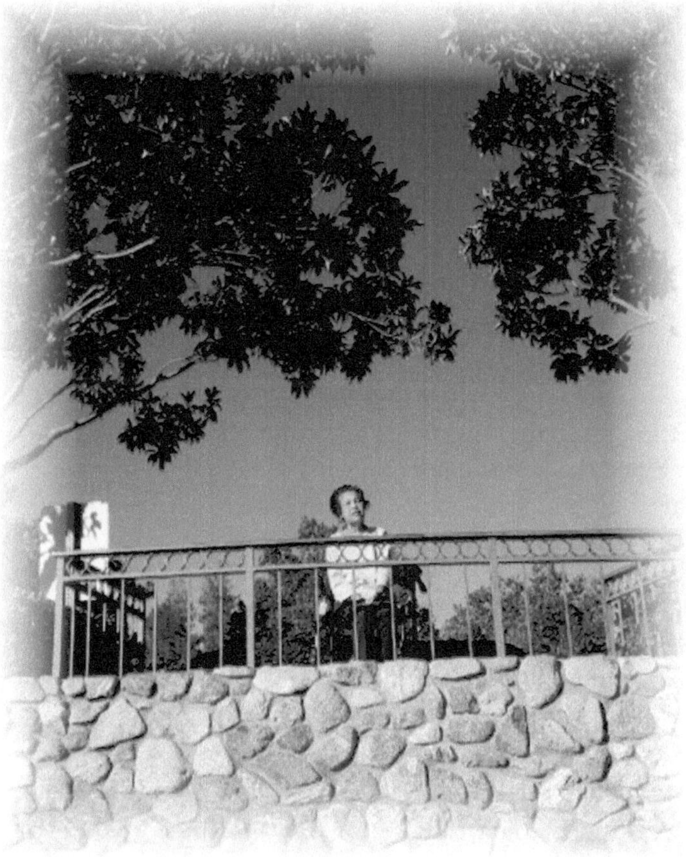

Amelia's Illness Had Worsened

I always improvised ways to make Amelia's life and mine as manageable as possible.

Getting on bed was fun. After dinner, I would have her sit on the edge of the bed, lay her down, and roll her towards the wall, the location she preferred. As I rolled her, she would hum a nursery song which she used to teach in school thus making us laugh together. For an unexplained reason when she was ready to get up, she would not roll back in reverse. She preferred to get up from the foot end of the bed, a move that was not difficult to do because the bed is mechanical. All I had to do was raise the head end of the bed and slide her towards the foot end, put her feet down, and gradually stand her up, another occasion to laugh early in the morning.

Before getting up in the morning, she would ask me to turn the stereo on. Since the bed is equipped with a speaker system we usually stayed on bed for a while, she listening to the music and I scanning my tablet for the early news of the day.

This morning, January 17, 2017 was different, however. Amelia's body did not appear to cooperate when I slid her from the bed, even when I raised the head end to the fullest. When she did slide, she was slumping, only prevented from dropping to the floor by my full body weight braced against the clothes chest.

I did not have the strength to raise her up to the bed. My only option was to grab two pillows, placed them on the floor, and had Amelia slide on them. Then I raced for a walker and had her sit on it. She appeared confused and was slurring heavily. I was seriously thinking that she was having another stroke. It was time for me to call the emergency hotline which dispatched an ambulance

Amelia's Illness Had Worsened

promptly. Amelia was taken to the hospital leaving no indication of extreme pain other than the usual difficulty on her right leg.

I guessed the hospital did not think that Amelia was having an emergency. The ambulance was about thirty minute ahead of me, yet when I arrived at the hospital Amelia was not in the emergency ward. I waited for approximately an hour before I was told that Amelia was now in the emergency ward. When I got in, there was no sense of urgency. No IV fluid was given to Amelia, so I thought that everything was all right. About an hour later the doctor came and examined Amelia. Then she told me that before any decision on whether or not to admit her, the internist would have to examine Amelia.

The internist came an hour or so later, and after examining Amelia, pulled me outside the ward and told me that Amelia was all right; there was nothing wrong with her. The doctor, I sensed, was trying to mildly break the sad news to me. Amelia's condition had worsened; the doctor appeared to indicate that Alzheimer's was overwhelming her.

That was the reason why Amelia was not admitted to the hospital. The doctor indicated to me that the case officer would be explaining my options. When the case officer came, she handed me some brochures of nursing facilities to which Amelia could be discharged at my choice. She then told me that the social worker would be coming by to discuss additional options.

In the meantime, I was told by the initial attending nurse that Amelia would be released to me on this same day depending on the options I would be making. That did not happen; hospital shift change had occurred and another nurse took over. It was getting late in the afternoon and Amelia was still in the emergency ward.

Amelia's Illness Had Worsened

Finally after inquiry about Amelia's status in the emergency ward, the nurse sought another hospital officer who later came by and told me that Amelia would be kept overnight at the emergency ward, and that I should be in the hospital at 8:00 AM the following morning to talk to another case officer.

I requested the nurse to order food for Amelia because it was very late in the afternoon and Amelia was very hungry, not having breakfast and lunch. I believed that had I not ordered food, Amelia would be missing dinner while the other patients were enjoying theirs, based on the ongoing activities in the emergency wards.

After feeding Amelia, I left and waited to be back the following morning as I promised.

VNA (Visiting Nurses Association) to the Rescue

I was not sure what the term "hospice" meant. If the internist who talked to me the previous day mentioned and described it, I may have forgotten its meaning owing to the number of medical professionals talking to me while I was in a very confused state. I was more worried about Amelia's uncertain status than trying to understand medical terms.

As promised though, I was at the hospital at 8:00 AM the following morning; Amelia was still in the emergency ward where I left her the previous day. A case officer came by about an hour later followed by an officer from VNA. Evidently from the hospital records, I committed to having hospice care for Amelia at home – I was not sure I did, but I let the hospital case officer and the VNA officer took control of the activities because I was still confused.

The VNA officer made a few phone calls including arrangement for the delivery of bed equipment and accessories to our house, while the hospital case officer contacted All-In-One Care Solutions, Inc. to request the service of a caregiver for the remainder of the day. Even while Amelia was still being prepared for release from the emergency ward of the hospital, I could observe (by remote camera) the flurry of activities going on in our house, which made me feel relieved and grateful.

Amelia was transported to our house by VNA, and was laid relaxed on a bed designed for hospice care. She was comfortably conversing with our children in very familial manner. Except for slight discomfort when the caregiver was repositioning her, there was nothing to indicate her soon-to-follow bouts with physical pain. She could rise from bed with slight assistance.

VNA (Visiting Nurses Association) to the Rescue

Hospice care was not frightful after all, as I originally and horribly thought. VNA personnel were on call anytime. Medical equipment and supplies were delivered to our house without being requested. Evidently, VNA anticipated what medications were important and necessary and in what frequency they had to be administered. They were packaged and left with us for emergency administration before the arrival of a medical practitioner, if we needed assistance.

Amelia was bathed three times a week or frequently if necessary. Through VNA, Eucharistic ministers came more than once to offer communion to Amelia. A catholic priest came more than once as well to offer prayers for Amelia and the family. Everything that helped to relieve the family of physical and emotional tension was being offered by VNA including after-funeral support for a year.

Owing to Amelia's Part B coverage under Medicare, VNA did not bill us for its services. I was able to fulfill my promise to Amelia that as long as I was able to take care of her, she would be home - not nursing home – bound. Although at this time her illness appeared to have worsened, the family was comfortable in the feeling that Amelia was not being exposed to potential neglect and maltreatment at nursing home facilities.

We were satisfied that after the confusion that occurred the previous day, hospice care at home was the best choice I made for Amelia after all, thanks to VNA.

Incessant Admiration for White Objects

Amelia's recent attraction towards white objects became more defined and somewhat mysterious. I was not certain what brought it along; I blithely attributed it to dementia and at first I kept ignoring it.

It was strange that while flowers were beautifully blooming along Peyton Drive and Grand Avenue at Chino Hills, California, Amelia's admiration was not directed towards them. Instead, her gaze and attention was focused on the white wooden fences. The first occasions that she acted this way did not arouse any unusual impression in me. But when she would specially request to drive along the same route every day, even on drizzly ones, just to admire the white fences, I knew that her mood was changing.

On the days of Christmas when shops and some homes were decorated and adorned with elegant multicolored lights, Amelia would prefer to watch those at corner of Peyton Drive and Grand Avenue where a series of white lights were stringed end to end. She never missed pointing them out to me, heaping praises on the lights that I did not even consider a color, while ignoring the beautiful twinkling ones on the Christmas tree at the Shoppe on the other corner. Often, I would openly despise her choice of color, a trick I employed to divert her attention. She would ignore me completely.

Then in the park where hundreds of birds and geese fly and feed themselves, Amelia's eyes would follow the flights and movements of the white ones for as long as they were in sight. With the snaps of her fingers, she would encourage the white birds that perched close by on the trees and on the fence to approach her. Calmly and peacefully, she watched the birds until we agreed to go home, again along the avenue of white wooden fences.

Pain and Suffering

The day that Amelia was released from the hospital at around 3:00 PM on January 18, 2017 did not carry signs of discomfort other than her difficulty to stand and walk. Pain was still at the tolerable level that she was used to during the past several months. Its sharpness would change though during the night and would carry over into the following day and gradually intensified until the end.

Every time that she was being moved and repositioned, she would scream of pain. At first the pain was concentrated mainly on her right leg, gradually spreading throughout her entire body as each day passed. Amelia became very sensitive to touch, suddenly jolting and often screaming when a hand was laid on her. Asked which part of her body was the source of the pain, she would point out everywhere like her neck, her sides, her head, her legs, so on so forth.

VNA firstly prescribed a milder form of medication to assuage the suffering. The first two or three administrations of the drugs worked, but as Amelia became addicted, the drug's potency became ineffective. In the meantime, complications ensued causing even more pain. Amelia was choking when she was swallowing her food or drinking fluids. She became constipated causing an even more intense pain.

The VNA doctor finally graduated Amelia's medication to the more potent morphine. Administered every two hours, the medication sedated Amelia. However, if timing was missed during the period, Amelia would wake up and complain of extreme pain, even more extreme than she was previously feeling.

At the middle of the night when perhaps everybody was soundly sleeping, Amelia, because of pain, would be praying, her prayers

Pain and Suffering

interspersed with moans and screams. Her prayers were a mixture of English versions and Filipino vernaculars.

Part of the improvised Filipino version of her prayers that would keep breaking my heart would run this way, "Diyos ko po, maawa ka sa akin. Tulongan mo po akooo. Tulungan mo po ang asawa ko. Tulongan mo po ang kapatid ko. Tulongan mo po ang mga anak ko." Roughly translated to English the prayer meant, "Dear God, have mercy on me. Please help me. Please help my husband. Please help my brother. Please help my children." The emphasis on "akooo" projected extreme pain coming from the lips of a dying human being, Amelia.

At my encouragement, she would repeat her prayers starting with the Lord's Prayer in English et al followed by her spontaneous creations in Filipino vernaculars. Despite Alzheimer's, Amelia would recite her prayers in clear and unmistakable sequence.

Amelia's fondness for classical music turned to gospel music. Holding her hand and crying in pity for her, I would softly play gospel music in the background hoping that it would alleviate and mitigate the pain and misery. Countless number of times did I play Amazing Grace and Rock of Ages that even when they were not on, I seemed to hear them.

For most of the last twenty three days that Amelia was living, the above midnight scene was repeated every night. Up to the termination of this book, I am still learning how to initiate a good night's sleep, trying to recover from the ordeal.

"I Am Going Home"

Amelia was not yet bedridden after Christmas of 2016. I was still accommodating her requests to drive around the city for no reason other than to get away from the confines of home. I liked being outdoor myself so it was our arrangement that after lunch every day, weather permitting, we would go to parks, malls, and other nearby places.

Frequently, she would ask about the time of the day. When I pointed out the car clock to her she would shrug her shoulders and casually accept her failure to realize that the time was just in front of her. Then she would ask about the day of the week. Challenging her ability to remember, I would offer wrong days to see if she could still recognize the days of the week. She could not and would just accept the day that I offered. She would not even try and would defer everything that needed remembering to me.

When she was in hospice at home and no longer easily driven around but still very cognizant of her surroundings, she would still ask about the time and the day of the week. In addition, she would ask how old she would be on her next birthday. I would honestly and frankly – no more challenges – tell her the right time, the right day of the week, and her age on her next birthday. She would look around and smile. On more than one occasion however, the following dialogue occurred after asking me about the time and day of the week.

Looking at me she said: "I am going home." When I told her that she was already at home, she repeated with an additional sentence: "I am going home. You will be left alone." Then she would calmly go to sleep when her medications started to take effect.

"I Am Going Home"

I did not attach any sad meaning to the conversation because I did not expect that Amelia was going to die soon. Her dementia, I made a fun of, was causing her desire to go home. It was naïve and foolish of me to be making fun of her plan to go home when she was already at home. In this case however, home appeared to have a different location and meaning to Amelia.

She was still communicative and able to move except for pain on certain parts of her body. She would still talk while feeding herself on the kitchen table. Besides, everybody was still fresh from the New Year's celebrations and had no time to regroup and get organized. Amelia was still in celebratory mood despite her immobility.

As Amelia's illness turned for the worse the dialogue carried on very significant and sad implication. In retrospect, Amelia appeared to have known that she was going to die, and that she would be leaving me a widower. Less than two weeks later she passed away.

Yes, she went home. She went to a different home! How insensitive I was not to recognize that Amelia was meaning to go to a different home, a home apart from where I now live – ALONE, as she indicated.

The Taunting

In our marriage, I never heard Amelia uttered profane language let alone words of defiance, aggression, and threats. She may have scowled in disagreements but never showed displeasure in the form of vulgar words coming out of her mouth. Perhaps out of pain the following incident happened.

Two days in a row at around 5:00 PM, in the midst of her extreme suffering from pain, she was saying in Filipino: "Yayariin kita." Translated to English the words mean: "I will do you." or "I will harm you." She would repeat the sentence until she was overcome by drowsiness due to the medication, the same medication that she was taking while praying to alleviate her pain.

The caregiver and I were dumbfounded to hear Amelia appearing to be talking to an invisible being. She was being taunted and threatened, it seemed. In response Amelia sounded to be defensive, defiant, protective, and retaliatory. Her hands would grip the side of the bed in a show of force and defiance. I never heard the words from her before.

I did not believe Amelia was hallucinating in the strict sense of the word, for if she was, her prayers could be interpreted as products of hallucinations too. She was not creating truths out of untruths. In her state of extreme pain, she was addressing her words in second person. She was in a state of quarrel and she seemed to be holding her ground. Whatever it was that created the incident, it will never be known. Amelia passed away a week later.

Finally the End Had Come

Each time that I was left alone with Amelia, now bedridden, and had to administer a dose of morphine every two hours, I would feel her pulse. It was still very distinct and unmistakable despite VNA's pronouncement that Amelia's life would terminate soon. The caregiver would do the same thing in the morning. We were amazed at how normal was Amelia's pulse even when she was not actively responding due to the medication. She was a fighter, we used to comment.

At 4:20 AM, February 9, 2017, I gave her the required dose of morphine. She bit on the syringe and ground her teeth. After I disengaged the syringe, she relaxed and as if feeling relieved, she went to sleep. Little did I realize that that designated time for her dose of morphine was the last time I would be holding her alive. Finally, Amelia succumbed to her illness against my hope and prayer that she remained alive a little longer.

Her death did not dawn on me until I tried to administer the next dose of morphine at 6:20 AM. Her forehead was still warm but her hands were cold and she was not breathing. I could no longer feel her pulse. I knew that the end had come. It was time to notify the members of the family and VNA.

Officially, VNA pronounced Amelia's death at 9:10 AM, February 9th, 2017. Although the sight of Amelia being wrapped in black and placed in a body bag was very disturbing, I could not help but watched her depart. She was now gone forever, leaving fifty-four years of our marriage! Only sad emotion is left with me!

With her loss, I lost a loving wife, our children lost a dear mother, and our grand children lost a caring grandmother.

What Comes After

Buried in Amelia's casket is a time capsule that contains copies of this book and its variations. For a symbolic gesture, Amelia's family does not object to having her casket exhumed to expose the time capsule several years from now, to celebrate a real breakthrough in the cure of Alzheimer's in particular, and the triumph of science over the other diseases that helped to fell Amelia, namely, diabetes, strokes, and congestive heart failure.

I am sure that at the rate progress is being made in the search for the cure of the diseases it will be decades more before real success can be declared. By then, I as the author of this book, and probably the next one or more generations after me, will have been gone. For now, we can only hope that no more members of any family fall victims to the dreaded diseases.

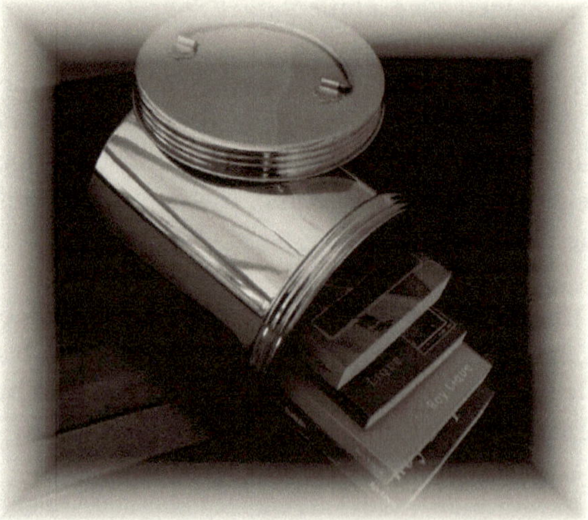

What Comes After

Chapter 22 – In Pictures

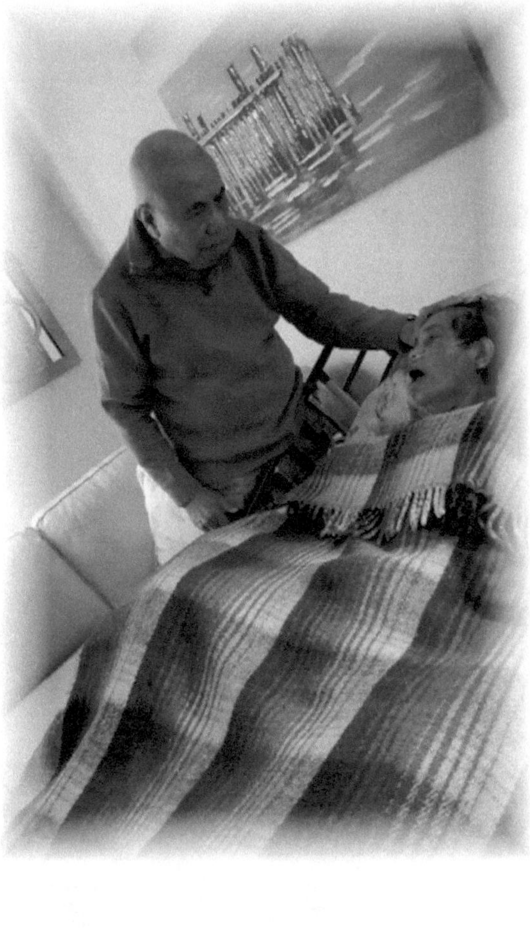

Amelia's Last Christmas

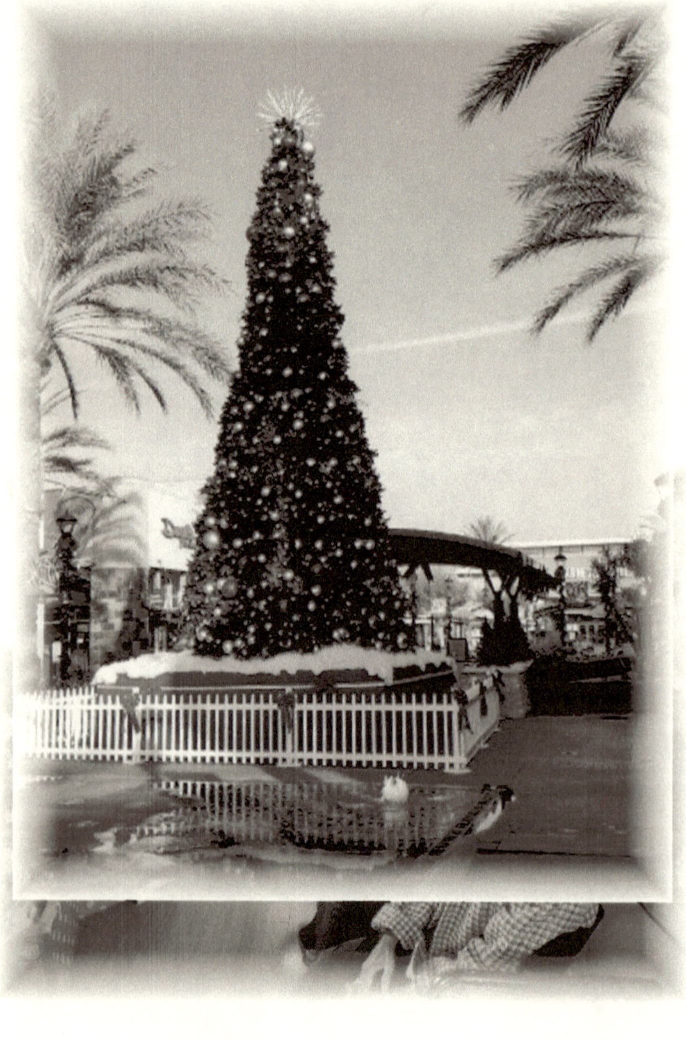

Amelia's Last Christmas

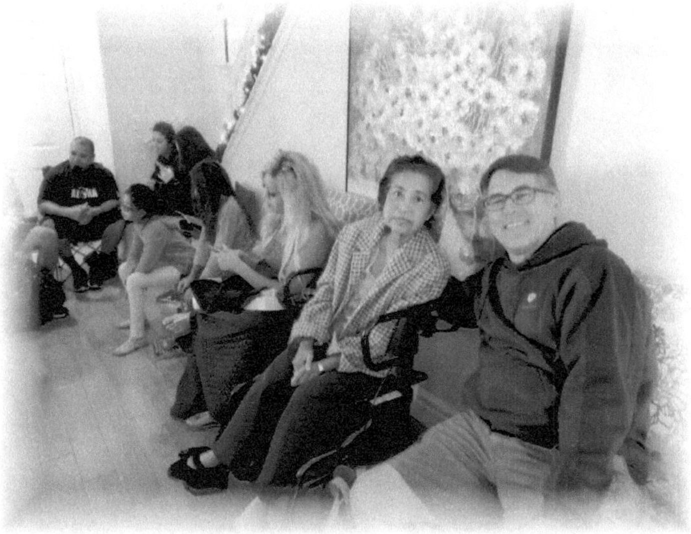

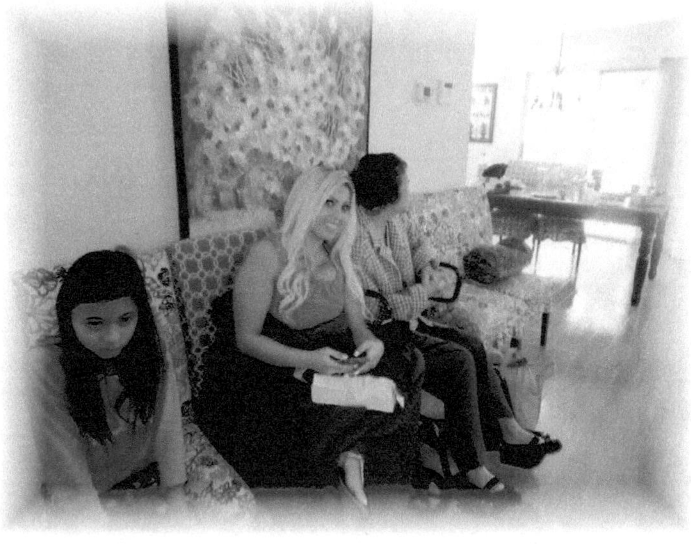

Amelia's Last Christmas

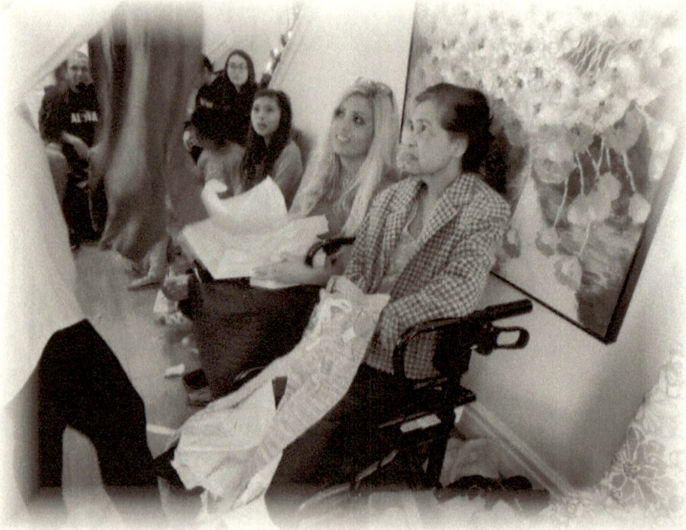

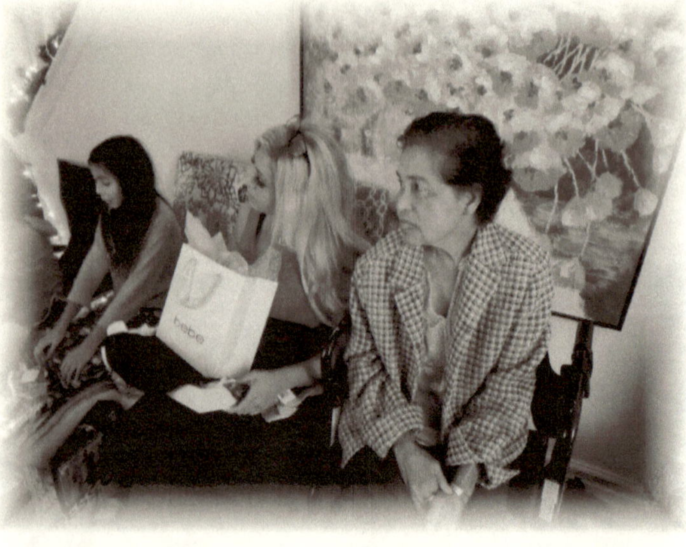

Amelia's Last Christmas

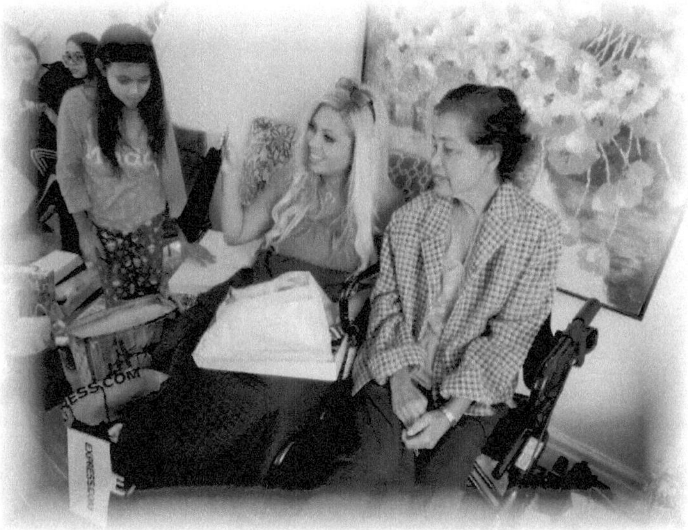

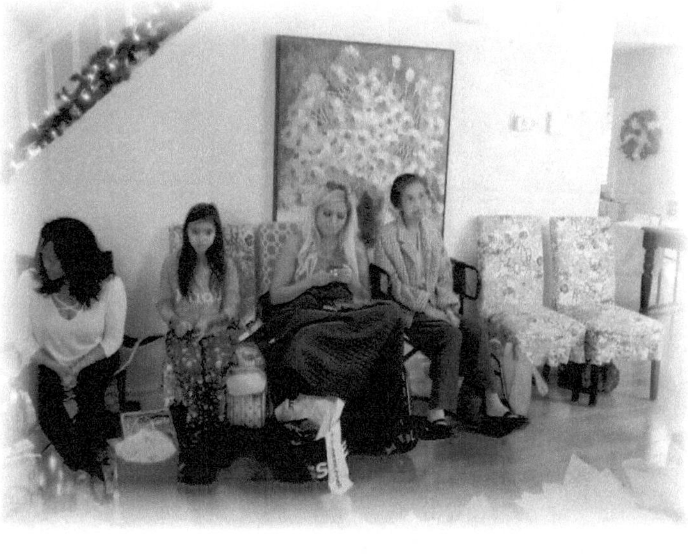

Amelia's Last Christmas

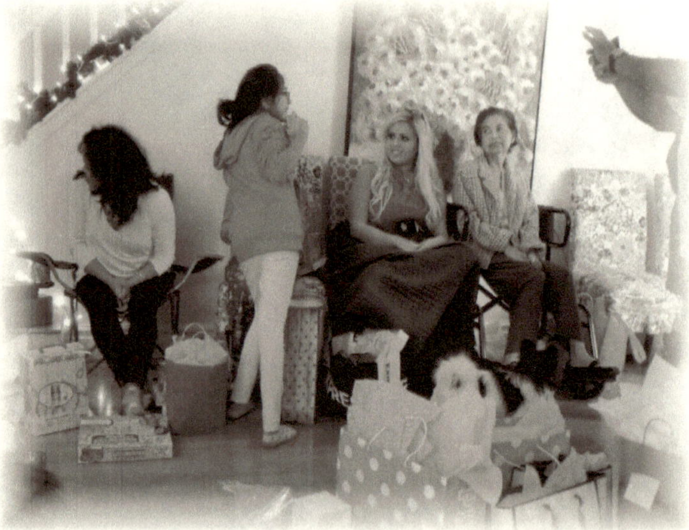

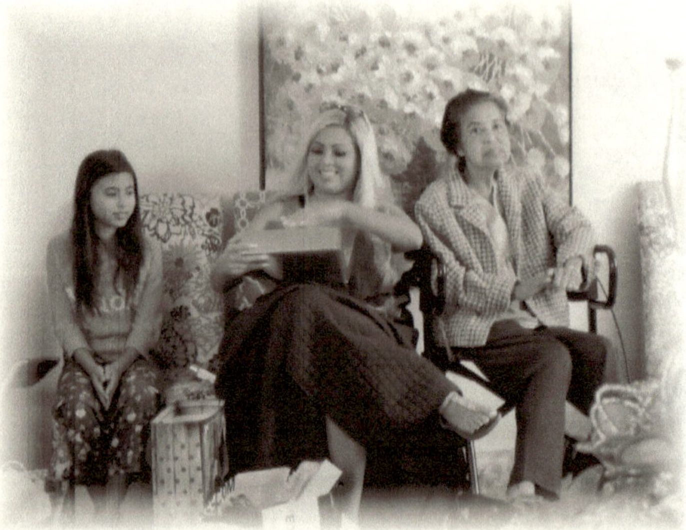

Amelia's Last Christmas

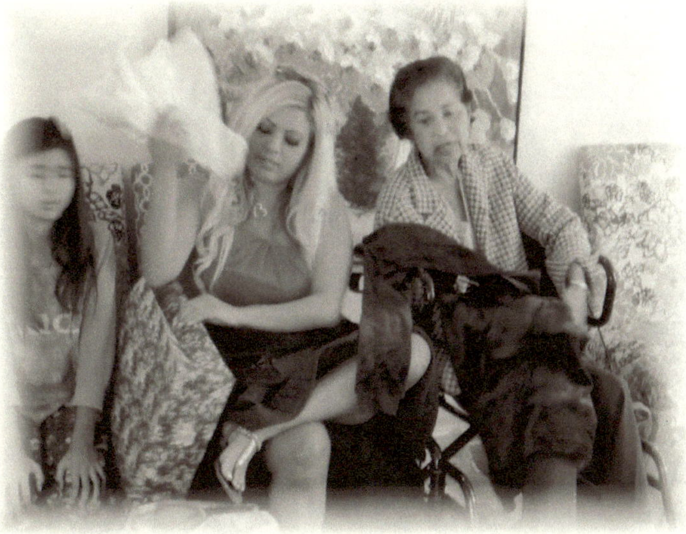

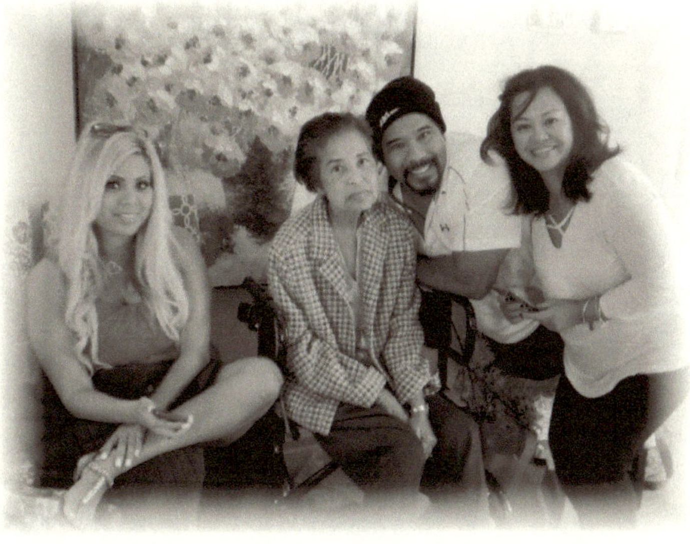

Amelia's Last Christmas

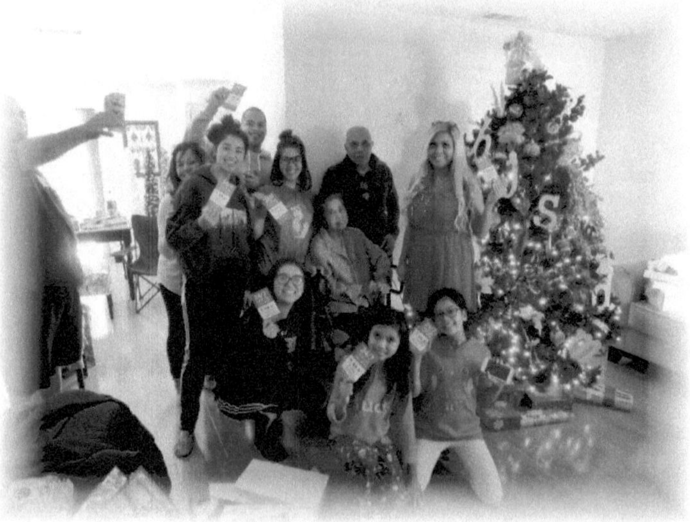

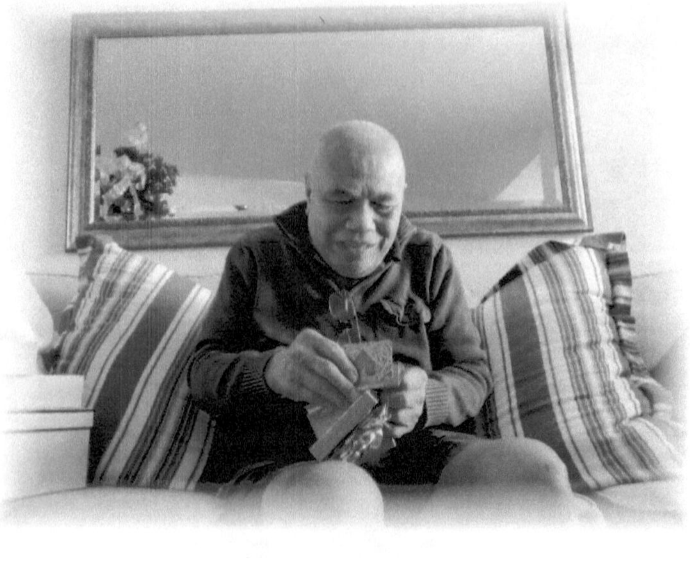

Amelia's Last Christmas

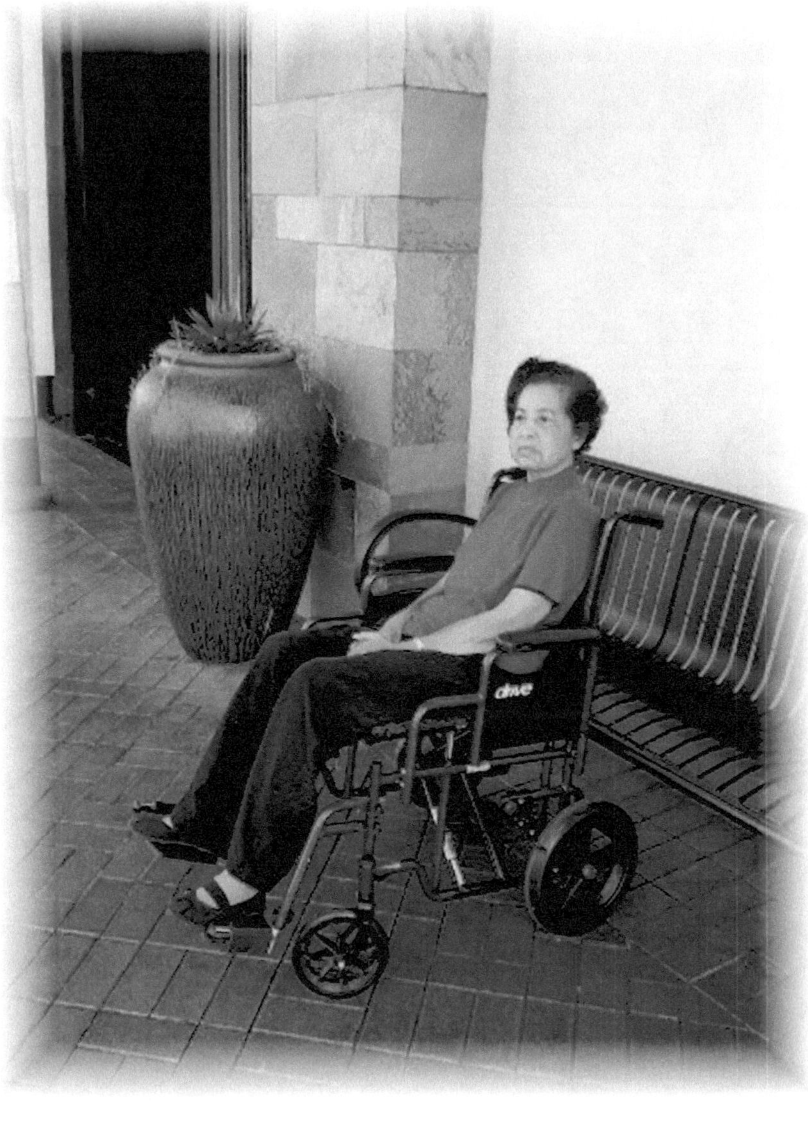

In Memory of Amelia Apalit Lique

In Memory of Amelia Apalit Lique

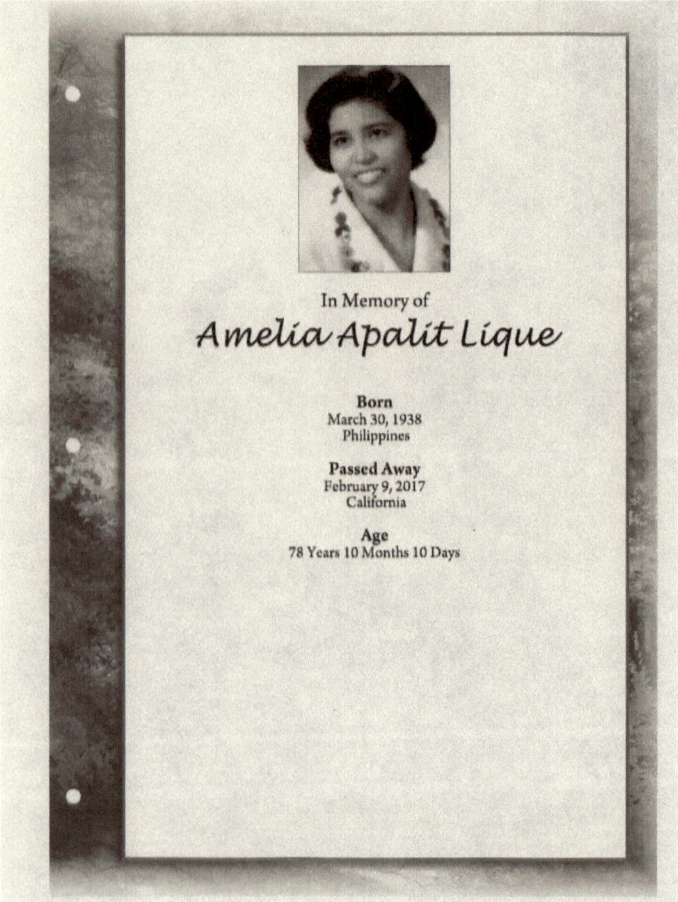
In Memory of
Amelia Apalit Lique
Born
March 30, 1938
Philippines
Passed Away
February 9, 2017
California
Age
78 Years 10 Months 10 Days

Death Certificate

Death Certificate

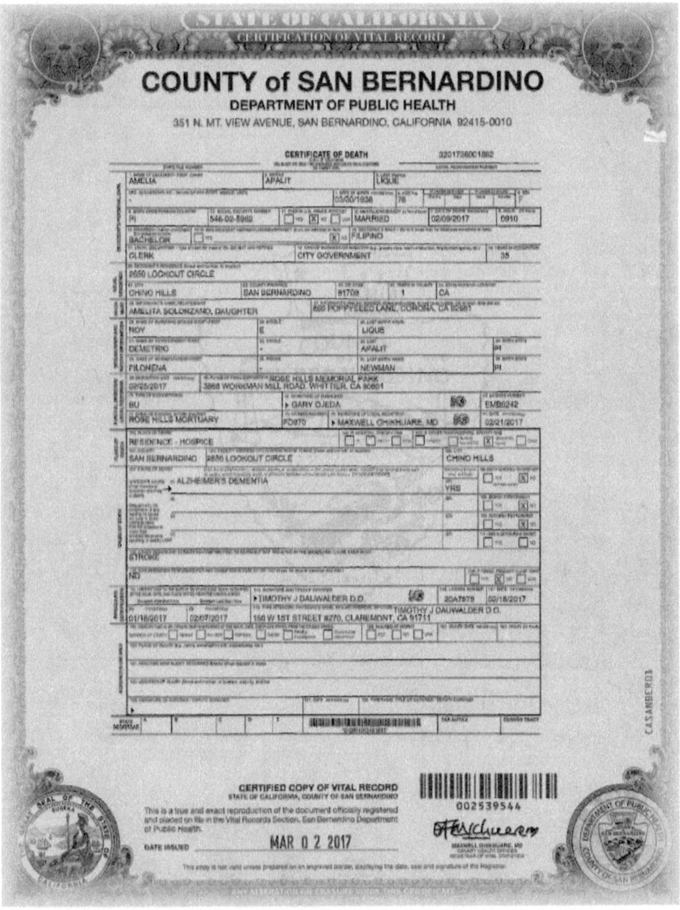

STATE OF CALIFORNIA
CERTIFICATION OF VITAL RECORD

COUNTY of SAN BERNARDINO
DEPARTMENT OF PUBLIC HEALTH
351 N. MT. VIEW AVENUE, SAN BERNARDINO, CALIFORNIA 92415-0010

CERTIFICATE OF DEATH
3201736001862

AMELIA
APALIT
LIQUE
03/30/1938
78
F
PI
546-02-5962
MARRIED
02/09/2017
0910
BACHELOR
FILIPINO
CLERK
CITY GOVERNMENT
35
2650 LOCKOUT CIRCLE
CHINO HILLS
SAN BERNARDINO
91709
1
CA
AMELITA SOLORZANO, DAUGHTER
ROY
E
LIQUE
DEMETRIO
APALIT
PI
FILOMENA
NEWMAN
PI
02/25/2017
ROSE HILLS MEMORIAL PARK
3888 WORKMAN MILL ROAD, WHITTIER, CA 90601
BU
GARY OJEDA
EMB0242
ROSE HILLS MORTUARY
FD970
MAXWELL OHIKHUARE, MD
02/21/2017
RESIDENCE - HOSPICE
SAN BERNARDINO
2650 LOOKOUT CIRCLE
CHINO HILLS
ALZHEIMER'S DEMENTIA
YRS
STROKE
NO
TIMOTHY J DAUWALDER D.O.
20A7875
02/16/2017
01/16/2017
02/07/2017
TIMOTHY J DAUWALDER D.O.
150 W 1ST STREET #270, CLAREMONT, CA 91711

CERTIFIED COPY OF VITAL RECORD
STATE OF CALIFORNIA, COUNTY OF SAN BERNARDINO

This is a true and exact reproduction of the document officially registered and placed on file in the Vital Records Section, San Bernardino Department of Public Health.

DATE ISSUED MAR 0 2 2017

002539544

This copy is not valid unless prepared on an engraved border, displaying the date, seal and signature of the Registrar.

The Lord's Prayer

The Lord's Prayer

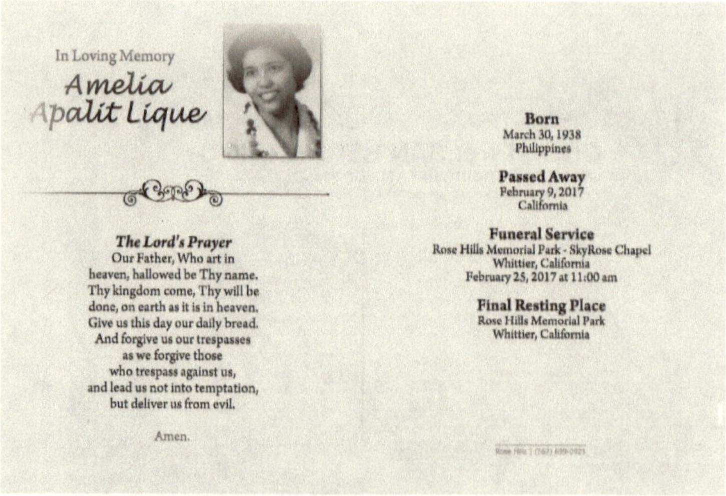

In Loving Memory

Amelia Apalit Lique

The Lord's Prayer

Our Father, Who art in heaven, hallowed be Thy name. Thy kingdom come, Thy will be done, on earth as it is in heaven. Give us this day our daily bread. And forgive us our trespasses as we forgive those who trespass against us, and lead us not into temptation, but deliver us from evil.

Amen.

Born
March 30, 1938
Philippines

Passed Away
February 9, 2017
California

Funeral Service
Rose Hills Memorial Park - SkyRose Chapel
Whittier, California
February 25, 2017 at 11:00 am

Final Resting Place
Rose Hills Memorial Park
Whittier, California

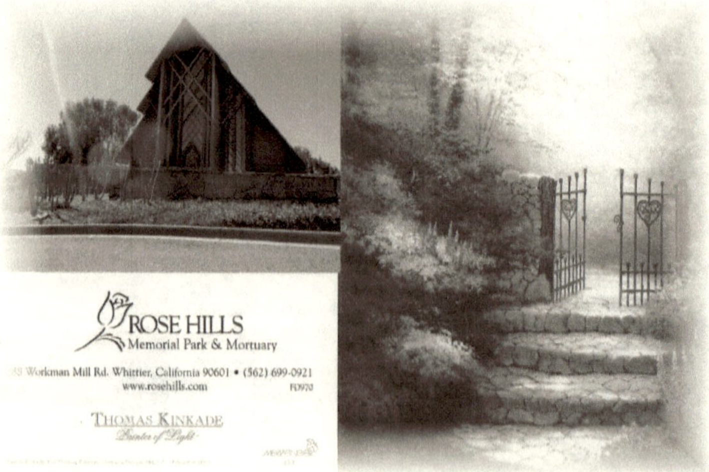

Heaven's Back Yard by Sherrie Bradley Neal

Heaven's Back Yard by Sherrie Bradley Neal

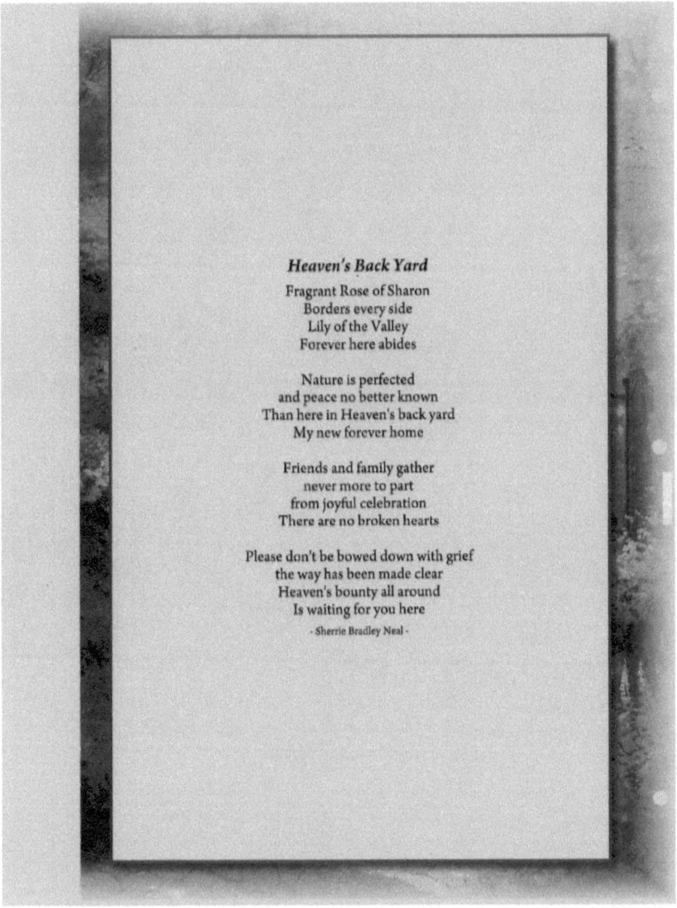
Heaven's Back Yard
Fragrant Rose of Sharon
Borders every side
Lily of the Valley
Forever here abides
Nature is perfected
and peace no better known
Than here in Heaven's back yard
My new forever home
Friends and family gather
never more to part
from joyful celebration
There are no broken hearts
Please don't be bowed down with grief
the way has been made clear
Heaven's bounty all around
Is waiting for you here
- Sherrie Bradley Neal -

The Garden of Prayer by Sherrie Bradley Neal

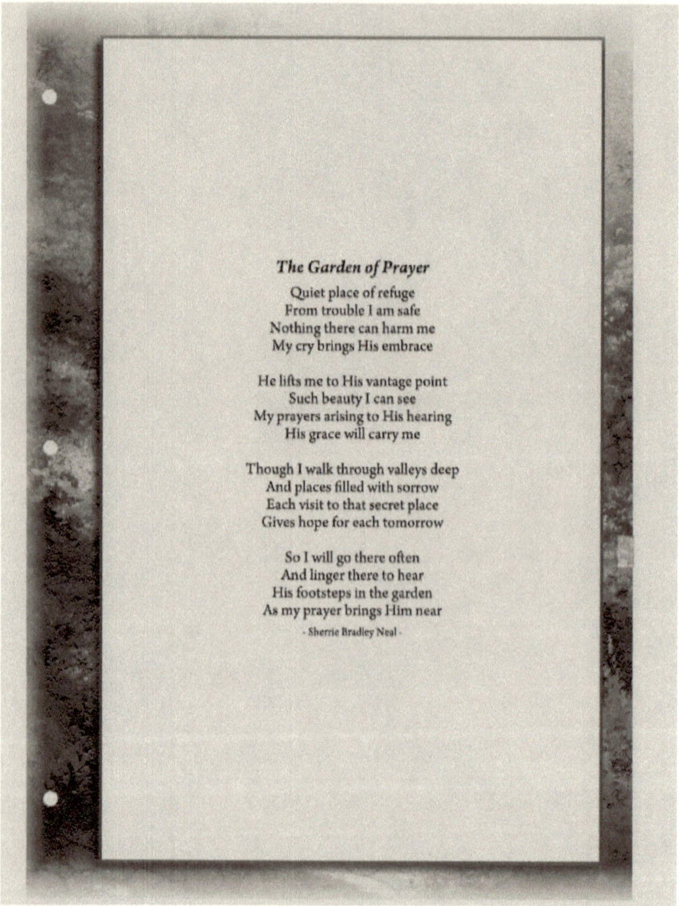

The Garden of Prayer

Quiet place of refuge
From trouble I am safe
Nothing there can harm me
My cry brings His embrace

He lifts me to His vantage point
Such beauty I can see
My prayers arising to His hearing
His grace will carry me

Though I walk through valleys deep
And places filled with sorrow
Each visit to that secret place
Gives hope for each tomorrow

So I will go there often
And linger there to hear
His footsteps in the garden
As my prayer brings Him near

- Sherrie Bradley Neal -

Creation's Song by Sherrie Bradley Neal

Creation's Song by Sherrie Bradley Neal

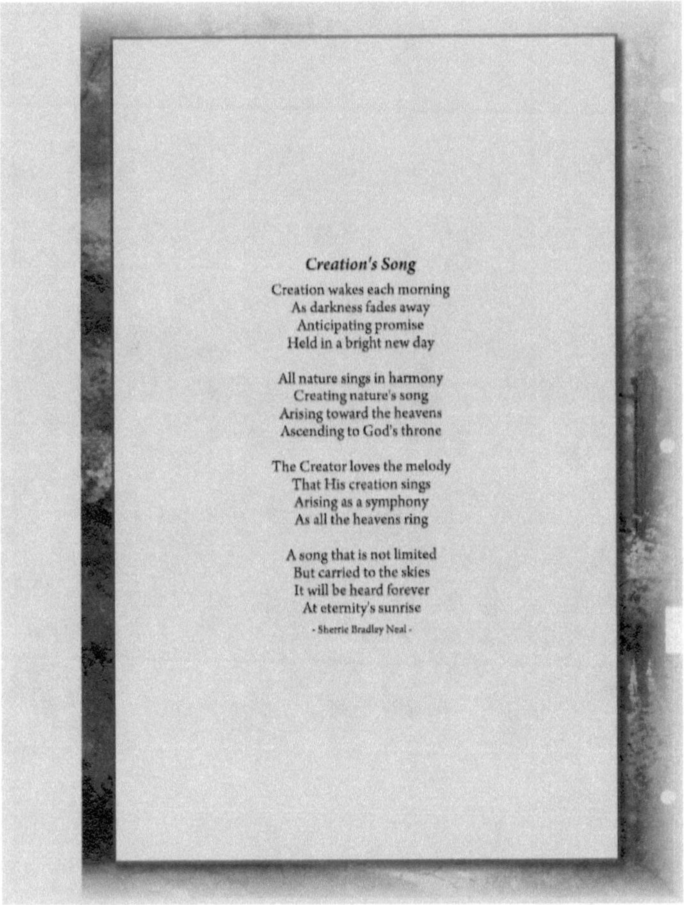
Creation's Song
Creation wakes each morning
As darkness fades away
Anticipating promise
Held in a bright new day
All nature sings in harmony
Creating nature's song
Arising toward the heavens
Ascending to God's throne
The Creator loves the melody
That His creation sings
Arising as a symphony
As all the heavens ring
A song that is not limited
But carried to the skies
It will be heard forever
At eternity's sunrise
- Sherrie Bradley Neal -

The Visitation

The Visitation

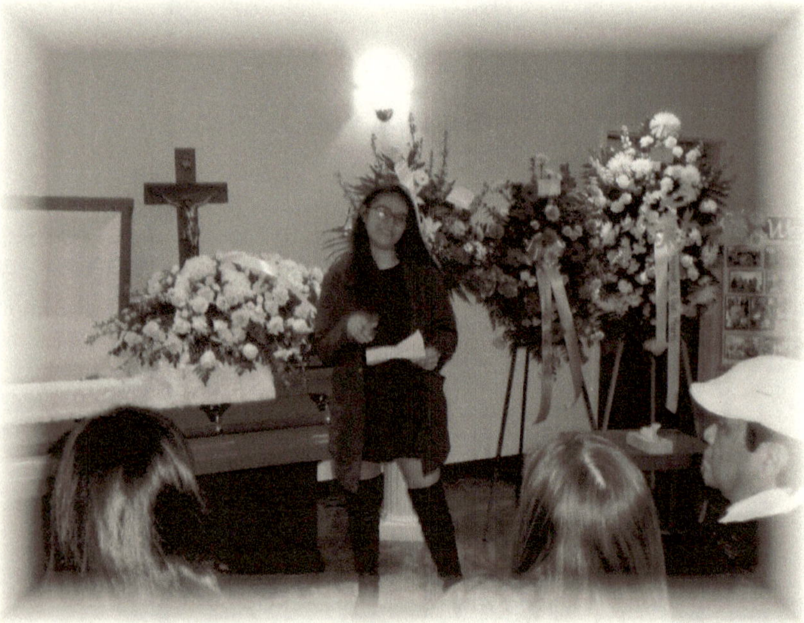

The Visitation

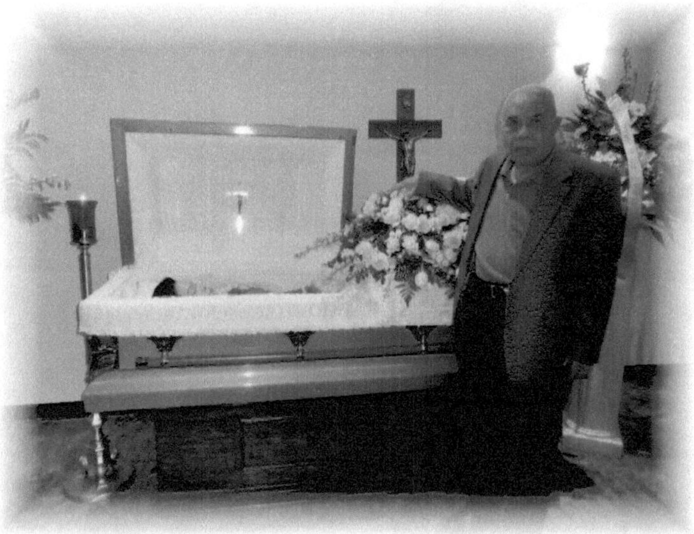

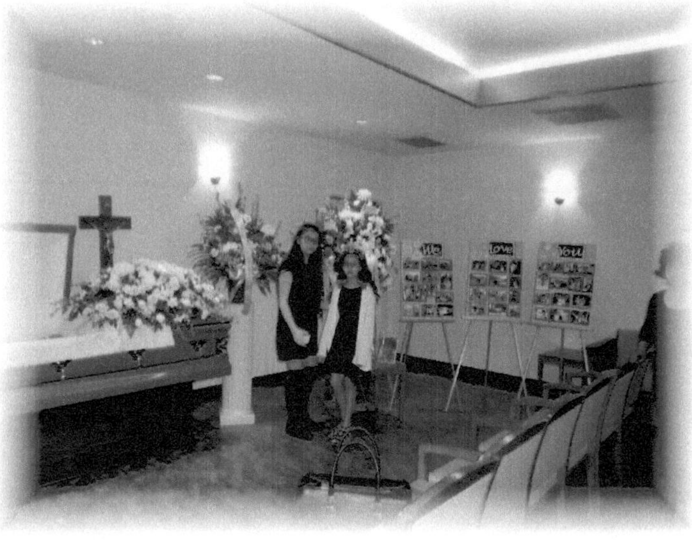

The Visitation

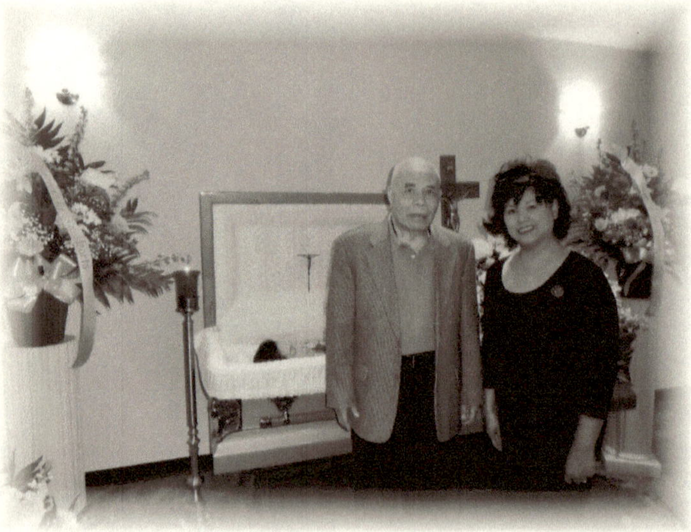

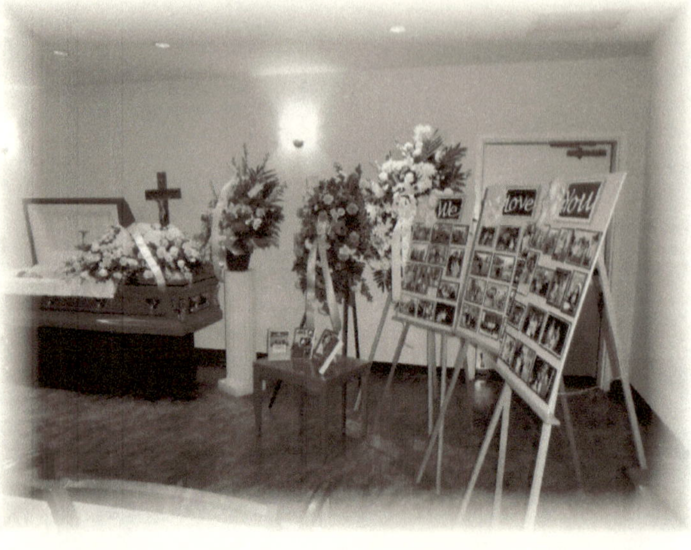

The Visitation

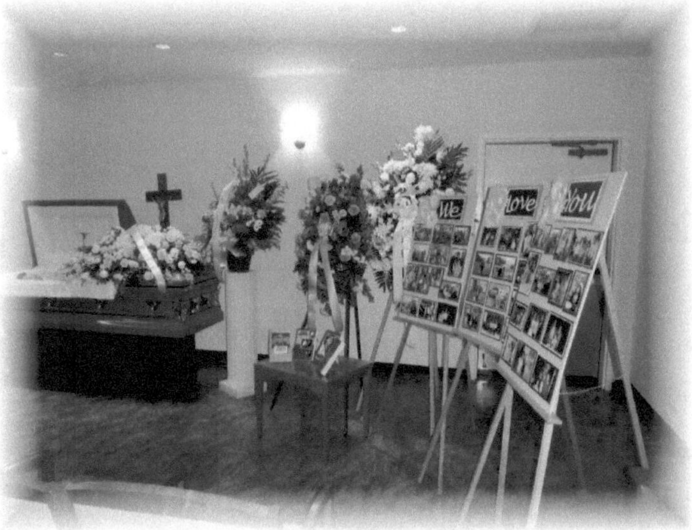

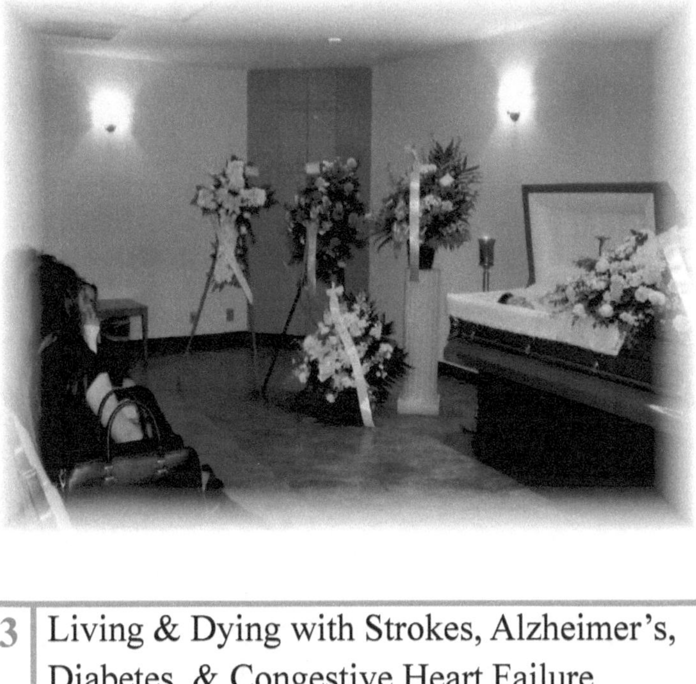

The Visitation

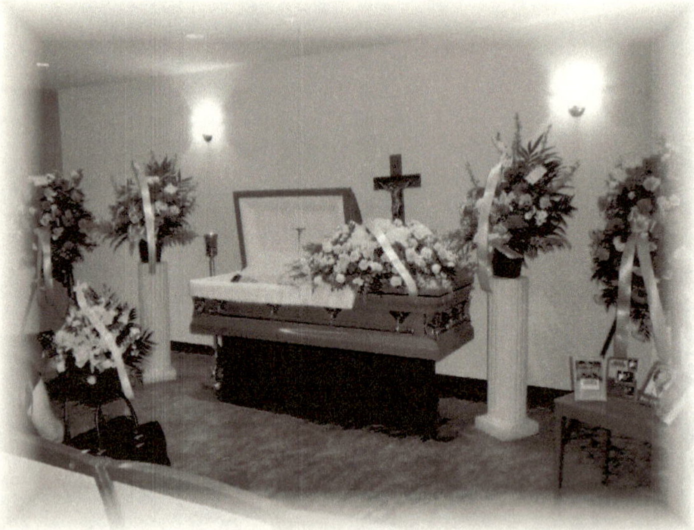

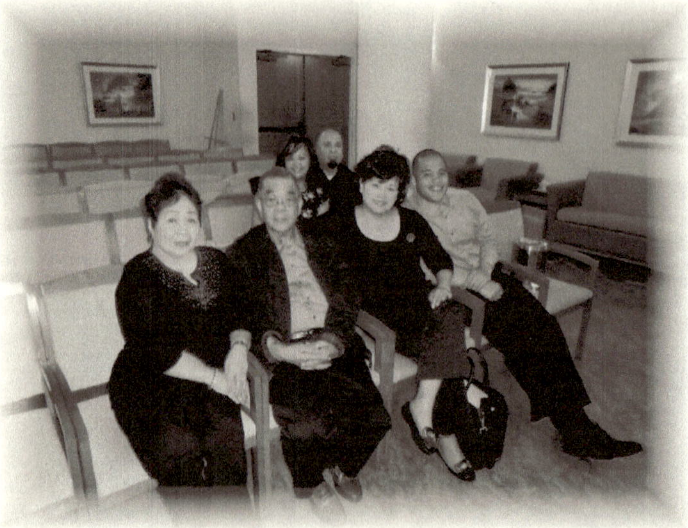

The Visitation

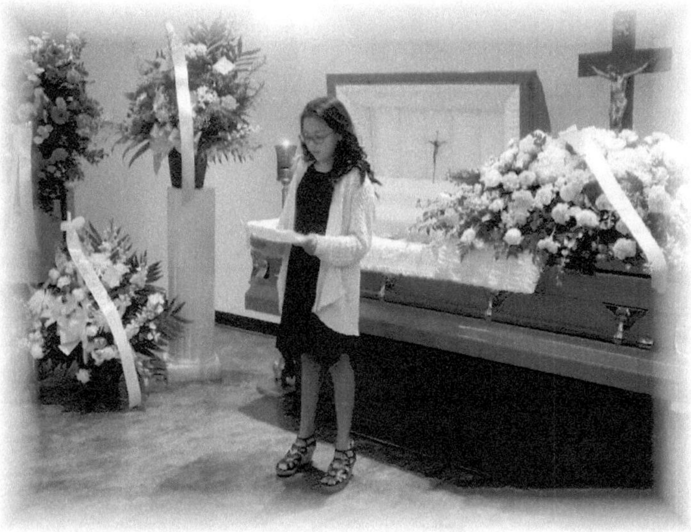

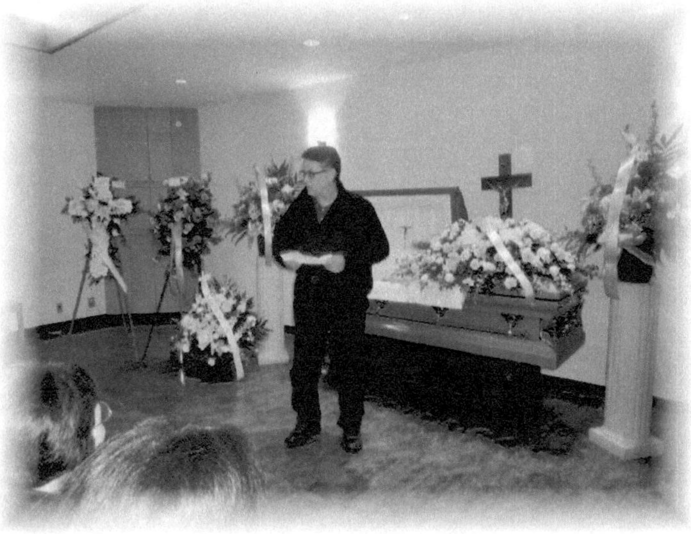

Relatives and Friends of Amelia Apalit Lique

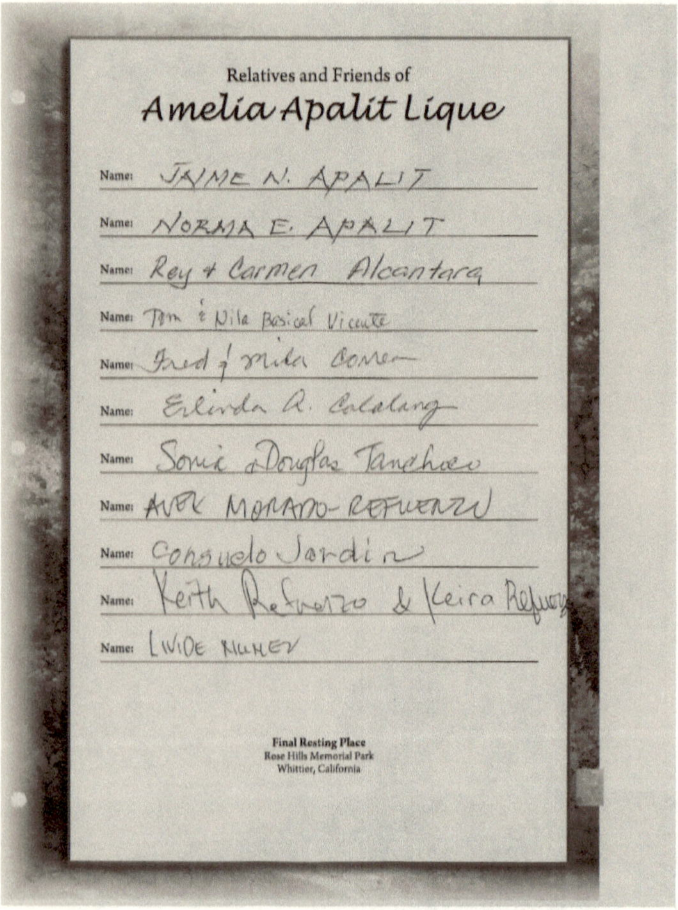

Relatives and Friends of

Amelia Apalit Lique

Name: JAIME N. APALIT

Name: NORMA E. APALIT

Name: Rey + Carmen Alcantara

Name: Tom & Nila Basical Vicente

Name: Fred & Mila Cerrer

Name: Erlinda R. Calalang

Name: Sonie & Douglas Tanchoco

Name: AVEL MORADO-REFUERZO

Name: Consuelo Jardin

Name: Keith Refuerzo & Keira Refuerzo

Name: LWIDE NUNEZ

Final Resting Place
Rose Hills Memorial Park
Whittier, California

Relatives and Friends of Amelia Apalit Lique

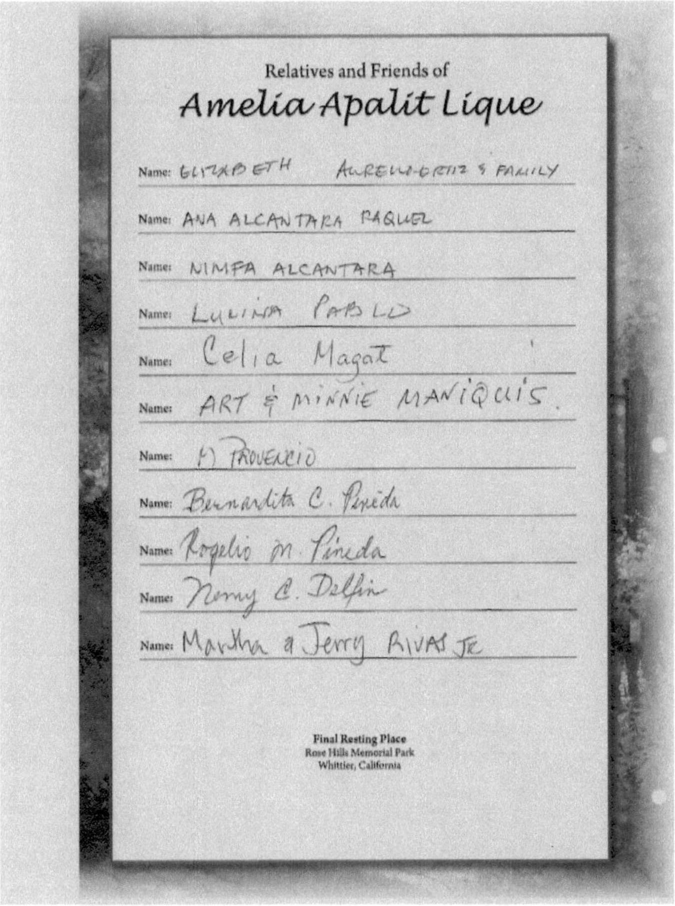

Relatives and Friends of

Amelia Apalit Lique

Name: ELIZABETH AURELIO-ORTIZ & FAMILY

Name: ANA ALCANTARA RAQUEL

Name: NIMFA ALCANTARA

Name: LULINA PABLO

Name: Celia Magat

Name: ART & MINNIE MANIQUIS.

Name: M PROVENCIO

Name: Bernardita C. Pineda

Name: Rogelio M. Pineda

Name: Nerry C. Delfin

Name: Martha & Jerry RIVAS JR

Final Resting Place
Rose Hills Memorial Park
Whittier, California

Relatives and Friends of Amelia Apalit Lique

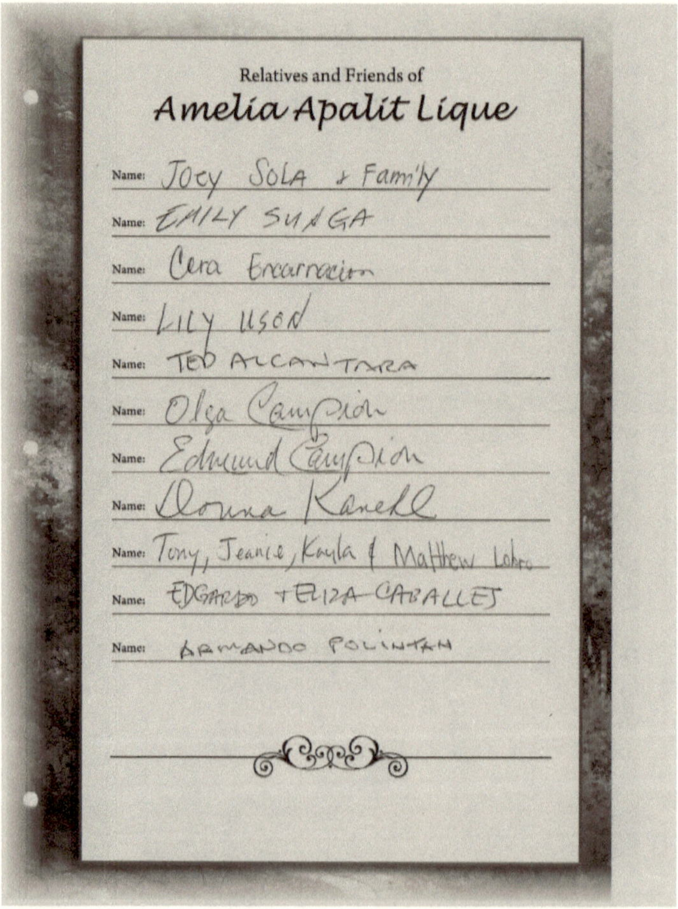

Relatives and Friends of

Amelia Apalit Lique

Name: Joey Sola & Family

Name: EMILY SUNGA

Name: Cera Encarnacion

Name: LILY USON

Name: TED ALCANTARA

Name: Olga Campion

Name: Edmund Campion

Name: Donna Karell

Name: Tony, Jeanie, Kayla & Matthew Lohr

Name: EDGARDO + ELIZA CABALLES

Name: ARMANDO POLINTAN

Relatives and Friends of Amelia Apalit Lique

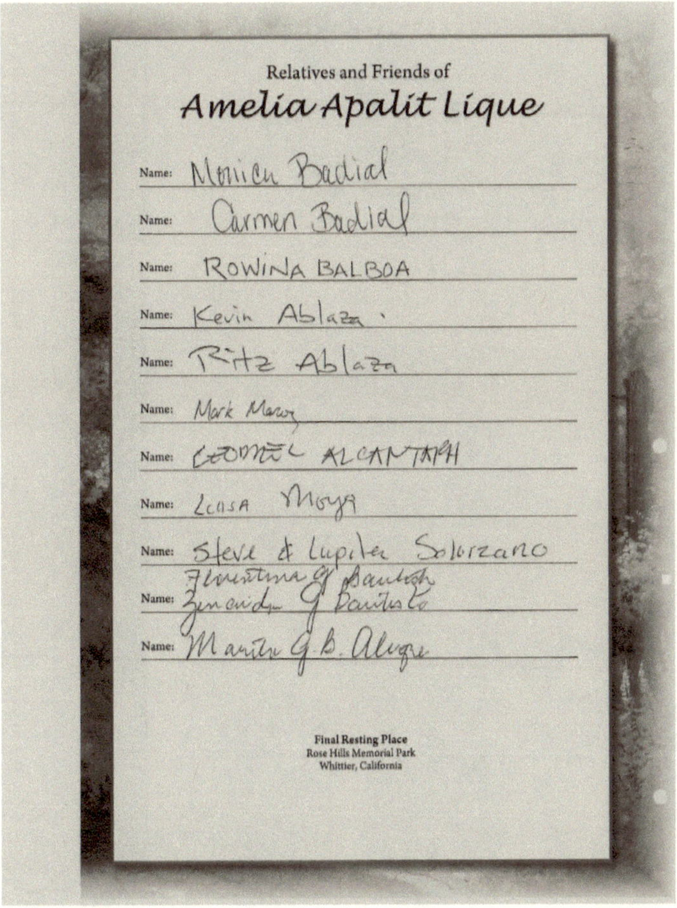

Relatives and Friends of

Amelia Apalit Lique

Name: Monica Badial

Name: Carmen Badial

Name: ROWINA BALBOA

Name: Kevin Ablaza

Name: Ritz Ablaza

Name: Mark Maru

Name: GODMEL ALCANTARA

Name: Luisa Moya

Name: Steve & Lupita Solorzano

Name: Florentina G Bautista Zenaida G Bautista

Name: Marita G.B. Alegre

Final Resting Place
Rose Hills Memorial Park
Whittier, California

Relatives and Friends of Amelia Apalit Lique

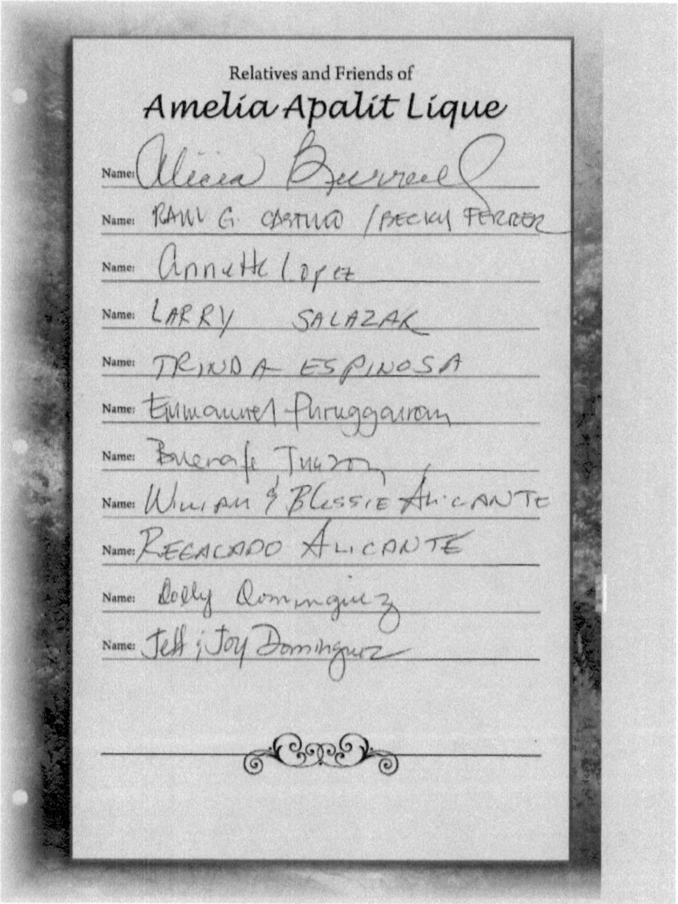
Relatives and Friends of

Amelia Apalit Lique

Name: Alicia Burrell

Name: RAMIL G. CASTILLO / BECKY FERRER

Name: Annette Lopez

Name: LARRY SALAZAR

Name: TRINIDA ESPINOSA

Name: Emmanuel Piruggaron

Name: Buenafe Tuazon

Name: William & Blessie ALICANTE

Name: REGALADO ALICANTE

Name: Dolly Dominguez

Name: Jeff & Joy Dominguez

Relatives and Friends of Amelia Apalit Lique

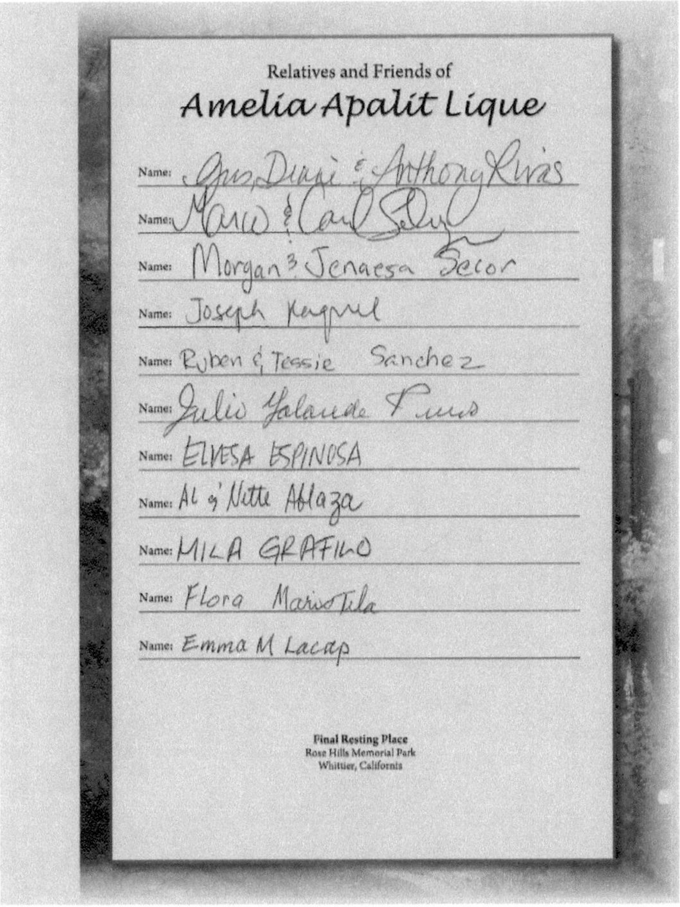

Relatives and Friends of

Amelia Apalit Lique

Name: [illegible] & Anthony Rivas

Name: [illegible]

Name: Morgan & Jenaesa Secor

Name: Joseph [illegible]

Name: Ruben & Tessie Sanchez

Name: Julio Yolanda [illegible]

Name: ELVESA ESPINOSA

Name: Al & Nitte Ablaza

Name: MILA GRAFILO

Name: Flora [illegible]

Name: Emma M Lacap

Final Resting Place
Rose Hills Memorial Park
Whittier, California

Relatives and Friends of Amelia Apalit Lique

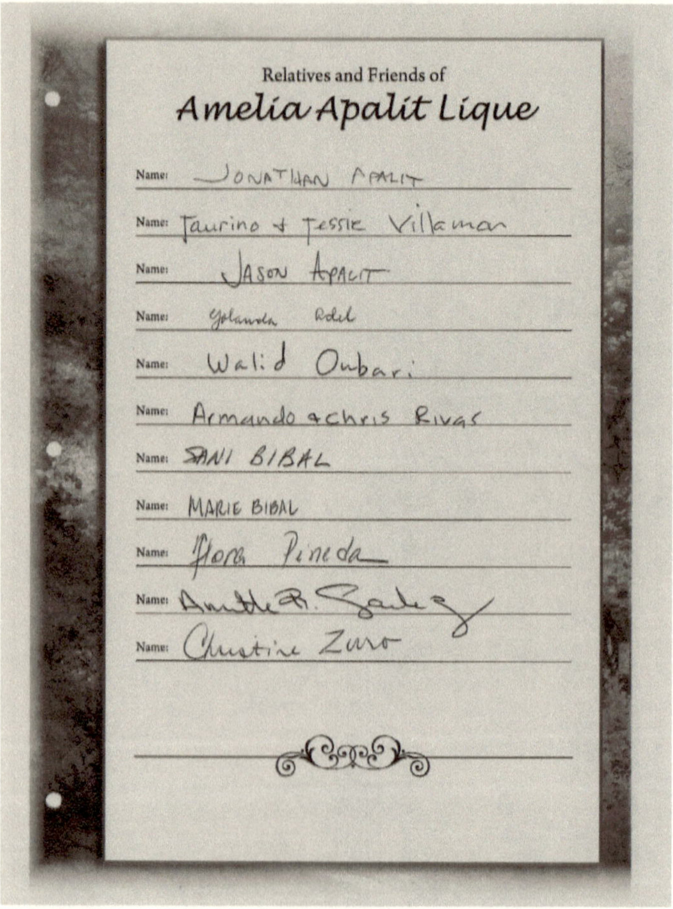
Relatives and Friends of
Amelia Apalit Lique

Name: JONATHAN APALIT
Name: Taurino + Tessie Villaman
Name: JASON APALIT
Name: Yolanda Rodel
Name: Walid Oubari
Name: Armando & Chris Rivas
Name: SANI BIBAL
Name: MARIE BIBAL
Name: Flora Pineda
Name: [illegible]
Name: Christine Zuro

Relatives and Friends of Amelia Apalit Lique

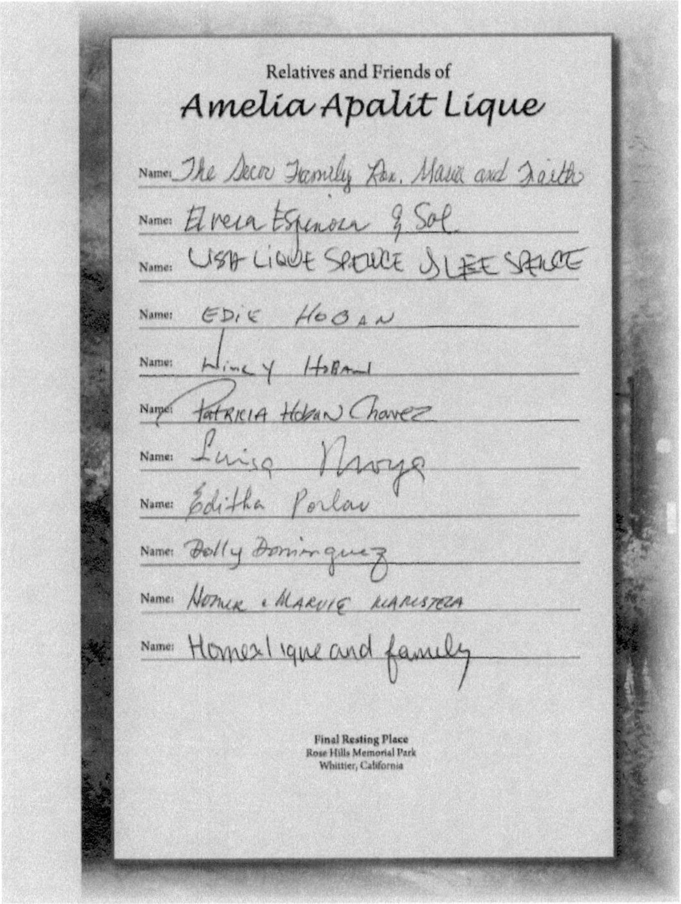

Relatives and Friends of

Amelia Apalit Lique

Name: The Secor Family Ron, Maria and Faith
Name: Elvera Espinoza & Sol
Name: LISA LIQUE SPENCE & LEE SPENCE
Name: EDIE HOGAN
Name: WINCY HOBAN
Name: PATRICIA HOGAN Chavez
Name: Luisa Noya
Name: Editha Porlar
Name: Dolly Dominguez
Name: HOMER & MARVIE MARISTELA
Name: Homer Lique and family

Final Resting Place
Rose Hills Memorial Park
Whittier, California

Relatives and Friends of Amelia Apalit Lique

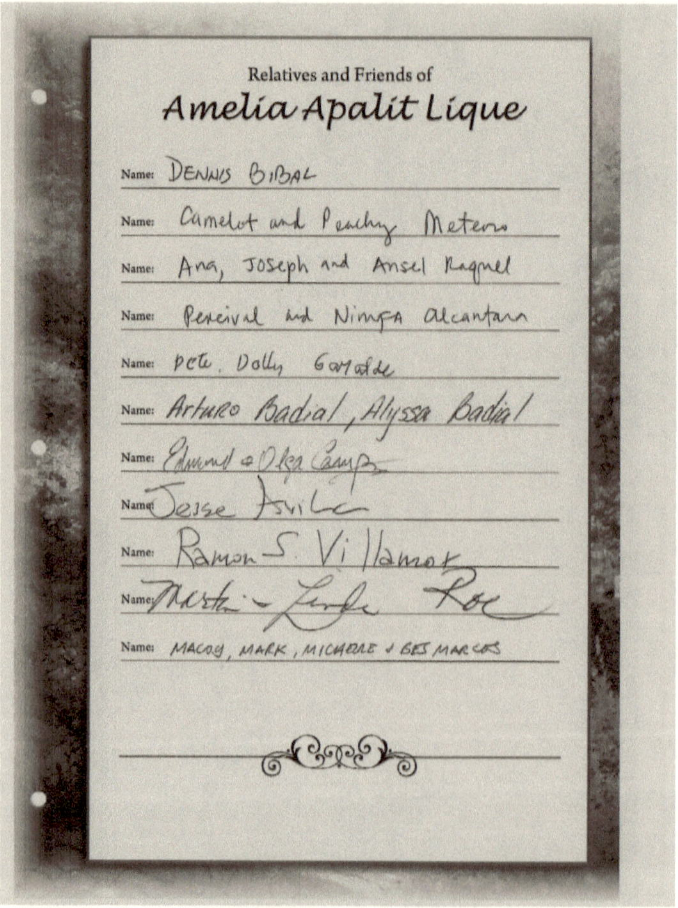

Relatives and Friends of

Amelia Apalit Lique

Name: DENNIS BIBAL

Name: Camelot and Peachy Metero

Name: Ana, Joseph and Ansel Raquel

Name: Percival and Nimfa Alcantara

Name: Pete, Dolly [illegible]

Name: Arturo Badial, Alyssa Badial

Name: Edmund & Olga Campos

Name: Jesse Avila

Name: Ramon S. Villamor

Name: [illegible]

Name: MACOY, MARK, MICHELLE + BES MARCOS

Relatives and Friends of Amelia Apalit Lique

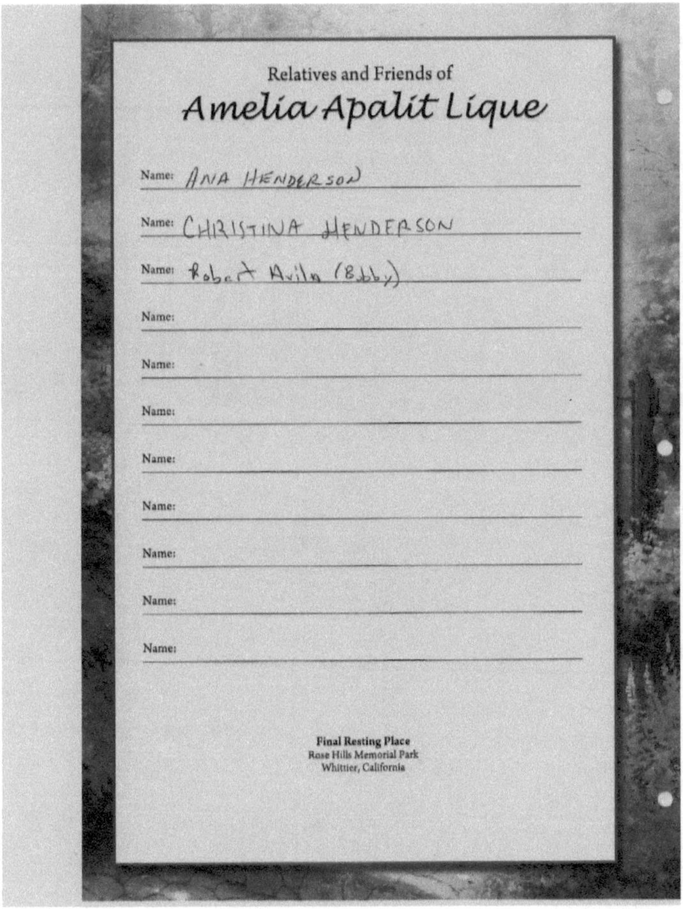

Relatives and Friends of

Amelia Apalit Lique

Name: ANA HENDERSON

Name: CHRISTINA HENDERSON

Name: Robert Avila (Bobby)

Name:

Name:

Name:

Name:

Name:

Name:

Name:

Name:

Final Resting Place
Rose Hills Memorial Park
Whittier, California

Relatives and Friends of Amelia Apalit Lique

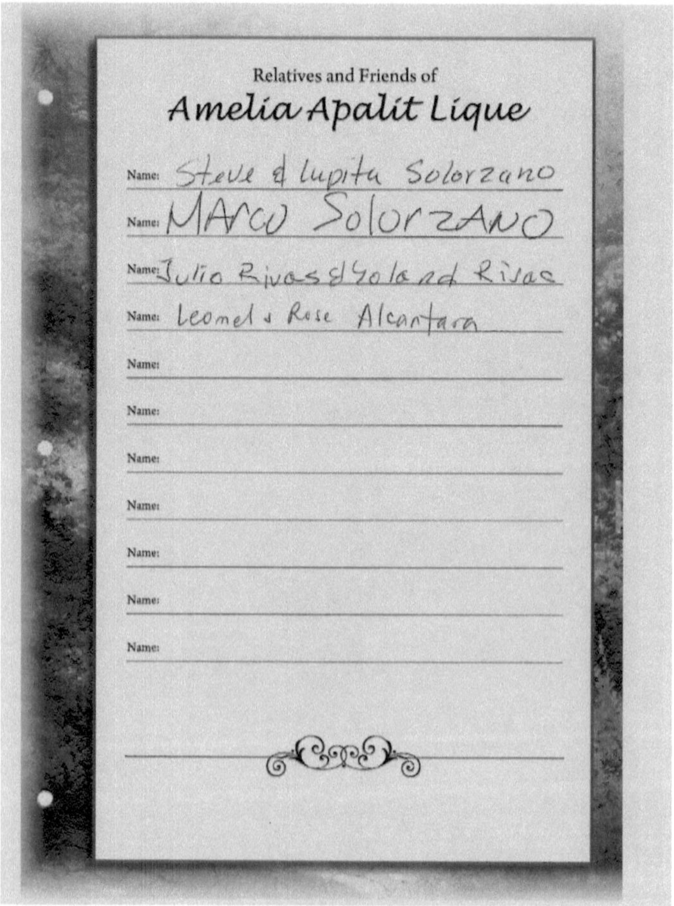

Relatives and Friends of

Amelia Apalit Lique

Name: Steve & Lupita Solorzano

Name: MARCO SOLORZANO

Name: Julio Rivas & Yoland Rivas

Name: Leonel & Rose Alcantara

Name:

Name:

Name:

Name:

Name:

Name:

Name:

Donors List

Donors List

lbert Ablaza 217 Porto Grande Drive iamond Bar, CA 91765	Albert Tolentino 18701 Greenbay Drive Rowland Heights, CA 91748	Armando Polintan 257 E Bort Street Long Beach, CA 90805
rt and Minnie Maniquis 404 Aline Street est Covina, CA 91792	Benjamin and Lolita Caceres 4111 Folsom Street San Francisco, CA 94110-6119	Camelot and Peachy Meteoro 2478 E. Mountain Street Pasadena, CA 91104
elia Magat 845 Earle Avenue osemead, CA 91770	Consuelo Jardin 419 N Mountain View Ave., Apt 207 Los Angeles, CA 90026	Doug and Sonia Tanchoco St. Elizabeth Church
d and Olga Campion 427 Millbury Avenue aldwin Park, CA 91706	Emma Lacap 9918 Via Monzon San Diego, CA 92129	Federico Cabatan and Family 27910 Agafantos Lane Valencia, CA 91350
lor and Pat Almoete 0 Eakins Cres Red Deer lbert, Canada T4R 2M9	Flor Maristela 114 Foxboro Avenue Chula Vista, CA 91911	Florentina Bautista 1629 Larkvane Road Rowland Heights, CA 91748
ancis and Tessie Villamor	Francis and Tessie St. Elizabeth Church	Homer and Marvelyn Maristela 695 E Naples Street Chula Vista, CA 91911-6838
ary Malig 2407 Griffin Lane ictorville, CA 9295	Leo and Rose Alcantara 542 N Walnut Avenue San Dimas, CA 91773	Lilia Espiloy
olita Bercasio 852 Hilo Street remont, CA 94538	Regalado Alicante/Ruben Sanchez P.O. Box 92935 City of Industry, CA 91715	Loreto Uson 4917 Townsend Avenue Los Angeles, CA 90041
ucina Pablo 536 New Avenue osemead, CA 91770	Luisa Moya 854 Pelancoini Ave. Glendale, CA 91202	Macoy/Bess/Mark/Michelle Marco 2655 Altamira Drive West Covina, CA 91792
aria Vivo 541 Welland Avenue emple City, CA 91780	Marlon Cabatan 28403 North Pinewood Court Santa Clarita, CA 91390	Mila Grafilo 4144 Van Buren Street Chino, CA 91710
orado/Refuerzo 19 N. Mountain View Ave Apt 103 os Angeles, CA 90026	Ningning 19522 Avenida del Campo Walnut, CA 91789	Nunez Family 2321 Highbury Avenue #51 Los Angeles, CA 90032
mmy Apalit 2900 Rio Lobos Diamond Bar, CA 91765	Percival and Nimfa Alcantara 3203 E Vermillion Street West Covina, CA 91792	Popoy Alda & Alen Cubacub 2187 Cimarron Way Addison, ILL 60101

Donors List

Raul Castillo
9110 Las Tunas Drive #D
Temple City, CA 91780

Ricardo and Elsie Letada
391 Guthries Green
Shackelfords, VA 91746

Seth and Endic Calalang
731 Judson Street
Los Angeles, CA 90033

Tom and Nila Vicente
656 Judson Street
Los Angeles, CA 90033

Reli Cayson
2638 27th Street Apt #2
Sacramento, CA 95818-2646

Roger and Bandit Pineda
13240 E Hoig Street
La Puente, CA 91746

Susa Family and Family
25517 Fitzgerald Avenue
Stevenson Ranch, CA 91381

Toto and Tessie Villamor
8400 Ranchito Avenue
Panorama City, CA 91402

Rey and Carmen Alcantara
480 Vista del Norte
Walnut, CA 91789

Rowena Balboa
9813 Hildreth Avenue
South Gate, CA 90280

Ted Alcantara
3028 Bellevue Avenue
Los Angeles, CA 90026

Vida Alfonso
921 S Trident Street Apt #5
Anaheim, CA 92804

The Funeral Service

The Funeral Service

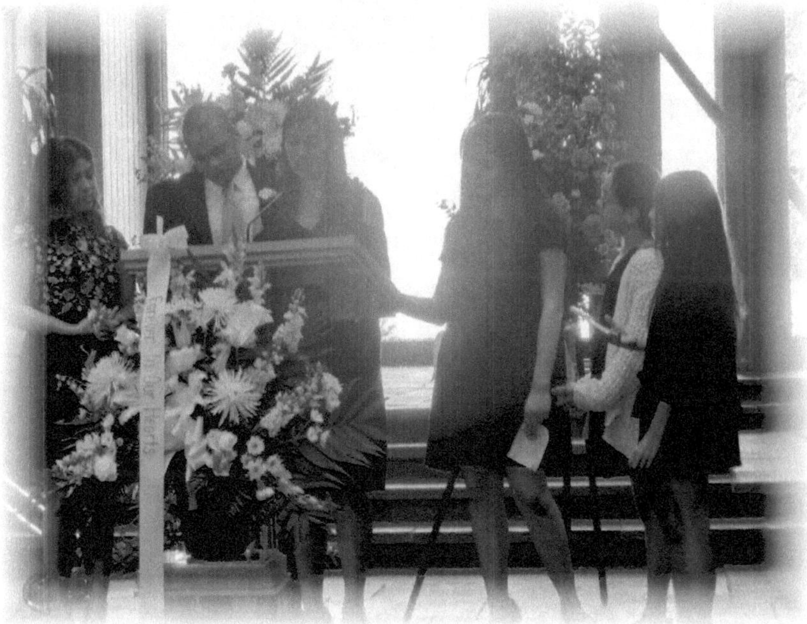

The Funeral Service

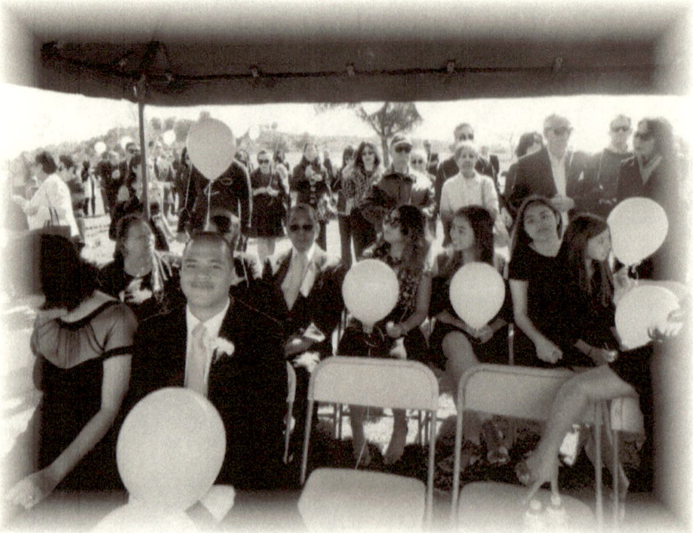

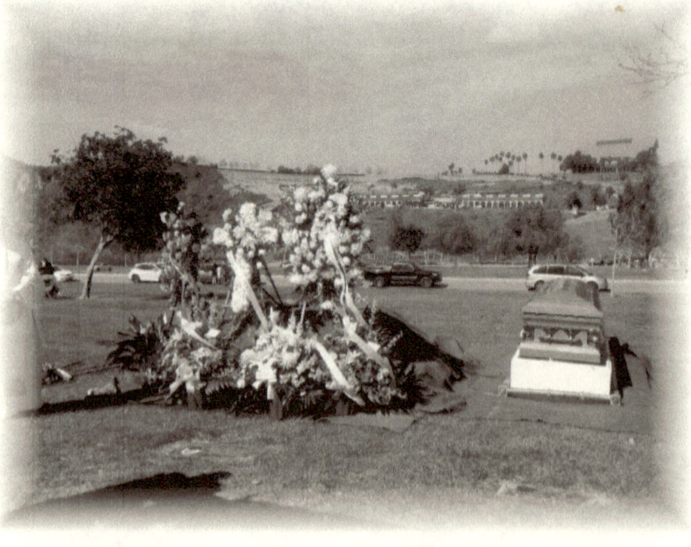

The Funeral Service

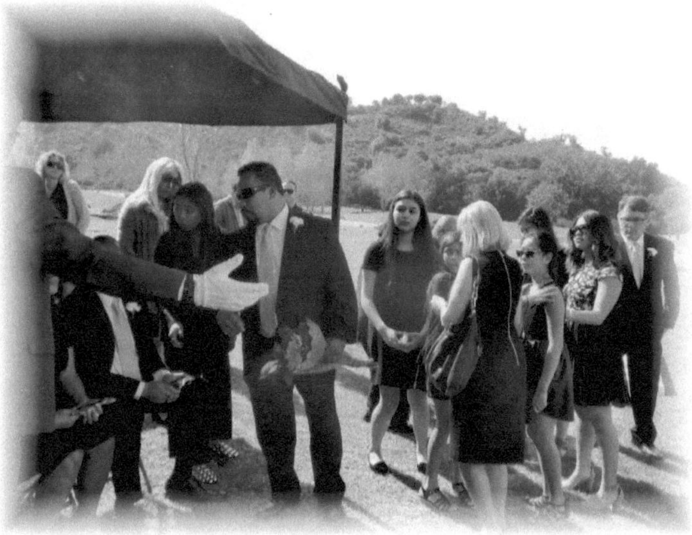

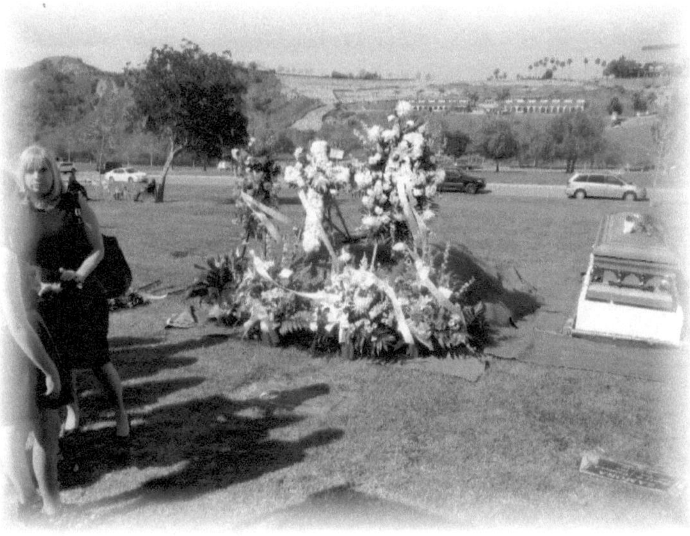

The Funeral Service

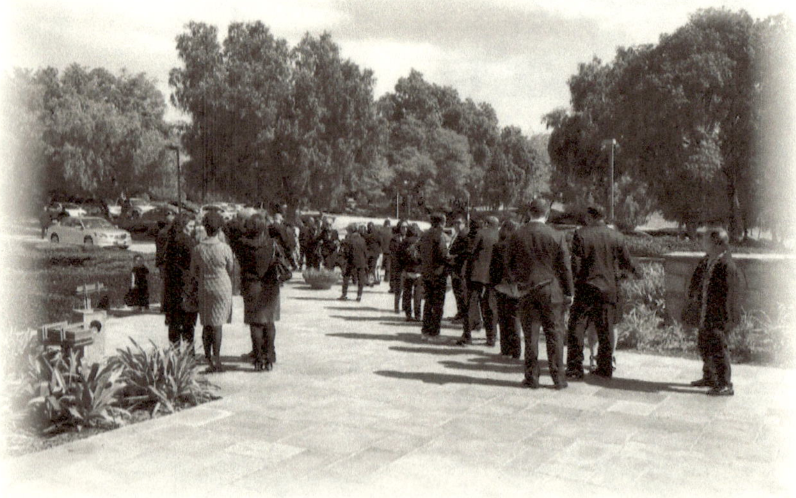

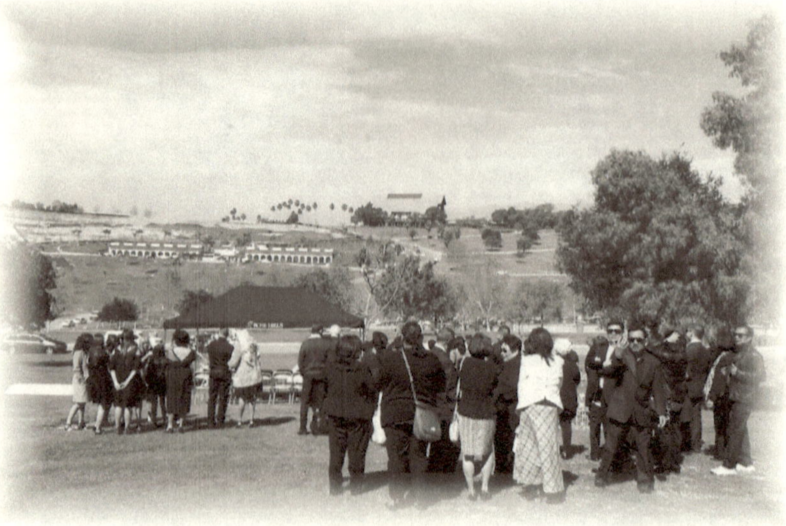

The Funeral Service

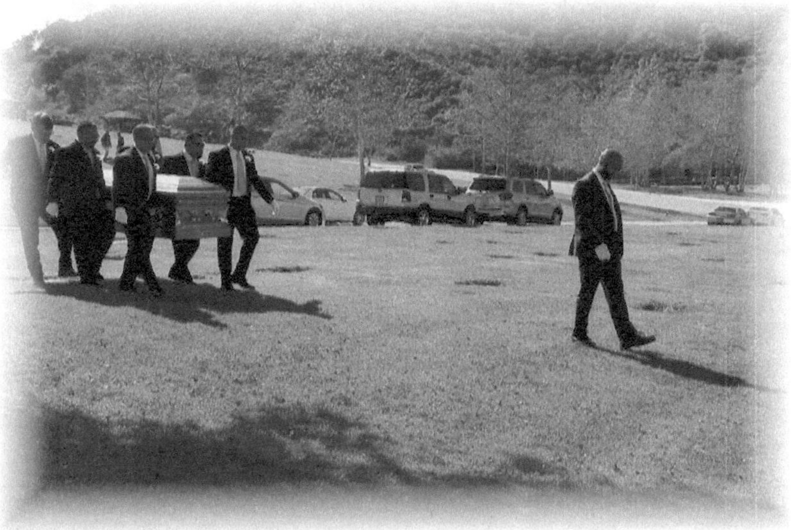

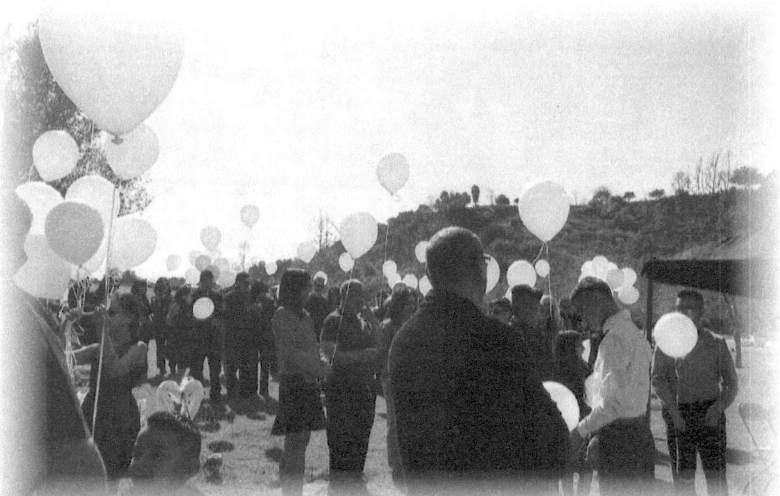

The Funeral Service

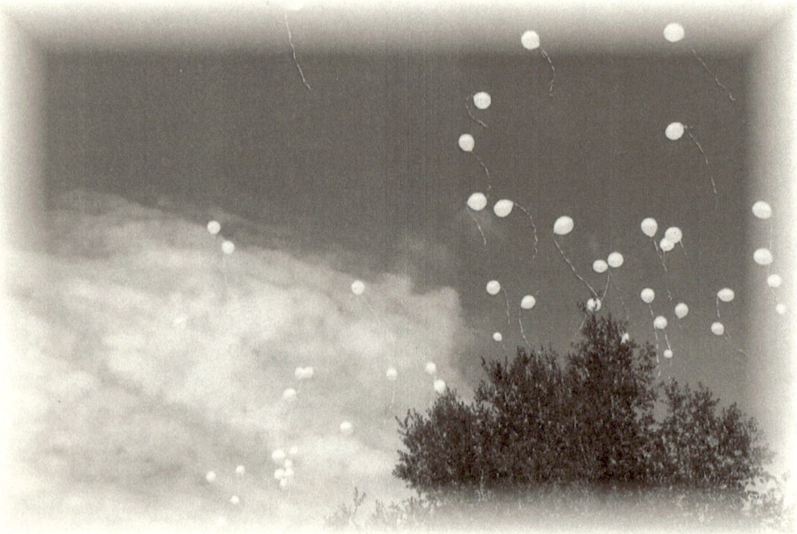

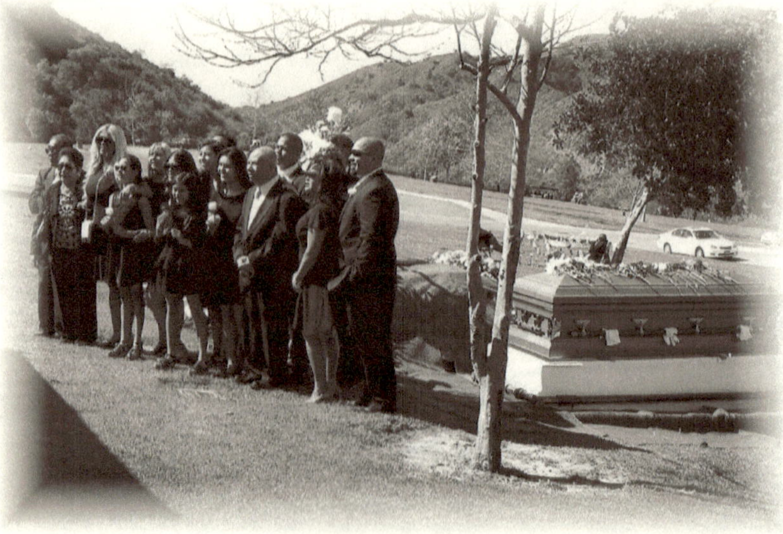

The Reception

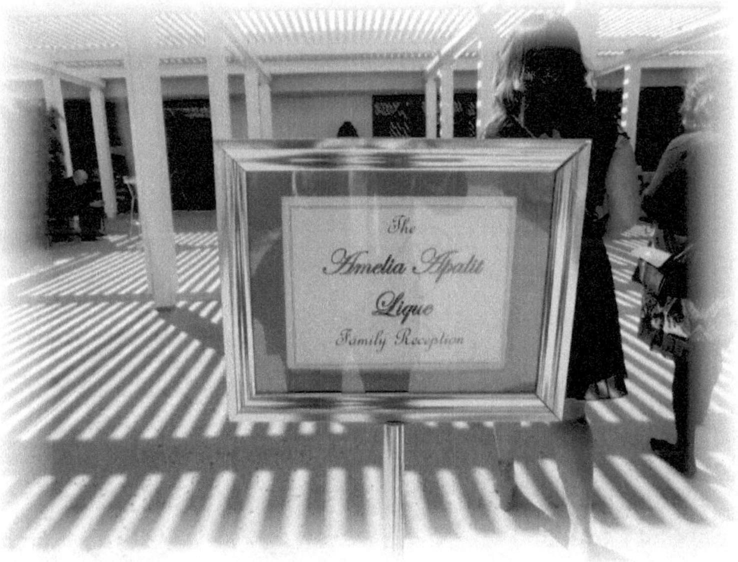

The Reception

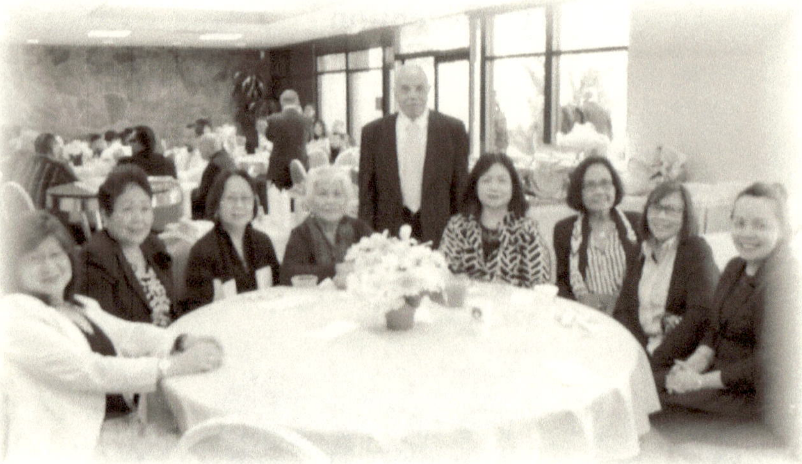

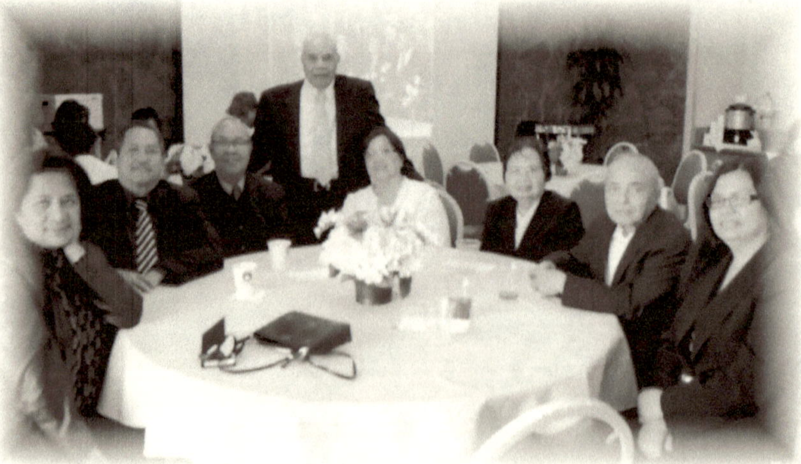

The Reception

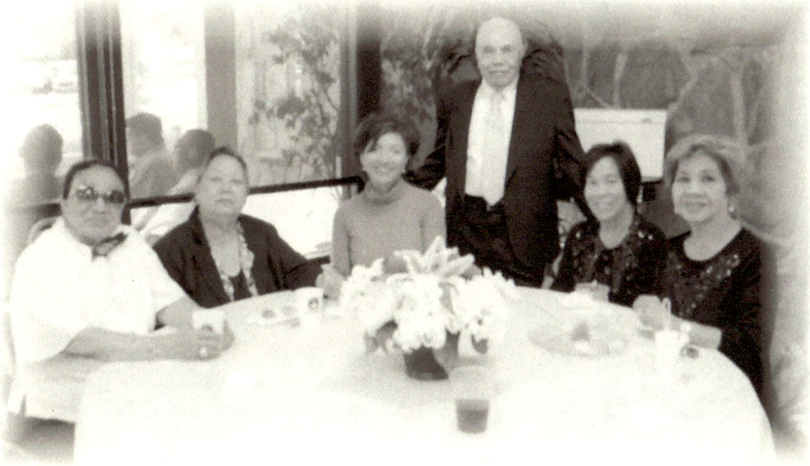

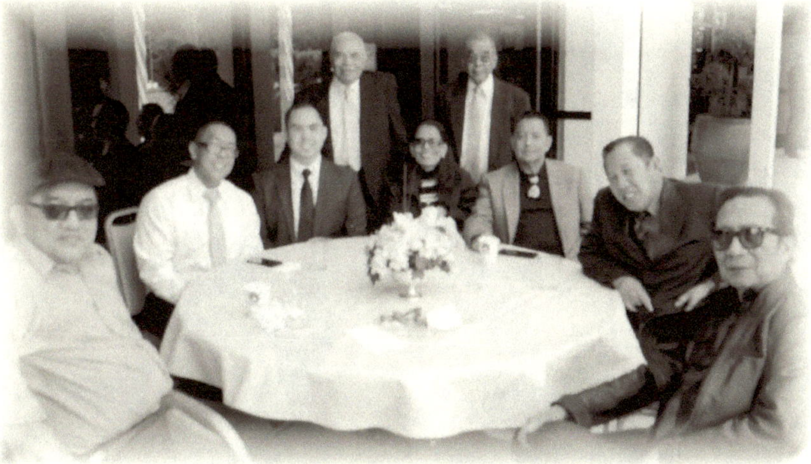

The Reception

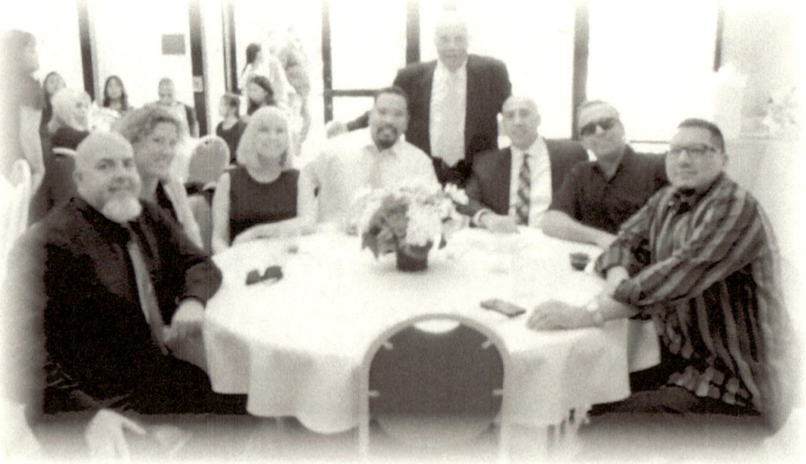

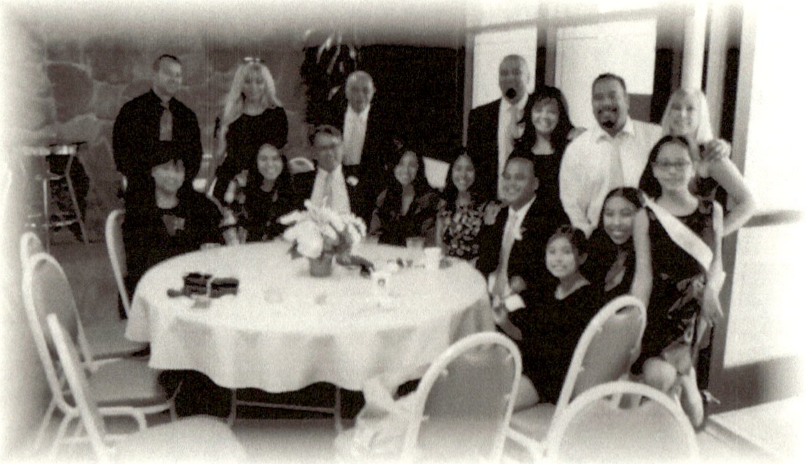

The Reception

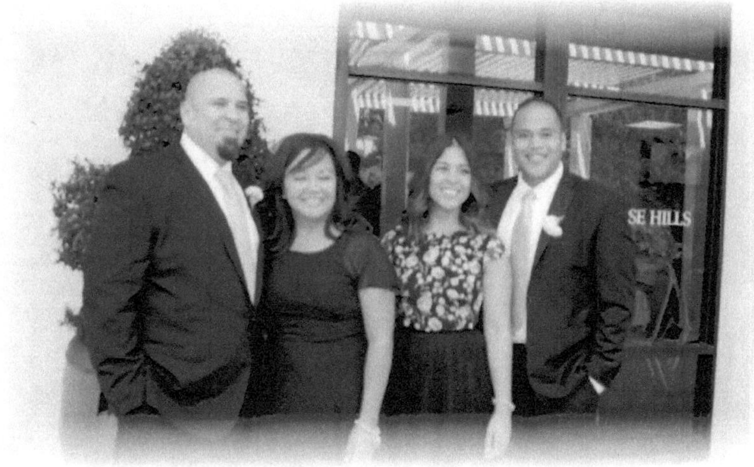

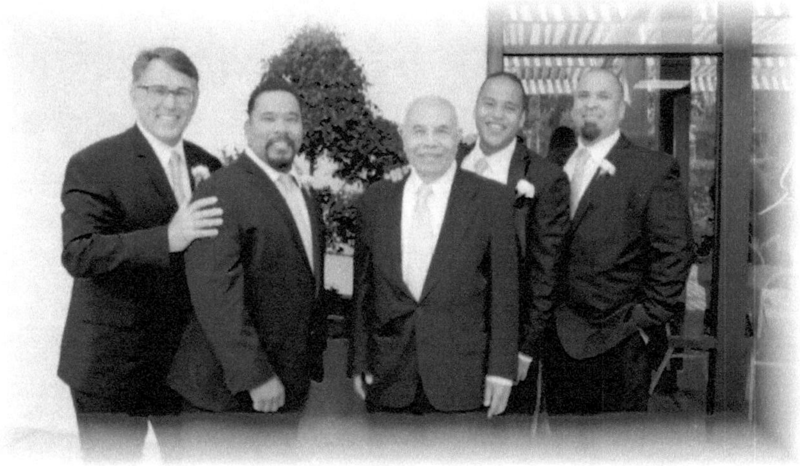

The Reception

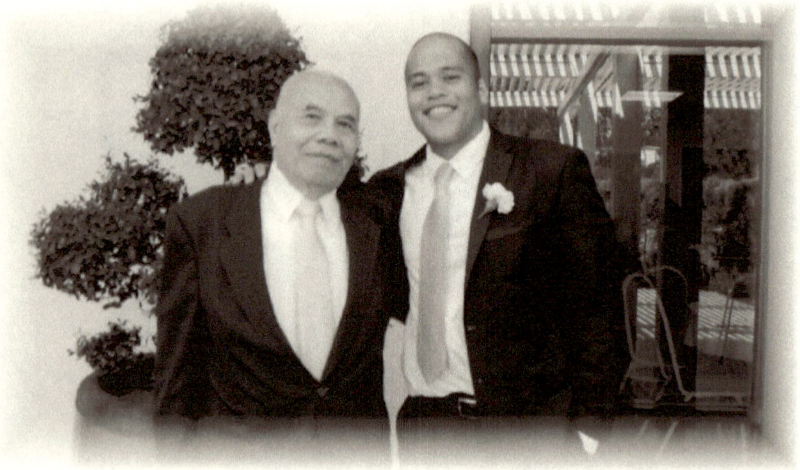

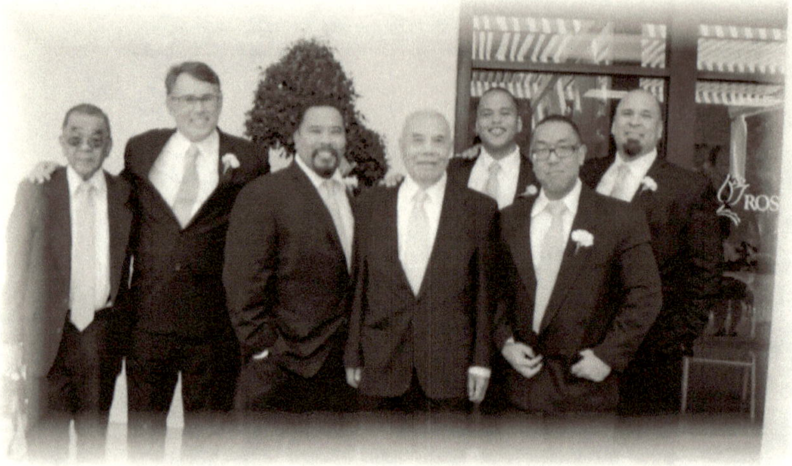

The Reception

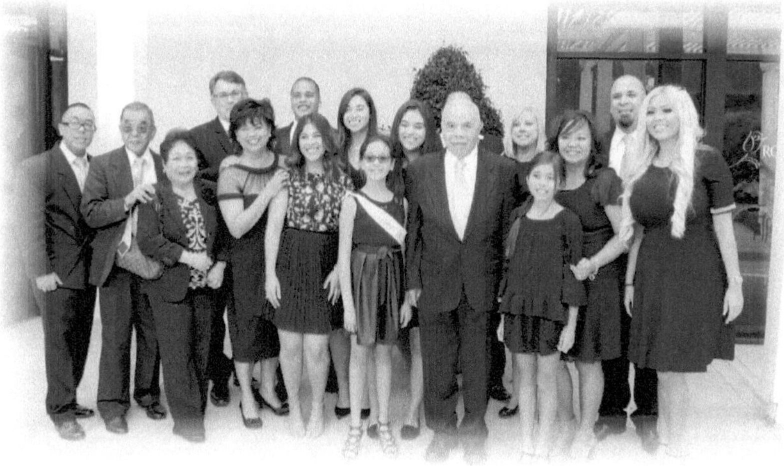

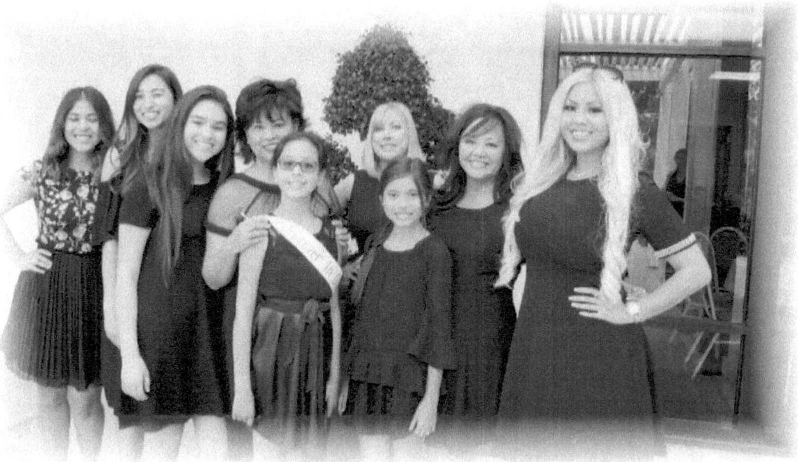

The Reception

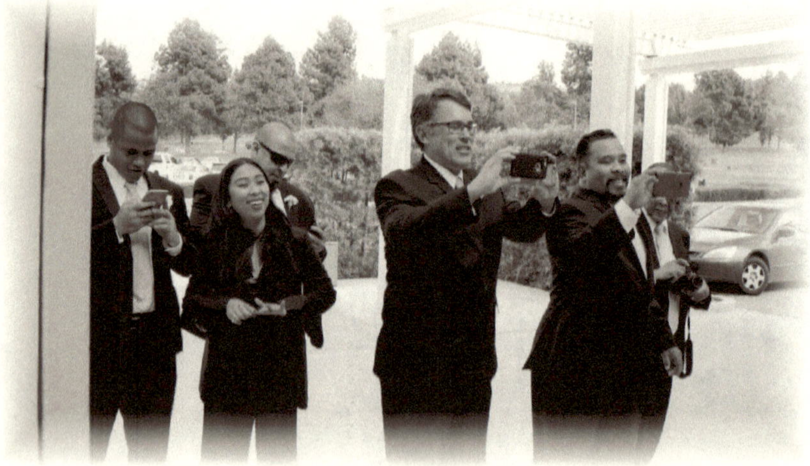

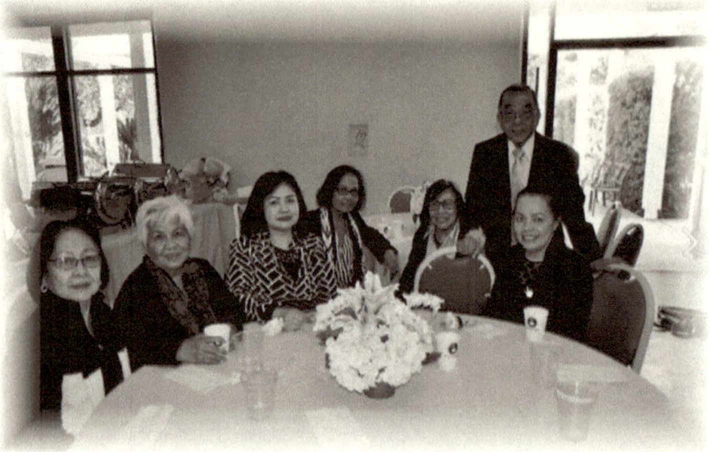

The Reception

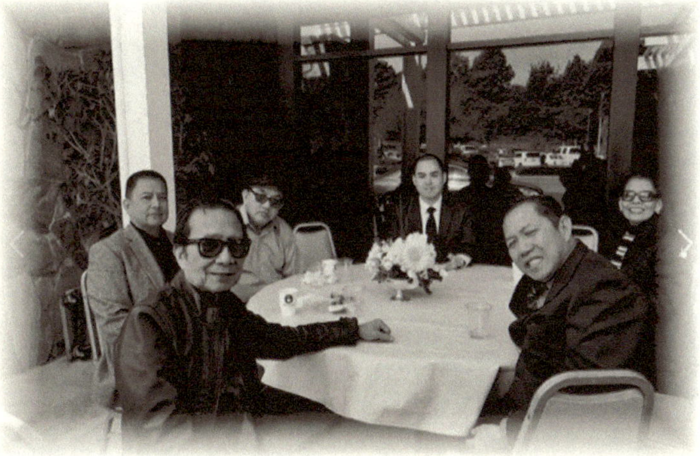

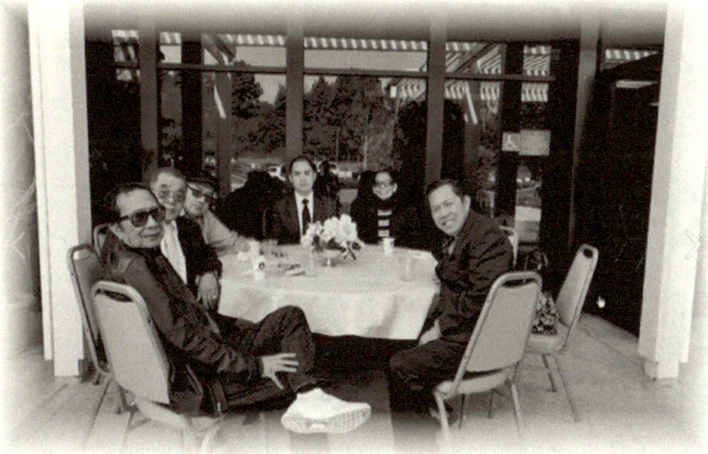

The Reception

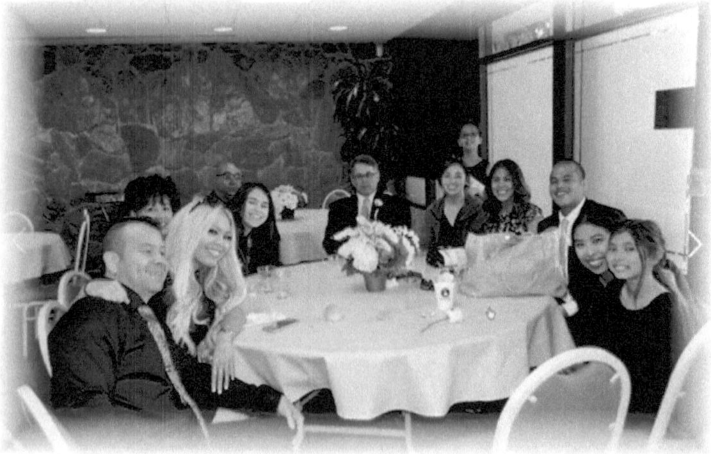

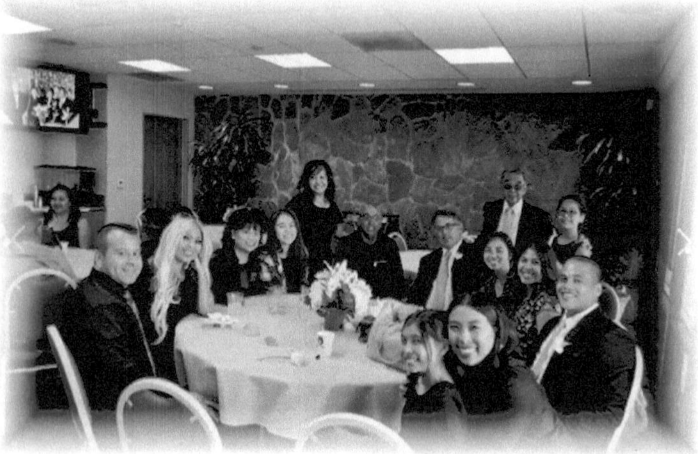

The Reception

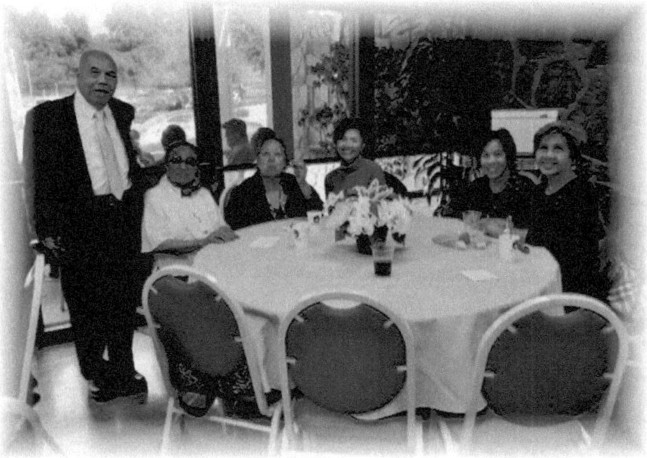

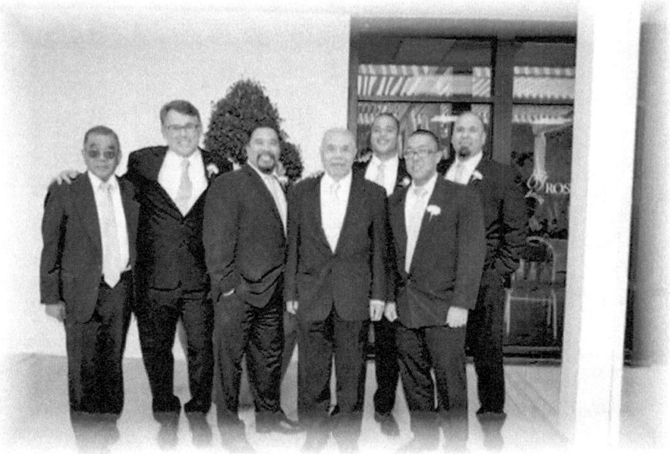

The Reception

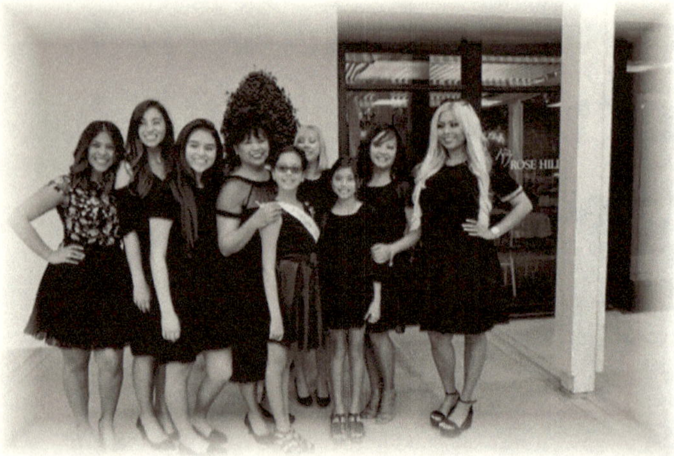

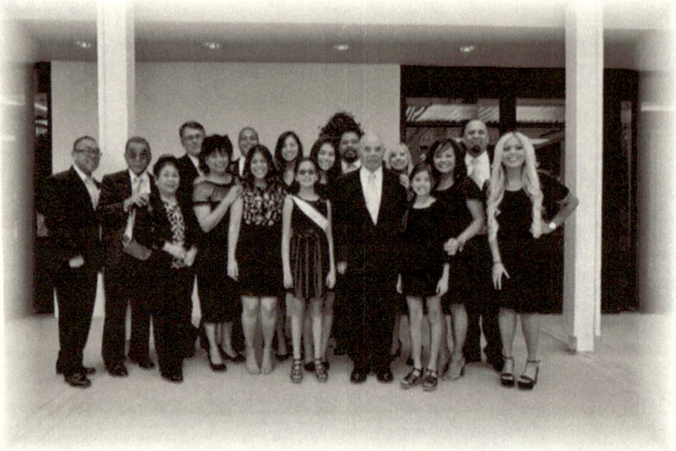

The Reception

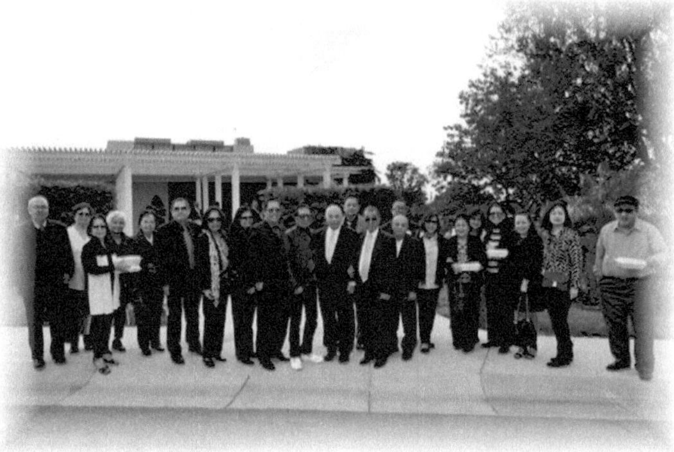

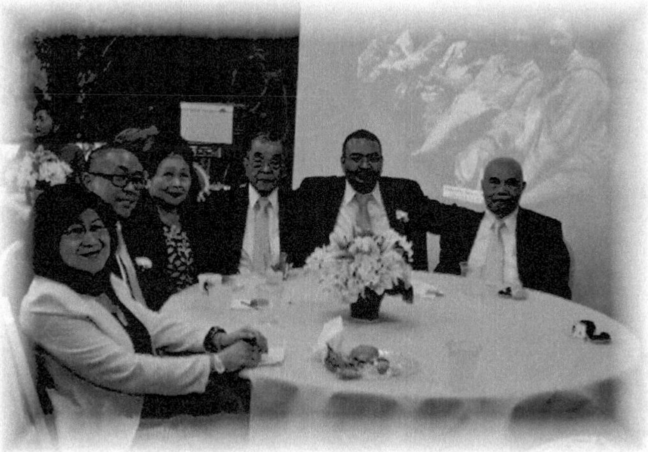

The Reception

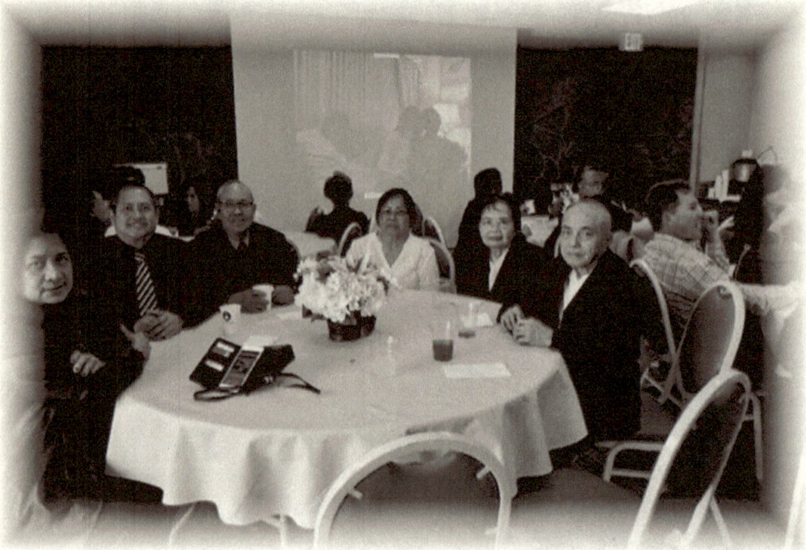

Farewell! Rest in Peace!

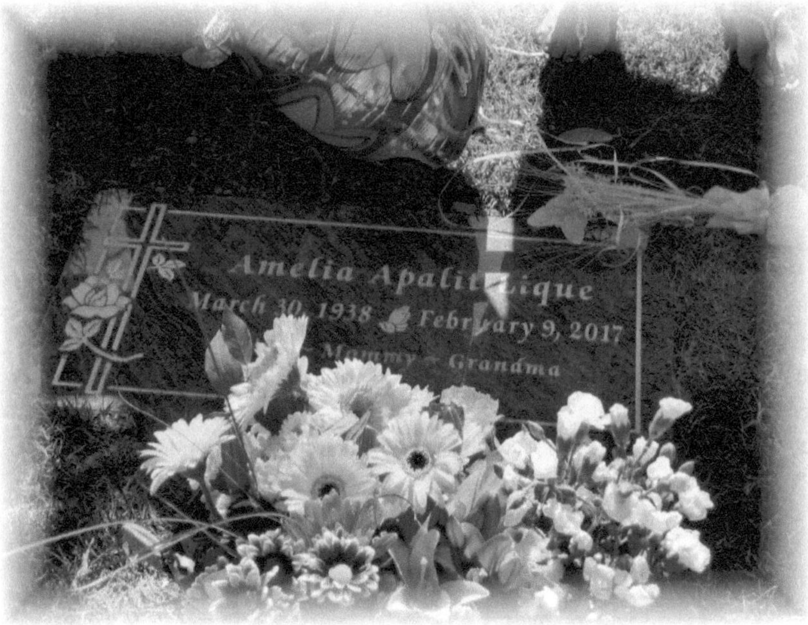

Chapter 23 – Where Terms Are Found

Index

Index

Index

Index

Index

Index

Index

Index

Index

Index

Index

T

Index

U

Index

www.ingramcontent.com/pod-product-compliance
Lightning Source LLC
Chambersburg PA
CBHW021418170526
45164CB00001B/4
* 9 7 8 1 5 3 6 8 3 3 9 4 2 *